PROGRESS IN OBSTETRICS AND GYNAECOLOGY
Volume Nine

EDITED BY

JOHN STUDD MD FRCOG

Consultant Obstetrician and Gynaecologist,
King's College Hospital and Dulwich Hospital;
King's College Hospital Medical School, London

CHURCHILL LIVINGSTONE
EDINBURGH LONDON MELBOURNE NEW YORK AND TOKYO 1991

CHURCHILL LIVINGSTONE
Medical Division of Longman Group UK Limited

Distributed in the United States of America by
Churchill Livingstone Inc., 650 Avenue of the Americas,
New York, 10011, and by associated companies, branches and
representatives throughout the world.

First published 1991
  Reprinted 1992 (twice)
  Reprinted 1994

ISBN 0-443-04412-0

ISSN 0261-0140

British Library Cataloguing in Publication Data
Progress in obstetrics and gynaecology.
  1. Gynaecology–Periodicals   2. Obstetrics
  –Periodicals
  618.05   RG1

Library of Congress Cataloging in Publication Data
Progress in obstetrics and gynaecology.
  Includes indexes.
  1. Obstetrics–Collected works.   2. Gynecology–
Collected works.   1. Studd, John [DNLM:
1. Gynecology–Periodicals.   2. Obstetrics–
Periodicals. W1 PR675PJ
RG39.P73   618   81-21699

Produced by Longman Singapore Publishers Pte Ltd
Printed in Singapore

PROGRESS IN OBSTETRICS AND GYNAECOLOGY

PROGRESS IN OBSTETRICS AND GYNAECOLOGY

Contents of Volume 8

Preface

During the 10 years since the first appearance of *Progress in Obstetrics &* *Gynaecology* there have been enormous advances in the areas of pre-natal diagnosis, fetal monitoring, infertility and gynaecological endocrinology including the menopause, osteoporosis and the hormonal treatment of depression in women. It is notable that the origin of much of this work is British but it is a source of great regret that there has been virtually no expansion of consultant numbers to cope with the increased clinical expectations or the greater clinical or laboratory research required to enable us to remain in the forefront of progress.

The realization that we have only about one-third of the consultant numbers per unit population compared with other Western Countries has been made before in these characteristically forthright prefaces but the problem goes on and the Government generously offers 200 extra consultants for the whole of medicine in the UK. Our speciality would quite like all of them! It is true that we do not suffer Italy's 70 000 unemployed doctors or even Germany's 30 000 but we do need adequate positions to enable us to do the job. This will not happen with the Government as the monopoly employer and some other means of funding consultant expansion must be employed.

The hope has to lie in the private sector for extra jobs but there must not be any double standard of the medical hierarchy enjoying the financial advantages of a private sector but being unwilling to recognize the specialist training available in some of these fine units. Private medical schools and hospitals function well in many parts of the world without any deleterious effect upon the State system. There is little doubt that British gynaecology (I am not so sure about obstetrics) has benefited from the skills of the private sector and belated official recognition of this would be in order.

Such is the shortage of consultant posts that the quick route through the ranks is perceived to be through clinical research. If the trainee emerges from a paper factory without comprehensive clinical skills but supported by the reputation of his supervisor he is more likely to get the job than a good clinical doctor who treats his/her patients well. Such may be one of the disadvantages of the abandonment of the FRCS by gynaecologists. *Mea culpa*. Part of the solution could be to make accredited (or even second-year) senior registrars eight-session consultants with the missing income being made up by private practice or research sessions. This will produce more consultants at little extra cost, and will reduce the bottleneck at the end of training which is already too long. If any consultant doubts whether this scheme would be attractive to the trainees I would challenge them to ask any registrar or senior registrar.

It is hard to predict what will be the relevant outcome for trust status hospitals. Will more appointments be made because of research and fund-raising ability, or will the good doctors have their day? Do we need the flexibility – and insecurity – of shorter contracts? Will the academics produce research and will the teachers teach? Above all can we produce sufficient posts to allow gifted and highly trained young doctors to maintain the clinical standards and innovative research that has characterized British medicine even within the crumbling ruin of the National Health Service?

London, UK
1991   J.S.

Contributors

Hossam Ibrahim Abdalla MB ChB MRCOG
Director, Fertility and Endocrine Centre, Lister Hospital, London, UK

L. Appleby BSc, MRCP, MRCPsych
Senior Lecturer in Psychiatry, University of Manchester, UK

Rod Baber MB BS BPharm MRCOG FRACOG
Visiting Obstetrician and Gynaecologist, The Royal North Shore Hospital of Sydney, St Leonards, New South Wales, Australia

C. G. W. Barnick MB BS
Registrar, Department of Obstetrics and Gynaecology, St Mary's Hospital, London; *Formerly* Research Registrar, Department of Obstetrics and Gynaecology, King's College Hospital, London, UK

Simon Barton BSc MB BS MD MRCOG
Senior Registrar in Genitourinary Medicine, Westminster Hospital, London, UK

T. Ariff Bongso DVM MSc PhD
Research Associate Professor, Department of Obstetrics and Gynaecology, National University Hospital, Singapore

P. J. Bowell FIMLS
Laboratory Patient Services Manager/Head of Ante Natal Serology, Regional Transfusion Centre, John Radcliffe Hospital, Oxford, UK

Gerard Burke MB BCh MRCOG
Research Registrar, Coombe Lying-in Hospital, Dublin; Tutor in Obstetrics and Gynaecology, University College, Dublin, Ireland

Linda Cardozo MD MRCOG
Consultant Obstetrician and Gynaecologist, King's College Hospital, London, UK

T. Chard MD FRCOG
Professor of Reproductive Physiology, St Bartholomew's Hospital, London, UK

G. Constantine BSc MB ChB MRCP MRCOG
Senior Registrar, Birmingham Maternity Hospital, Queen Elizabeth Medical Centre, Birmingham, UK

Sarah Creighton MRCOG
Research Fellow, Urodynamic Unit, Department of Obstetrics and Gynaecology, St George's Hospital, London, UK

Niall M. Duigan MD MAO FRCOG
Associate Professor of Obstetrics and Gynaecology, University College, Dublin; Consultant Obstetrician and Gynaecologist, Coombe Lying-in Hospital and St Vincent's Hospital, Dublin, Ireland

John A. Eden MD MRCOG FRACOG
Senior Lecturer in Reproductive Endocrinology, Royal Hospital for Women, Paddington, New South Wales, Australia

Jonathan Frappell FRCS FRCS(Ed) MRCOG
Consultant in Obstetrics and Gynaecology, Freedom Fields Hospital, Plymouth; *Formerly* Senior Registrar, Department of Obstetrics and Gynaecology, St George's Hospital, London, UK

Jennifer M. Higham MB BS
Research Fellow, Academic Department of Obstetrics and Gynaecology, Royal Free Hospital, London, UK

R. J. Lilford MRCOG MRCP PhD
Professor, and Head, Department of Obstetrics and Gynaecology, St James's University Hospital, Leeds, UK

I. Z. MacKenzie MA MD FRCOG
Clinical Reader in Obstetrics and Gynaecology, University of Oxford, Oxford, UK

Peter McParland MRCOG MRCPI
Assistant Master, National Maternity Hospital, Dublin, Ireland

Adam L. Magos BSc MD MRCOG
Senior Lecturer, and Honorary Consultant, Academic Department of Obstetrics and Gynaecology, Royal Free Hospital, London, UK

J. C. Montgomery MB BS MRCOG
Senior Registrar in Obstetrics and Gynaecology, University College Hospital, London, UK

Robert Morrow MD MRCOG
Assistant Professor, Department of Obstetrics and Gynaecology, Mount Sinai Hospital, Toronto, Ontario, Canada

Soon-Chye Ng MB BS MMed MD MRCOG
Associate Professor, Department of Obstetrics and Gynaecology, National University Hospital, Singapore

Colm O'Herlihy MD FRCPI FRCOG FRACOG
Professor, and Head, Department of Obstetrics and Gynaecology, University College, and National Maternity Hospital, Dublin, Ireland

David Oram FRCOG
Consultant Gynaecological Oncologist, Gynaecology Oncology Unit, The Royal London Hospital (Whitechapel), London, UK

J. Malcolm Pearce MD FRCS MRCOG
Senior Lecturer, Department of Obstetrics and Gynaecology, St George's Hospital Medical School, London, UK

Ann Prys Davies MRCOG
Research Fellow, Gynaecology Oncology Unit, The Royal London Hospital (Whitechapel), London, UK

S. S. Ratnam MB BS MD FRCS FRCS(Ed) FRCS(G) FRACS FRCOG
FRACOG(Hon) FWACS(Hon) FACOG(Hon)
Professor, and Head, Department of Obsterics and Gynaecology, National University of Singapore, Singapore

F. Reader MRCOG, Diploma of Human Sexuality
Honorary Senior Lecturer in Human Sexuality, St George's Hospital Medical School, London, UK

C. W. G. Redman MA MB BChir FRCP
Clinical Reader, Nuffield Department of Obstetrics and Gynaecology, John Radcliffe Maternity Hospital, Oxford, UK

Felicity Reynolds MD FFARCS
Reader in Pharmacology applied to Anaesthesia, and Honorary Consultant Anaesthetist, St Thomas's Hospital, London, UK

A. Henry Sathananthan BSc PhD
Senior Lecturer, La Trobe University, Bundoora; Senior Research Associate, Monash Medical Centre, Melbourne, Victoria, Australia; Visiting Senior Research Fellow, National University Hospital, Singapore

Mark Selinger DM MRCOG
Lecturer, Department of Obstetrics and Gynaecology, John Radcliffe Hospital, Oxford, UK

Robert W. Shaw MD MRCOG FRCS(Ed)
Professor of Obstetrics and Gynaecology, Royal Free Hospital School of Medicine, London, UK

Albert Singer PhD DPhil FRCOG
Consultant Gynaecologist, Royal Northern and Whittington Hospitals, London, UK

C. M. Stacey MB BS MRCOG
Registrar, Department of Obstetrics and Gynaecology, Whittington Hospital, London, UK

Stuart L. Stanton FRCS FRCOG
Consultant Gynaecologist, and Honorary Senior Lecturer, St George's Hospital, London, UK

John Studd MD FRCOG
Consultant Obstetrician and Gynaecologist, King's College Hospital, and Dulwich Hospital, London, UK

Michael Turner MAO MRCPI MRCOG
Clinical Lecturer, University College, Dublin; Consultant Obstetrician and Gynaecologist, Coombe Lying-in Hospital, Dublin, Ireland

Jos van Roosmalen MD PhD
Obstetrician, Department of Obstetrics and Gynaecology, Leiden University Hospital, Leiden, The Netherlands

Judith B. Weaver MD FRCS FRCOG
Consultant Obstetrician, Birmingham Maternity Hospital, Queen Elizabeth Medical Centre, Birmingham, UK

Martin J. Whittle MD FRCOG FRCP(Glas)
Consultant Obstetrician/Perinatologist, The Queen Mother's Hospital, Glasgow, UK

Contents

PART THREE: GYNAECOLOGY

PART ONE

General

1. How useful is a test?

T. Chard   R. J. Lilford

Mrs X is 32 weeks pregnant. Umbilical artery bloodflow patterns measured by Doppler ultrasound are below the 2nd centile of the population range. What is the risk that this baby is asphyxiated?*

Clearly the answer to this question is not simple. On the one hand the abnormal result does not guarantee that fetal outcome will be unsatisfactory. On the other hand it shows that the fetus is at greater risk than if the test result were normal. The aim of this chapter is to demonstrate how test results of this type should be interpreted. What is the risk to the fetus, and how should it be expressed to yield maximum clinical usefulness? In addition, how should clinicians read and interpret the literature on such tests? Here we attempt to provide an understanding of the jargon used (and all too often misused) in describing the result of research studies on diagnostic procedures.

TEST ERRORS: THE CONCEPT OF TRUE POSITIVES, FALSE POSITIVES, ETC.

There is virtually no such thing as a perfect test in clinical medicine. All tests have an error rate and on occasion will either fail to identify an abnormality, or identify an abnormality which is not present. This error rate is described by the terms 'true and false positive', and 'true and false negative'. These terms are defined in Table 1.1 and shown diagrammatically in Figure 1.1.

Some pitfalls in the use of true positives, false positives, etc.

Superficially, the use of these terms seems straightforward. However, there are many pitfalls for the unwary. With most tests there is considerable argument as to what feature constitutes an abnormal or 'positive' result (or,

---

* The reader may immediately say, I need more information about the case. That is quite justifiable. The interpretation of multiple items of information is reserved for later in the chapter, after the discussion of isolated results.

Table 1.1 The definition of true and false positives, and true and false negatives. Each of these terms is also associated with a 'rate'. Thus the false positive rate is the proportion of unaffected individuals yielding a positive result

True positive (TP): the test result is positive in the presence of the clinical abnormality
True negative (TN): the test result is negative in the absence of the clinical abnormality
False positive (FP): the test result is positive in the absence of the clinical abnormality
False negative (FN): the test result is negative in the presence of the clinical abnormality

Practical hint. Even with close attention these figures are often misdefined and miscalculated. A simple test is to check that all four add up to the same as the total number of observations (100 if percentages are used).

conversely, what constitutes a negative result). Many supposed differences between the findings of research studies can be explained by differences in the way in which a positive result is defined rather than in any fundamental difference in the test itself. The manner in which this can occur is illustrated diagrammatically in Figure 1.2. Similarly, changing the definition of the abnormality can have a substantial effect on the apparent error rate, as shown in Figure 1.3.

CLINICAL EFFICIENCY: THE MEANING OF SENSITIVITY, SPECIFICITY, PREDICTIVE VALUE, AND OTHER PARAMETERS

Because the presentation of test results as true and false positives and true and false negatives can be misleading, or at least difficult to comprehend, it is now customary to describe the efficiency of a clinical test by the terms sensitivity, specificity, and predictive value. Other commonly used parameters are relative risk and likelihood ratio. All of these parameters have been used by professional statisticians for many decades, but their introduction to clinical medicine was largely as a result of the publication in 1975 of a highly influential book (see Galen & Gambino 1975).

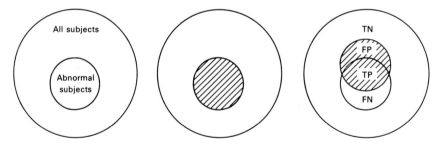

Fig. 1.1 The concept of true and false positives, and true and false negatives. On the left, the total population studied, including the abnormal subjects. In the centre, a perfect test, illustrated by the hatched area: all abnormals have a positive result, all normals have a negative result. On the right, the results of a typical test in real life. The positive test results (hatched area) are strongly associated with the abnormality, but the two are not completely coincident. This situation illustrates the concept of true positives (TP), false positives (FP), true negatives (TN) and false negatives (FN).

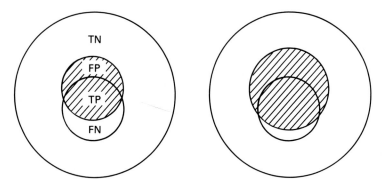

Fig. 1.2 Diagram to show how the definition of the cut-off point between positive and negative results can affect the error rate. On the left is the situation shown in Figure 1.1. On the right is the same clinical situation, but the definition of a positive test result is made less restrictive. As a result, there are more true positives and fewer false negatives, but this is at the expense of an increase in false positives and a reduction in true negatives. If the test were being described solely on the basis of the true-positive rate (a very common situation in the literature), then the results shown on the right would appear superior to those on the left.

The definition of these and a few other commonly used terms are set out in Table 1.2 and illustrated in Figure 1.4. In words, they can be described as follows:

Sensitivity. This is the proportion of all cases of the clinical abnormality which have an abnormal test result. It is equivalent to the statement '40% of cases of stillbirth have an abnormal umbilical artery blood-flow'.

Specificity. This is the proportion of cases with no clinical abnormality

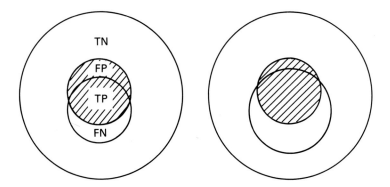

Fig. 1.3 Diagram to show how the definition of the clinical abnormality can affect the error rate. On the left is the situation shown in Figure 1.1. On the right is the same situation, but the definition of the clinical abnormality is broadened (an excellent example in obstetrics would be defining small-for-dates as being below the tenth centile of the population rather than below the fifth centile). This leads to an increase in true positives and a decrease in false positives, but at the expense of a decrease in true negatives and an increase in false negatives.

Table 1.2   The definition of various terms used to describe the clinical efficiency of a test (TP, TN, etc. are defined in Table 1.1)

Sensitivity[a]	$TP/(TP+FN)$
Specificity	$TN/(FP+TN)$
Predictive value (positive)[b]	$TP/(FP+TP)$
Predictive value (negative)	$TN/(TN+FN)$
Relative risk	$\dfrac{TP/(TP+FP)}{FN/(FN+TN)}$
Likelihood ratio	$\dfrac{TP/(TP+FN)}{FP/(TN+FP)}$ or $\dfrac{\text{Sensitivity}}{1\text{-Specificity}}$
Odds	Probability (1-probability)
Accuracy	$(TP+TN)/\text{total}$
Non-error rate (Youden's index)	Specificity + sensitivity-1

[a] Also known as 'detection rate'
[b] Also referred to as 'odds of being affected given a positive result'

which have a normal test result. It is equivalent to the statement '90% of women with a normal child have a normal umbilical artery blood-flow'.

Predictive value (positive). This is the proportion of cases with an abnormal test result which have the clinical abnormality. It is equivalent to '30% of all women with an abnormal umbilical artery blood-flow have a stillbirth'. Unlike sensitivity, predictive value is dependent on the prevalence of the disease as well as the properties of the test.

Predictive value (negative). This is the proportion of cases with a normal test result which do not have the clinical abnormality. It is equivalent to '90% of all women with a normal umbilical artery blood-flow have a normal outcome'.

Relative risk. This is a slightly more difficult concept but one which can be very useful in comparing the value of different tests. A relative risk of

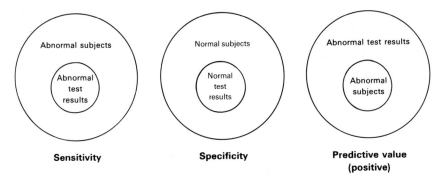

Fig. 1.4   Diagram to illustrate the concepts of sensitivity, specificity and predictive value.

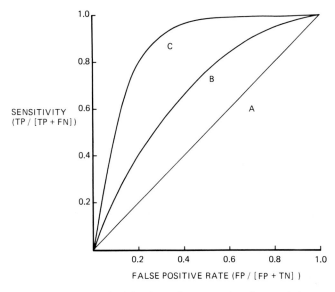

Fig. 1.5 Diagram to show the principle of a receiver-operating characteristic curve (ROC curve). In its commonest form this is a plot of sensitivity versus false-positive rate. As the sensitivity of a test is increased by changing the cut-off point between normal and abnormal, there will be an inevitable increase in the false-positive rate. If the test has no discriminatory power whatsoever, the ROC curve will be a straight line (line A). However, with a good test a high level of sensitivity can be achieved at the expense of only a small increase in false positives (line C). Line B demonstrates a test with some discriminatory power, but obviously less than that of line C. A single value measure of the accuracy of a test is proved by the proportion of the whole area of the graph which lies below the ROC curve (Swets 1988). This value will range from 0.5 (equivalent to A on this figure) up to 1.0 for a perfect test.

1 indicates that the observation does not distinguish a risk which is any different from that in the population as a whole; below 1 the observation indicates a reduced risk, above 1 an increased risk. For example, the statement that an elevated maternal serum AFP level carries a relative risk of 2 in respect of low birthweight implies that a woman with a raised AFP has twice the chance of delivering a growth-retarded child as a woman with a normal AFP. Relative risk can also be used as the basis of a weighting system for different clinical features. Thus, it can provide the quantitative basis for calculating a total risk from a group of features each of which carries a different risk.

Likelihood ratio (also known as odds ratio). This is a similar concept to relative risk. The main value is in combining the results of a series of tests.

Receiver-operating characteristic (ROC) curve. The ROC curve is a rather cumbersome term which describes a useful and widely used device for assessing and comparing the value of tests. It usually takes the form of a graph of sensitivity versus the false-positive rate. The principles of this are shown in Figure 1.5.

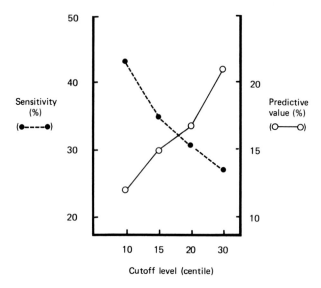

Fig. 1.6   Diagram to show how sensitivity and predictive value can be influenced by the choice of cut-off point of a test. In this example, it is assumed that the test gives a numeric answer, that the dividing line between normal and abnormal can thus be expressed as a percentile of the normal range (horizontal axis), and that low values are generally associated with the abnormality. Increasing the cut-off level increases sensitivity. This is self-evident, because it must increase the number of true positives and reduce the number of false negatives. But the predictive value is automatically decreased, because there is an inevitable increase in the number of false positives.

Some pitfalls in the use of sensitivity, specificity, predictive value and other parameters

Alterations in cut-off point

Even though terms such as sensitivity, etc., give a more meaningful clinical picture than the raw data from which they are derived, they can easily be misleading unless interpreted with care. In particular, they can be much influenced by the definition of positive and negative test results, and by the definition of the abnormality. This is illustrated in Figures 1.6 and 1.7, which demonstrate how sensitivity can be apparently increased by increasing the cut-off level at which the test is defined as positive. The fallacy of this approach is immediately apparent on inspection of predictive value, which shows a concomitant fall. The reverse applies equally, if it is intended to show predictive value in a favourable light. Unfortunately, the medical literature, and especially the obstetric literature, is replete with examples of over-optimistic interpretation as a result of reporting indices of clinical efficiency in isolation: in other words, sensitivity alone or predictive value alone. The solution is very simple: editors and readers should demand that all three major parameters be reported together, together with the

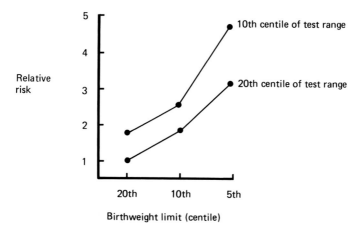

Fig. 1.7 Diagram to show how relative risk can be manipulated by the choice of cut-off points for both the test and the abnormality. The situation is the same as that described in Figure 1.6. It is apparent that using more stringent cut-off points for both the test and abnormality increases the relative risk.

relative risk. The necessity of this is illustrated by the 'absurd' cases shown in Tables 1.3 and 1.4. Even better, results should be demonstrated graphically as an ROC to show the relative changes in sensitivity and specificity with alterations in cut-off levels.

Biased reporting

Another common error is to report sensitivity alone under circumstances in which it is actually *impossible* to calculate clinical efficiency; and to give a favourable view of predictive value by pre-selection of a population. These pitfalls are illustrated by specific examples in Tables 1.5 and 1.6.

Table 1.3 The reductio ad absurdum: predicting fetal sex from maternal sex. The question asked is: 'If the mother is female, what are the chances that the fetus is female?'. This shows very clearly why it is necessary to see *all* parameters of clinical efficiency at the same time

	%
True positives (mother female, fetus female)	50
True negatives (mother male, fetus male)	0
False positives (mother female, fetus male)	50
False negatives (mother male, fetus female)	0
Sensitivity TP/TP+FN	100
Specificity TN/FP+TN	0
Predictive value TP/FP+TP	50

Table 1.4 Another reductio ad absurdum: predicting fetal sex by tossing a coin (heads = male; tails = female). What is the clinical efficiency of 'heads'? Taken individually, the figures for sensitivity etc., look impressive—but the relative risk is 1, i.e. the test has no value

	%
True positives (heads, male fetus)	25
True negatives (tails, female fetus)	25
False positives (heads, female fetus)	25
False negatives (tails, male fetus)	25
Sensitivity (TP/TP+FN)	50
Specificity (TN/FP+TN)	50
Predictive value (TP/FP+TP)	50
Relative risk ((TP/TP+FP)/(FN/FN+TN))	1

'Optimizing' predictive value by pre-selection is, of course, acceptable provided that no attempt is made to extrapolate the findings to a low-risk population.

Failure to allow for prevalence

Predictive value is very sensitive to the prevalence of the condition which the test is designed to detect and will vary greatly according to whether a high- or low-risk population is under investigation. Lack of specificity and a lower predictive value are inevitable when a population cut-off point (e.g. 2 standard deviations) is used to detect a rare condition. For example, the predictive value of maternal serum alphafetoprotein (MSAFP) in detecting spina bifida falls from 10% in high-risk populations to 5% in low prevalence areas. However, sensitivity and specificity do **not** change according to prevalence, unless the condition becomes more (or less) severe as its prevalence increases (or declines).

Table 1.5 Inappropriate use of the term 'sensitivity'. A test is performed in 10 cases of stillbirth; 5 cases are found to be positive, and the conclusion reached is that the sensitivity of the test is 50%. This is highly misleading, because the study includes no normal cases. Thus it is impossible to give figures for false positives and true negatives, or for specificity and predictive value

True positives = 5		
False negatives = 5	Sensitivity	= 50%
False positives = ?	Predictive value = ?	
True negatives = ?	Specificity	= ?

Table 1.6 How the apparent predictive value can be improved by pre-selection of a group of cases. Two tests are applied, both of which detect the same risk, with a sensitivity and predictive value of 50%. However, if test 2 is applied to a group of subjects already shown to be positive by test 1, then the predictive value will be much enhanced. This is equivalent to saying that a test for growth-retardation would have a greater predictive value in patients with severe pre-eclampsia, a defined risk group, than in the population as a whole

	Sensitivity (%)	Predictive value (%)
Test 1	50	50
Test 2	50	50
Test 2 in subjects with positive test 1	50	75

Treatment paradox

If a test is truly predictive and the clinician acts appropriately on test results, then the harmful outcome that the test is designed to predict will be pre-empted. This paradox has bedevilled attempts to describe the test efficiency of intrapartum cardiotocography.

THE MEANING OF MULTIPLE TEST RESULTS

Bayes' theorem

Another way to calculate the predictive value of test results is by the procedure known as Bayes' theorem (The Reverend Thomas Bayes was an eighteenth century mathematician.) In its simplest form, this compares the probability of a given abnormality *before* a test is done (the 'prior probability') with the probability of the abnormality *after* the test has been done (the 'posterior probability'). This can be expressed by the following equation:

$$P(A:PT) = \frac{P(PT:A)P(A)}{P(PT:A)P(A)+P(PT:\text{not }A)P(\text{not }A)}$$

where P is probability, A is the abnormality, and PT is a positive test result. Thus, the expression on the left, P(A:PT), is equivalent, in words, to 'the probability P of abnormality A given the positive test result PT'. This is often described as the 'posterior probability'.

Needless to say, since it is based on the same underlying data, this equation has a direct relation to the indices of clinical efficiency already described. Thus, the equation above could be re-written as:

Predictive value
$$= \frac{(\text{sensitivity})(\text{prevalence})}{(\text{sensitivity})(\text{prevalence})+(1-\text{specificity})(1-\text{prevalence})}$$

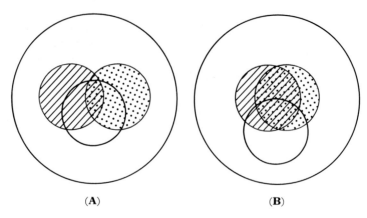

(A)   (B)

Fig. 1.8   Diagram to show the operation of Bayes' theorem in reaching a diagnosis on the basis of multiple pieces of non-definitive information (e.g. a group of test results). (**A**) The outer circle is the whole population, the inner circle (heavy border) delineates patients with a given abnormality. Two tests are applied (hatched and dotted circles), each of which gives some true and some false results. Taken together, a rather larger proportion of cases of the abnormality are identified (both hatched and dotted areas) than with either test alone. A similar combination is achieved mathematically by Bayes' theorem. (**B**) This shows the situation in which the tests are not completely independent. There is now very substantial overlap between the two sets of results, and relatively little is gained by combining them.

Some believe that this is easier to understand when presented on the basis of odds, where:

$$\text{Posterior odds} = \text{prior odds} \times \frac{\text{sensitivity}}{1 - \text{specificity}} \text{(i.e. likelihood ratio)}$$

It would be fair to admit that the purpose and meaning of Bayes' theorem, as set out above, is sometimes difficult to grasp. However, Bayes' theorem is especially useful in situations in which there are multiple test results (or, for that matter, multiple abnormalities) to analyse (Fig. 1.8). The equation can then be expanded by the inclusion of further terms for each of the test results (and/or diagnoses) and generates an overall probability for the complete set of test results. This, of course, is the situation most commonly encountered in clinical obstetrics, where a management decision has to be made against the background of many pieces of information, some positive and some negative. For example, the situation described at the beginning of this chapter (Mrs X) included only one test result—Doppler ultrasound measurement. But typically other data would be available. If she was also known to have severe pre-eclampsia and to have had a growth-retarded child in a previous pregnancy, it would obviously further increase the probability of fetal problems in the current pregnancy. Similarly, current attempts to increase the effectiveness of screening for Down's syndrome with multiple biochemical and biophysical tests require risk calculations using this type of methodology.

This process of summing risk factors, none of them absolute, to yield an overall conclusion is very similar to the process known as 'intuition' in the human. Bayes' theorem might therefore qualify for designation as 'artificial intelligence'. Desirable though this may seem, there are two main problems with the mathematical approach (and for that matter the human, though less frequently admitted). The first is that the actual probabilities are often not known— what is the exact probability that a woman with a previous growth-retarded child will have another one in the current pregnancy? The second problem is that Bayes' theorem can only be applied if the various diagnostic features are relatively independent. But this is often not the case. Mrs X may have essential hypertension, in which case the growth retardation and the pre-eclampsia are all *related* manifestations of the same underlying process, not independent at all. Clinical obstetric diagnosis is replete with observations which are likely to be mutually dependent (Lilford & Chard 1983, Rose & Lamb 1988) (see Fig. 1.8B). Test results are usually combined intuitively in obstetric decision-making.

Describing test results

Optimally, clinical tests should be described in the following terms:

 a. Their clinical efficiency expressed as sensitivity, specificity and predictive value;
 b. Their performance in high-, medium- and low-risk populations;
 c. Their clinical efficiency over a range of test cut-off points [receiver-operating characteristic (ROC) curves].

To further demonstrate these concepts let us look at the description of a new test—Doppler ultrasound. Take a high-risk population in which 100 of 1100 babies are destined to be born dead or with unequivocal biochemical and/or clinical evidence of hypoxia. Consider different cut-off points (reversal of flow, no flow, reduced flow, and normal flow) in respect of the outcome in a study in which clinicians are not given the test findings. In Table 1.7 we present estimates of true and false positives and true and false negatives for each cut-off level. The trade-off between sensitivity and specificities is clearly shown in Figure 1.9. Note that as the cut-off becomes more stringent, so the likelihood ratio (LR) rises.

The true worth of a test

Finally, the true clinical worth of a test depends not only on its efficiency but also on its effectiveness. Will knowing the results of the test lead to management which will improve the outcome for the patient, without imposing extra risks due to the occurrence of false-positive and false-negative results? The likely clinical impact of a test can be examined by

Table 1.7 Calculation of the likelihood ratio (LR) associated with various umbilical artery flow patterns ascertained by Doppler ultrasound using hypothetical but plausible results. The population consists of 1100 high-risk women of whom 100 will have an asphyxiated or dead baby

	Test positive	Test negative
Reversed flow		
Disease positive	20	80
Disease negative	1	999
Sensitivity	20% — LR 200	
Specificity	99.9%	
Predictive value	> 90%	
No diastolic flow		
Disease positive	50	50
Disease negative	25	975
Sensitivity	50% — LR 20	
Specificity	97.5%	
Predictive value	66%	
Reduced diastolic flow		
Disease positive	80	20
Disease negative	200	800
Sensitivity	80% — LR 4	
Specificity	80%	
Predictive value	29%	

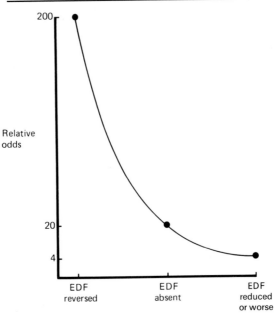

Fig. 1.9 Diagram to show that as the cut-off point for a test—in this case Doppler ultrasound measurement of umbilical artery resistance—becomes more stringent, so the specificity and the likelihood ratio (relative risk) increases, but the number of cases identified (sensitivity) decreases. EDF = end diastolic flow. This is an alternative method for presenting a ROC curve.

decision analysis, a process by which the overall utility of a test can be calculated on the basis of its clinical efficiency and the probabilities and values of the various outcomes. But the final measure of the value of a new test should be the results of a randomized controlled trial to determine the overall effects of its use. An analysis by decision theory should always be part of the design of such trials, particularly in obstetrics, because this will often show that the potential benefits are small and that vast sample sizes would be required to confirm these differences.

REFERENCES AND RECOMMENDED FURTHER READING

Galen R S, Gambino S 1975 Beyond normality: the predictive value and efficiency of medical diagnosis. John Wiley, New York

Grant A, Mohide P 1982 Screening and diagnostic tests in antenatal care. In Enkin M, Chalmers I (eds) Clinics in developmental medicine, nos 81/82. Effectiveness and satisfaction in antenatal care. Spastics International Medical Publications. Heinemann, London. J B Lippincott, Philadelphia pp 22–59

Knill-Jones R P 1987 Diagnostic systems as an aid to clinical decision making. Br Med J 295: 1392–1396

Lilford R J, Chard T 1983 Problems and pitfalls of risk assessment in antenatal care. Br J Obstet Gynaecol 90: 507–510

Lilford R J, Obiekwe B C, Chard T 1983 Maternal blood levels of human placental lactogen in the prediction of fetal growth retardation: choosing a cut-off point between normal and abnormal. Br J Obstet Gynaecol 90: 511–515

Polansky F F, Lamb E J 1989 Analysis of three laboratory tests used in the evaluation of male infertility: Bayes' rule applied to the post-coital test, the in vitro mucus migration test, and the zona-free hamster egg test. Fertil Steril 51: 215–228

Rose B I, Lamb E J 1988 Multiple simultaneous predictors of gestational age. Am J Perinatol 5: 44–50

Simel D L 1985 Playing the odds. Lancet i: 329–330

Swets J A 1988 Measuring the accuracy of diagnostic systems. Science 240: 1285–1293

Wald N, Cuckle H 1989 Reporting the assessment of screening and diagnostic tests. Br J Obstet Gynaecol 96: 389–396

PART TWO

Obstetrics

2. Doppler ultrasound—is it any use?

M. J. Whittle   R. J. Morrow

Antenatal tests of fetal wellbeing depend indirectly on changes in fetal physiology an aspect of the fetus which, until recently, has been relatively inaccessible to study. For several decades the measurement of fetal heart rate changes provided the only insight into fetal condition but ultrasound has allowed the direct observation of fetal activities such as movement and breathing and the estimation of amniotic fluid volume all of which have been combined together as the biophysical profile, an important method of fetal assessment in current practice.

Doppler ultrasound is an innovation in fetal testing which may indicate the state of the fetoplacental vascular bed from which implications about the fetal condition can be drawn. Although the technique has potential value its exact role remains to be assigned and its relation to currently available techniques of evaluation is unclear.

The two main objectives of antenatal tests are to provide firstly a screening method to help identify at-risk pregnancies and secondly a technique to evaluate a pregnancy already complicated by some clinically recognized condition such as hypertension or fetal growth retardation. The extent to which currently available methods of fetal evaluation fulfil these objectives is a little difficult to judge and considerable debate surrounds the preferred endpoints to be used. Some obvious ones are perinatal death and the delivery of the small-for-dates baby but the former is too crude, and nowadays too infrequent, and many of the latter are perfectly normal. The use of 'condition at birth' is also unsatisfactory and long-term follow up of the developing baby is extremely costly and difficult to organize. In addition to its ability to predict perinatal problems it is also important that any test system does not lead to either an inappropriate, elective, premature delivery or excessive numbers of Caesarean sections.

In spite of the reservations concerning these endpoints they have been used, to a greater or lesser extent, to evaluate existing methods of fetal assessment. Ironically Doppler has come under closer scrutiny than most other tests in current use although, partly because of the wide range of techniques, instruments and measurements used, its value in clinical practice is still difficult to discern. Indeed for the test to be of obvious value it must be shown to provide information which is either additional to, or complements, existing methods, a feature which will be explored in this chapter.

TECHNIQUE OF MEASUREMENT

The technique of Doppler measurement has been extensively described elsewhere and only the salient features will be mentioned. The principle is that the frequency of the sound reflected from moving objects is related to their speed and direction. The frequency shift is proportional to the velocity of the blood but calculation is complicated and angle-dependent. The quantification of blood flow is unreliable using current technology as vast errors can be produced both from small changes in the angle of incidence of the Doppler beam and in calculation of the cross-sectional area of the vessel.

Semiquantitative analysis of the characteristic waveforms is used which involves the measurement of three main indices, namely the systolic/diastolic (S/D or A/B) ratios, the resistance index (RI) and the pulsatility index (PI). These indices are relatively crude but they have been used extensively clinically although undoubtedly more information is available from the waveform if suitable mathematical descriptions could be developed.

Either continuous or pulsed wave Doppler equipment can be used, the former being relatively cheap and simple with the disadvantage of being nondiscriminant so that all moving structures in the beam will cause a Doppler shift. In contrast, pulsed Doppler can be range-gated allowing a vessel to be examined without interference from surrounding structures. Pulsed Doppler equipment is expensive and certainly is not necessary if only the umbilical artery is to be examined. However, if the target is more discrete, for example the fetal aorta or cerebral vessels, pulsed equipment is vital not just because of the gating facility but also the ability to visualize the vessel while the Doppler examination is in progress.

Considerable concern has been raised relating to the power output of the Doppler equipment, especially the pulsed apparatus. The recommendation is that it should not exceed $100 \, \mathrm{mW/cm^2}$ and it is also becoming mandatory that such information is available from the manufacturer at the time of purchase.

DOPPLER AND THE MEASUREMENT OF UTERINE AND FETAL BLOOD FLOW

The uterine arterial tree has proved difficult to examine using Doppler techniques. Firstly it is hard to establish which part of the circulation should be assessed and certainly once the uterine artery has commenced branching, vessel identification becomes unreliable (Bewley et al 1989). A further problem relates to the extent of the contribution from the extensive anastomoses not only with the contralateral uterine artery but also the ovarian arteries. Finally it has been shown that healthy spiral arteries themselves open and shut intermittently (Ramsey et al 1963).

The fetal vasculature, in contrast, provides more discrete targets to study. Thus umbilical artery, aorta, umbilical vein and the cerebral and renal arteries can all be identified and Doppler waveforms measured with reasonable reproducibility (Hastie et al 1988, Pearce et al 1988).

Umbilical artery

This is the most commonly examined vessel and much of the work in the literature relates to it. The umbilical artery feeds the usually low resistance circulation of the placental vessels and the waveform, easily detected using a continuous wave instrument, has a characteristically high velocity diastolic component which increases as gestational age advances. In contrast, in an abnormal waveform the diastolic velocity is reduced, absent or even reversed, changes which probably result from increased downstream resistance.

Fetal aorta

Several groups have reported the changes in the fetal aorta Doppler waveforms (Griffen et al 1984, Eik-Nes et al 1982) which follow a similar pattern to those in the umbilical artery. Quantification of fetal blood flow has been attempted but the inherent difficulties have led most to settle on the semiquantitative analysis of the waveforms as in the umbilical artery. It remains uncertain whether the aorta is a more sensitive guide to the fetal condition than the umbilical cord.

Whether or not attempts are made to quantify blood flow in the aorta, pulsed equipment is required because of the problems of vessel identification and the need to control the range of the Doppler beam by gating. Because of the expense of the equipment, study of the aorta remains essentially a research tool restricted to the larger perinatal centres.

Other vessels

Cerebral

With the further development of imaging systems, the combination of pulsed Doppler equipment and colour flow mapping has made it possible, with care, to identify the fetal internal carotid, middle and anterior cerebral arteries (Mari et al 1989). When the fetus is hypoxic the resitance to flow in these vessels appears to fall and thus diastolic velocities increase.

Renal

Research is currently at an early stage but the fetal kidney also appears to have a low resistance vascular bed, the pulsatility index falling with gestational age (Vyas et al 1989).

AIMS OF DOPPLER IN PREGNANCY ASSESSMENT

Tests of fetal condition can be divided into those which are most efficient at screening and those which perform best as diagnostic tests (Whittle 1987). The exact role for Doppler has yet to be defined but it might be expected to function well as a screening test because alterations in umbilical flow, and also probably uterine flow, may represent changes in impedance in the placental vasculature which should predate problems in the fetus. The most likely perceptible clinical consequence would be growth problems in the fetus and these are certainly difficult to identify using either clinical or ultrasound techniques.

The use of Doppler, specifically as a test of fetal wellbeing, relates less to the umbilical velocity changes and more to alterations in other vessels such as the aorta and the cerebral circulation. The data available are fewer than for the umbilical velocities and therefore it is impossible to judge the current role of the technique.

The detection of fetal growth and the evaluation of fetal condition remain crucial problems in obstetrics and the possible value of Doppler in relation to these issues needs to be compared with existing techniques (Table 2.1).

DOPPLER AS A SCREENING TEST FOR FETAL GROWTH RETARDATION

Currently both clinical and ultrasound methods are used in the assessment of fetal growth. Clinical diagnosis of intra-uterine growth retardation tends to be inaccurate with a sensitivity of around 40%. Conflicting reports exist

Table 2.1   Comparison of methods for screening for the small-for-dates fetus

	Sensitivity %	Positive predictive value %	Reference
Clinical	27–73	17–60	Numerous
Ultrasound	83	45	Neilson et al 1980
Doppler Umbilical artery	40	9	Beattie & Dornan 1989
	16.7	23	Newnham et al 1990
	40	61	Dempster et al 1989
Uterine artery	10	16.7	Newnham et al 1990
	43	18	Steel et al 1990

concerning the value of symphysial height measurements with positive predictive values for the identification of the small-for-dates fetus ranging from 17% to 60% and a sensitivity of between 27% and 73%. However in general, and certainly in an unselected population, the method appears to be unreliable.

Ultrasound in the assessment of fetal growth has proved to be of surprisingly limited value although the predictive value for the small-for-dates fetus is better than with clinical methods alone. Geirsson et al (1985) found that measurement of the fetal abdominal circumference was about 70% sensitive for the baby less than 10th centile and this figure is close to the 83% reported by Neilson et al (1980). The head/trunk ratio which was proposed as being an effective way of identifying the asymmetrically growth retarded baby (Campbell & Thoms 1977) was found to have a sensitivity of only 44% when used in a low risk population (Neilson et al 1980).

Several studies have investigated the use of ultrasound as a screening test for the small-for-dates fetus, but even when the test used was very sensitive and specific, detection of affected pregnancies had no impact on outcome (Neilson et al 1984). In fact, general disillusionment with the value of a 'late' scan for fetal assessment (Neilson & Grant 1989) has led to this approach being largely abandoned.

The reasons for these rather disappointing findings are probably two-fold. Firstly many of the severely growth retarded fetuses may already have perished by the third trimester. Secondly the concept of growth retardation has to move beyond a simple assessment of weight since some babies of average size may, in fact, be growth retarded and many babies who are statistically small are perfectly normal.

Doppler assessment of the fetoplacental vessels should identify the vascular disorder which is a prelude to the development of fetal growth problems and hence isolate an at-risk group some time before the problem becomes clinically manifest. However many of the initial studies on umbilical artery Doppler flow velocity waveforms (Erskine & Ritchie 1985, Berkowitz et al 1988) and fetal aortic flow (Griffen et al 1984) were conducted on pregnancies already complicated by severe growth problems. Not surprisingly, these clearly showed an association between abnormal Doppler and poor outcome although they gave no indication of the predictive value of the test.

Studies of the uterine artery waveforms likewise suggest an association between abnormal results and the development of pre-eclampsia and growth retardation, although current prospective studies are too small to be useful.

Umbilical artery

Currently only one large prospective study has been reported (Beattie & Dornan 1989) in which just over 2000 patients were examined consecutively at 28, 34 and 38 weeks using continuous wave Doppler. Most of those cases with abnormal Doppler (A/B ratio >90th centile) had a normal outcome and the predictive value was low for the various outcome measures used, including evidence of growth retardation. However 3 of the unexplained stillbirths, and a further stillbirth which occurred as a result of abruption, were found in the pregnancies with abnormal Doppler. The unexplained losses were at 28, 33 and 38 weeks and it remains unclear whether knowledge of the Doppler results would have successfully influenced outcome. Further it is not clear how reliably the 3 could have been separated from the approximately 200 patients with abnormal Doppler who had a satisfactory pregnancy outcome. When the waveform was grossly abnormal and end-diastolic velocities absent, as was found in 6 cases, only 3 had a normal outcome.

Data (Hanretty et al 1989) from the pilot study of a much larger randomized study which is nearing completion also indicate little difference in outcome between those babies with normal or abnormal Doppler in the umbilical artery although it is interesting that babies in the latter group appear to be smaller, but not necessarily small-for-dates. As in other studies more babies with abnormal Doppler were admitted to the neonatal intensive care nursery.

When the identification of the small-for-dates fetus has been the end-point chosen Doppler has been found generally to perform unsatisfactorily in a low risk population (Sijmons et al 1989) and, in fact, even in high risk, 'normal', groups such as twins (Hastie et al 1989). Even in a preselected high risk population Doppler, as a method of identifying the small-for-dates fetus, has been shown to have a sensitivity of only 40% (Dempster et al 1989) which is comparable with simple clinical methods. Of course size alone is not the most important factor (Sarmandal et al 1989) and in a comparison between ultrasound biometry and Doppler, although the former more reliably identified the small baby, the latter was superior at indicating the one likely to be compromised (Chambers et al 1989).

Aorta

A reduction in diastolic velocity has been confirmed in growth retardation (Laurin et al 1987). It has also been suggested that abnormal aortic waveforms are predictive of the development of severe neonatal problems (Hackett et al 1987a) and in the babies with birthweights less than 2000 g absent end-diastolic velocity was associated with a more adverse outcome in terms of necrotizing enterocolitis, intraventricular haemorrhage and perinatal death. Unfortunately the groups were not well matched and the babies with the worst outcome appeared smaller and more premature.

The use of aortic waveforms to assess conditions such as severe oligohydramnios to help identify the growth retarded fetus have been described (Hackett et al 1987b) normal waveforms being most likely to be associated with either renal agenesis or premature rupture of the membranes. Conversely abnormal results occurred in all growth retarded fetuses and in about 25% of those chromosomally abnormal. Knowledge of the uterine flow contributed, it being most commonly abnormal when the fetus was growth retarded.

Uterine arteries

The use of Doppler studies of the uterine arteries in pregnancy evaluation remains doubtful although Schulman et al (1987) did find that when the S/D ratios on either side of the uterus differed significantly that the pregnancy outcome appeared to be less satisfactory. In a study involving 126 cases abnormal uterine artery waveforms appeared to be more frequently associated with the development of fetal growth problems and maternal hypertension (Campbell et al 1986). A small randomized study of the Doppler waveforms in the uterine arteries (Steel et al 1990) appeared to confirm this in pregnancies screened at about 18 weeks and again at about 24 weeks. However Hanretty et al (1989), in a study which included over 300 patients, found screening the uterine arteries to be unhelpful as a means of identifying the at-risk pregnancy.

DOPPLER IN THE ASSESSMENT OF FETAL HEALTH

When Doppler is used to evaluate a population already selected because of a high risk feature such as hypertension or the suspicion of fetal growth problems, abnormal waveforms seem to be more reliably associated with an adverse outcome. Comparisons with other forms of fetal monitoring, however, are not easy not least because their efficacy is also uncertain.

Umbilical artery

Farmakides et al (1988) suggested that abnormal Doppler in a group of patients referred for non-stress cardiotocography (CTG) predated the appearance of a non-reactive test and seemed to identify a group of pregnancies at particular risk. Hastie et al (1990) found the combination of a non-stressed CTG and Doppler studies, in a group preselected because of a non-reactive CTG, to be a powerful indicator of outcome providing the results were in concordance. Others have also found the combination of Doppler with standard tests of fetal evaluation to provide a potentially powerful, predictive system although the studies are small (Lowery et al 1990). On the other hand Doppler evaluation of the umbilical artery has also been found to be no more effective than standard methods of evaluation, such as cardiotocography, in the identification of the severely sick fetus (Villar et al 1989).

Trudinger et al (1987) used Doppler in a randomized study of high risk pregnancies, in which about half were complicated by either hypertension or suspected fetal compromise. Knowledge of the Doppler findings appeared to make no significant difference to perinatal outcome but did seem to allow more successful identification of the pregnancies which would achieve a vaginal delivery; 35% of those in which Doppler was unknown required emergency Caesarean section compared with 13% in which the clinician was aware of the Doppler.

Whether Doppler is a useful method with which to identify the hypoxic fetus remains uncertain. Abnormal waveforms per se are not produced by hypoxia (Morrow et al 1990) but their presence, particularly in association with serious obstetric complications, is likely to indicate severe compromise. Conversely normal waveforms should be reassuring and allow the pregnancy to continue. The association between abnormal waves and fetal hypoxia and acidosis at the time of delivery has been described (Tyrell et al 1989) as well as the fact that normal waveforms were associated with a good outcome even in the presence of a small-for-dates fetus, an observation which has recently been confirmed (Burke et al 1990a). Often lacking is information about other assessment parameters, such as the biophysical profile and cardiotocography, with which to compare the Doppler results. However in a letter Burke et al (1990b) did indicate that both fetal smallness and changes in the biophysical profile were important independent indications for delivery.

The use of Doppler in specific conditions such as diabetes mellitus has been studied (Bracero et al 1986) and found to aid in the identification of the at risk fetus. These preliminary data have been confirmed (Landon et al 1989) but only in the pregnancy of a diabetic with known microvascular disease when abnormal Doppler in the umbilical artery was strongly associated with severe fetal growth problems.

The most severely abnormal waveform is when there is absent end-diastolic velocity which probably arises from high placental resistance and, certainly in early work, appeared to be associated with very poor perinatal outcome. Rochelson et al (1987) found only 3 intact survivors out of 10 babies with absent end diastolic flow. Woo et al (1987) have suggested that the finding of absent end diastolic flow indicates the need for immediate delivery. The implication has been that this is an irreversible change related to imminent death and indeed some objective evidence does suggest that these fetuses may be hypoxic and acidotic (Tyrell et al 1989, Nicolaides et al 1988). However the reappearance of diastolic velocities has been noted (Hanretty et al 1988), an observation confirmed by Brar & Platt (1989) and associated with a less adverse outcome.

In general it would seem that absent end diastolic flow indicates a pregnancy at considerable risk and one which requires careful scrutiny (Johnstone et al 1988). However in most cases it is not an indication for immediate delivery and in any case the rather high proportion of abnormal babies reported by some groups makes detailed ultrasonography mandatory and blood sampling possibly desirable.

Aorta

A reduction in diastolic flow has been described in the presence of asphyxia (Soothill et al 1986) but reversed diastolic flow has been associated with death within a day of recognition (Illyes & Gati 1988) and it presumably may indicate the final stages of circulatory collapse.

Other vessels

Study of the other fetal vessels is currently at an early stage but an increase in the end-diastolic velocity in the internal carotid artery in the growth retarded fetus has been observed (Wladimiroff et al 1986). In addition, Rizzo et al (1989) suggested an association between abnormal velocities in the internal carotid and post-asphyxial encephalopathy.

Doppler assessment of the renal arteries may also prove of value. Preliminary data suggest that the growth retarded fetus may have reduced diastolic velocities (Vyas et al 1989) presumably related to changes in resistance in the renal vascular bed and it has been speculated that this may be associated with oligohydramnios.

WHAT USE DOPPLER?

The introduction of new tests into obstetrics has always been greeted with great, and sometimes uncritical, enthusiasm and certainly Doppler seemed a test of considerable promise. Any new test should be evaluated using large, randomized prospective trials with a clear view of the various end-points to be tested, an approach which has not been frequently used in the past so making comparisons between current monitoring methods and Doppler difficult.

The most important question to answer is whether Doppler contributes useful additional information for the management of a particular pregnancy which is not available using the existing, accepted techniques. The data presented in this chapter suggest a theoretical role for Doppler as a screening test but although the concept is attractive evidence from the literature is lacking. That said, it would seem likely that abnormal umbilical artery waveforms do help to identify an at-risk group which warrants further surveillance. Whether this approach would improve perinatal outcome, however, is uncertain.

The value of Doppler in the assessment of the already identified high risk pregnancy is also unclear. Usually these pregnancies will already have other pointers to indicate impending trouble and even though the Doppler may be abnormal this information may not help clinical decision-making. Nevertheless there is a suggestion from the literature that Doppler may be of help in a negative way in that, even in the presence of pregnancy complications such as hypertension and growth retardation, a normal result may outweigh all else. If this is confirmed in further studies it might mean that Doppler will have an important reassuring role.

CONCLUSIONS

Doppler provides a potentially useful method of fetal evaluation but evidence as to its efficacy is still patchy. The key issue about whether or not it provides superior information to that already available from existing tests remains uncertain. Further work is required using properly constructed randomized studies to establish the role of Doppler in obstetrics today.

REFERENCES

Beattie R B, Dornan J C 1989 Antenatal screening for intrauterine growth retardation with umbilical artery Doppler ultrasonography. Br Med J 298: 631–635

Berkowitz G S, Mehalek K, Chitkara U, Rosenberg J, Cogswell C, Berkowitz R L 1988 Doppler umbilical velocimetry in the prediction of adverse outcome in pregnancies at risk for intrauterine growth retardation. Obstet Gynecol 71: 72–746

Bewley S, Campbell S, Cooper D 1989 Uteroplacental Doppler flow velocity waveforms in the second trimester. A complex circulation. Br J Obstet Gynaecol 96: 1040–1046

Bracero L, Schulman H, Fleischer A, Farmakides G, Rochelson B 1986 Umbilical artery velocimetry in diabetes and pregnancy. Obstet Gynecol 68: 654–658

Brar H S, Platt L D 1989 Antepartum improvement of abnormal umbilical artery velocimetry; Does it occur? Am J Obstet Gynecol 160: 36–39

Burke G, Stuart B, Crowley P, Scanaill S N, Drumm J 1990a Is intrauterine growth retardation with normal umbilical artery blood flow a benign condition? Br Med J 300: 1044–1045

Burke G, Stuart B, Crowley P, Scanaill S N, Drumm J 1990b Letter. Br Med J 300: 1525

Campbell S, Thoms A 1977 Ultrasonic measurements of the fetal head to abdomen ratio in the assessment of growth retardation. Br J Obstet Gynaecol 83: 165–174

Campbell S, Pearce J M F, Hackett G, Cohen-Overbeek T, Hernandez C 1986 Qualitative assessment of uteroplacental blood flow: early screening test for high risk pregnancies. Obstet Gynecol 68: 649–653

Chambers S E, Hoskins P R, Haddad N G, Johnstone F D, McDicken W N, Muir B B 1989 A comparison of fetal abdominal measurements and Doppler ultrasound in the prediction of small for dates babies and fetal compromise. Br J Obstet Gynaecol 96: 803–808

Dempster J, Mires G J, Patel N, Taylor D J 1989 Umbilical artery velocity waveforms: poor association with small for gestational age babies. Br J Obstet Gynaecol 96: 692–696

Eik-Nes S H, Brubbakk A O, Ulstein M K 1982 Measurement of fetal blood flow. Lancet i: 283–285

Erskine R L A, Ritchie J W K 1985 Umbilical artery blood flow characteristics in normal and growth retarded fetuses. Br J Obstet Gynaecol 92: 605–610

Farmakides G, Schulman H, Winter D, Ducey J, Guzman E, Penny B 1988 Prenatal surveillance using nonstress testing and Doppler velocimetry. Obstet Gynecol 71: 184–187

Geirsson R T, Patel N B, Christie A D 1985 Intrauterine volume, fetal abdominal area and biparietal diameter measurements with ultrasound in the prediction of small for dates babies in a high risk obstetric population. Br J Obstet Gynaecol 92: 936–940

Griffen D, Bilardo K, Masini L et al 1984 Doppler blood flow waveforms in the descending thoracic aorta of the human fetus. Br J Obstet Gynaecol 91: 997–1006

Hackett G A, Campbell S, Gamsu H, Cohen-Overbeek T, Pearce J M 1987a Doppler studies in the growth retarded fetus and prediction of neonatal necrotising enterocolitis, haemorrhage and neonatal morbidity. Br Med J 294: 13–16

Hackett G A, Nicolaides K H, Campbell S 1987b Doppler ultrasound assessment of fetal and uteroplacental circulations in severe second trimester oligohydramnios. Br J Obstet Gynaecol 94: 1074–1077

Hanretty K P, Whittle M J, Rubin P C 1988 Reappearance of end-diastolic velocity in a pregnancy complicated by severe pregnancy induced hypertension. Am J Obstet Gynecol 158: 1123–1124

Hanretty K P, Primrose M H, Neilson J P, Whittle M J 1989 Pregnancy screening by Doppler uteroplacental and umbilical artery waveforms. Br J Obstet Gynaecol 96: 1163–1167

Hastie S, Howie C A, Whittle M J, Rubin P C 1988 Daily variability of umbilical and lateral uterine wall artery blood velocity waveform measurements. Br J Obstet Gynaecol 95: 571–574

Hastie S J, Danskin F, Neilson J P, Whittle M J 1989 Prediction of the small for gestational age twin fetus by Doppler umbilical artery waveform analysis. Obstet Gynecol 74: 730–733

Hastie S J, Brown M F, Whittle M J 1990 Predictive values of umbilical artery waveforms and repeat cardiotocography in pregnancies complicated by nonreactive cardiotocography. Eur J Obstet Gynecol, Reprod Biol 34: 67–72

Illyes M, Gati I 1988 Reverse flow in the human fetal descending aorta as a sign of severe fetal asphyxia preceding intrauterine death. J Clin Ultrasound 16: 403–407

Johnstone F D, Haddad N G, Hoskins P, McDicken W, Chambers S, Muir B 1988 Umbilical artery Doppler flow velocity waveform; the outcome of pregnancies with absent end diastolic flow. Eur J Obstet Gynecol, Reprod Biol 28: 171–178

Landon M B, Gabbe S G, Bruner J P, Ludmir J 1989 Doppler umbilical artery velocimetry in pregnancy complicated by insulin dependent diabetes. Obstet Gynecol 73: 961–965

Laurin J, Marsal K, Persson P-H, Lingman G 1987 Ultrasound measurement of fetal blood flow in predicting outcome. Br J Obstet Gynecol 94: 940–948

Lowery C L, Henson B V, Wan J, Brumfield C G 1990 A comparison between umbilical artery velocimetry and standard antepartum surveillance in hospitalized high risk patients. Am J Obstet Gynecol 162: 710–714

Mari G, Moise K J, Deter R L, Kirshon B, Carpenter R J, Huhta J C 1989 Doppler assessment of the pulsatility index in the cerebral circulation of the human fetus. Am J Obstet Gynecol 160: 698–703

Morrow R J, Adamson S L, Bull S B, Ritchie K 1990 Acute hypoxemia does not affect the umbilical artery flow velocity waveform in fetal sheep. Obstet Gynecol 75: 590–593

Neilson J P, Grant A 1989 Ultrasound in obstetrics: effective care in pregnancy and childbirth. Chalmers I, Enkin M, Keirse M J N C (eds) Oxford University Press

Neilson J P, Whitfield C R, Aitchison T C 1980 Screening for the small for dates fetus: a two stage ultrasonic examination schedule. Br Med J 280: 1203–1206

Neilson J P, Munjanja S, Whitfield C R 1984 Screening for small for dates fetus: a controlled trial. Br Med J 289: 1179–1182

Newnham J P, Patterson L L, James I R, Diepeveen D A, Reid S E 1990 An evaluation of the efficacy of Doppler flow velocity waveform analysis as a screening test in pregnancy. Am J Obstet Gynecol 162: 403–410

Nicolaides K H, Bilardo C M, Soothill P W, Campbell S 1988 Absence of end diastolic frequencies in umbilical artery: a sign of fetal hypoxia and acidosis. Br Med J 297: 1026–1027

Pearce J M, Campbell S, Cohen-Overbeek T, Hackett G, Hernandez J, Royston J P 1988 Reference ranges and sources of variation for indices of pulsed Doppler flow velocity waveforms from the uteroplacental and fetal circulation. Br J Obstet Gynaecol 95: 248–256

Ramsey E M, Corner G W, Donner M W 1963 Serial and cineradioangiographic visualisation of maternal circulation in the primate placenta. Am J Obstet Gynecol 86: 213–222

Rizzo G, Arduini D, Luciano R et al 1989 Prenatal cerebral Doppler ultrasonography and neonatal neurological outcome. Ultrasound Med 8: 237–240

Rochelson B, Schulman H, Farmakides G et al 1987 The significance of absent end-diastolic velocity in umbilical artery velocity waveforms. Am J Obstet Gynecol 156: 1213–1218

Sarmandal P, Bailey S M, Grant J M 1989 A comparison of three methods of assessing inter-observer variation applied to ultrasonic fetal measurement in the third trimester. Br J Obstet Gynaecol 96: 1261–1265

Schulman H, Ducey J, Farmakides G et al 1987 Uterine artery Doppler velocimetry: the significance of divergent systolic/diastolicratios. Am J Obstet Gynecol 157: 1539–1542

Sijmons E A, Reuwer P J H M, Van Beek E, Bruinse H W 1989 The validity of screening for small for gestational age and low weight for length infants by Doppler ultrasound. Br J Obstet Gynaecol 96: 557–561

Soothill P W, Nicolaides K H, Bilardo C M, Campbell S 1986 Relation of fetal hypoxia in growth retardation to mean blood velocity in the fetal aorta. Lancet ii: 1118–1120

Steel S A, Pearce J M, McParland P, Chamberlain G V P 1990 Early Doppler ultrasound screening in the prediction of hypertensive disorders of pregnancy. Lancet 335: 1548–1551

Trudinger B J, Cook C M, Giles W B, Connelly A, Thompson R S 1987 Umbilical artery flow velocity waveforms in high-risk pregnancy. Lancet i: 188–190

Tyrell S, Obaid A H, Lilford R J 1989 Umbilical artery Doppler velocimetry as a predictor of fetal hypoxia and acidosis at birth. Obstet Gynecol 74: 332–336

Villar M A, Sibai B M, Gonzalez A R, Emerson D P, Anderson G D 1989 Plasma volume, umbilical artery Doppler flow and antepartum fetal heart testing in high-risk pregnancies. Am J Perinatol 6: 341–346

Vyas S, Nicolaides K H, Campbell S 1989 Renal artery flow-velocity waveforms in normal and hypoxemic fetuses. Am J Obstet Gynecol 161: 168–171

Whittle M J 1987 An overview of fetal monitoring. In: Whittle M J (ed) Clinical obstetrics and gynaecology. Baillière, London, pp 203–218

Wladimiroff J W, Tonge H M, Stewart P A 1986 Doppler ultrasound assessment of cerebral blood flow in the human fetus. Br J Obstet Gynaecol 93: 471–475

Woo J S K, Liang S T, Lo R L S 1987 Significance of an absent or reversed end diastolic flow in Doppler umbilical artery waveforms. J Ultrasound Med 6: 291–297

3. Management of red cell isoimmunization in the 1990s

I. Z. MacKenzie   M. Selinger   P. J. Bowell

There is a real possibility that rhesus incompatibility radically altered the course of English history by denying Henry VIII a male heir. If Catherine had been sensitized by her first husband, Arthur, Henry VIII's brother, this could have explained the several miscarriages and preterm labours which resulted in five babies all of whom died within a few days or weeks of delivery (Maclennan 1967). This suggestion could not have been made until 50 years ago, when Levine et al (1941) first recognized the existence of the rhesus factor. Consequently the repeated pregnancy losses could have been due to an incompatibility between the maternal and fetal rhesus types—rhesus alloimmunization. Wallerstein (1946) and Diamond (1947) showed how exchange transfusion improves survival of babies suffering from haemolytic disease of the newborn (HDN) and Bevis (1952, 1956) described how amniocentesis could be used to predict whether the fetus was being affected by the incompatibility. In 1963, Liley (1963) published his revolutionary idea of fetal intraperitoneal transfusion to try to improve the outlook for affected pregnancies and his basic principle is still the cornerstone of treatment today in the most severely affected cases.

Clarke et al (1963) demonstrated the protective effect of maternal administration of anti-D immunoglobulin against the development of rhesus-D [Rh(D)] alloimmunization; by the late 1960s, it had been widely adopted and the incidence of Rh(D) alloimmunization dramatically decreased. The majority of rhesus negative women need no longer be at risk of developing anti-D antibodies, but in the few who still become sensitized, the rarity of the disease and consequent lack of experience in its management by obstetric and neonatal paediatric units around the country has led to some potentially avoidable fetal and neonatal morbidity and mortality. A renewed interest in rhesus disease occurred at the beginning of the 1980s with the introduction of new technologies into obstetric practice. The present approaches to management of pregnancies complicated by rhesus incompatibility are an amalgam of ideas explored over the past 10 years which have been integrated into treatment strategies developed during the 1960s.

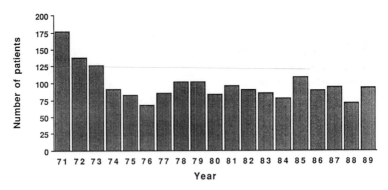

Fig. 3.1   Incidence of anti-D sensitization in the Oxford Health Region since the introduction of prophylaxis 1971–1989.

INCIDENCE

Following the introduction of anti-D prophylaxis in the late 1960s, there was a rapid decline in the number of mothers who became sensitized but since 1973 the incidence has remained relatively stable (Fig. 3.1). Women who showed evidence of rhesus sensitization during the 1970s include a large cohort who had developed antibodies before the introduction of prophylaxis and the size of this group has decreased and will constitute an even smaller proportion of the total problem in the 1990s. As this group has decreased, the proportion of women who have had inadequate or no prophylaxis due to an oversight at sensitizing events, and those developing an unprovoked antenatal sensitization have become more significant (Table 3.1).

Prophylaxis has had a considerable impact on the consequences of rhesus incompatibility. The incidence of perinatal death due to Rh(D) allo-immunization was 15 per 10 000 births before the introduction of prophylaxis when it accounted for 4·3% of all perinatal deaths (Butler & Bonham 1963). By 1983, the incidence of death from this cause had fallen to

Table 3.1   The changing aetiology of Rh(D) sensitization: 1969–1987

	1969[a]	1973[b]	1977[a]	1979[b]	1983[c]	1987[c]
n cases	164	117	71	60	34	38
Prior to prophylaxis	85%	43%	39%	13%	12%	13%
Omitted prophylaxis	0%	45%	10%	35%	26%	16%
Failure of prophylaxis	3%	6%	27%	37%	44%	53%
Mismatched transfusion	3%	0%	6%	0%	0%	0%
Antenatal sensitization	9%	6%	18%	15%	18%	18%

[a] Eklund (1978)
[b] Tovey & Taverner (1981)
[c] Tovey (1988)

0·54 per 10 000 births accounting for 0·3% of all perinatal deaths (Whitfield 1983). It is important to note that these figures under-estimate the true magnitude of the problem since therapeutic abortion performed because of severe rhesus disease, which amounted to twice the number of registered deaths from rhesus disease in 1984 and 1985 (Office of Population, Censuses and Surveys 1985, 1986, Clarke et al 1987), and spontaneous fetal losses before 28 weeks gestation are not generally recorded among perinatal death statistics and thus go unnoticed (Bowell et al 1985). The overall reduction in numbers of Rh(D) sensitized pregnancies has however resulted in a relative increase in the proportion of blood group incompatibilities due to other red cell antigens (see later).

ANTENATAL ASSESSMENT

Routine antenatal screening

In a recent study, it was shown that about one third of those women who become alloimmunized do not have demonstrable antibody in the first sample of blood taken in pregnancy (Bowell et al 1986a). It is recommended therefore, that all women, regardless of Rh(D) status should have at least two samples of blood taken during pregnancy with the second one (and third if Rh negative or previously transfused) being tested in the third trimester (Bowell et al 1986a). It was also shown that there is a correlation between the time antibody is first detected and the severity of any resulting HDN: thus antibodies detected in the booking blood sample are likely to cause more serious problems than those found for the first time late in pregnancy. Nevertheless antibodies detected near the end of gestation are capable of causing severe transfusion reactions and are likely to lead to delays in the provision of matched donor blood if required.

The most important part of the management of pregnancies at risk of rhesus alloimmunization is serial monitoring of maternal serum antibody levels throughout pregnancy. Over the past 30 years this principle has remained unaltered. However by the mid-1960s, automated systems to quantify anti-D levels were introduced (Rosenfield et al 1964) and more reproducible values compared with those obtained by manual titration were then available. It now seems inappropriate for units managing cases of Rh(D) alloimmunization to rely upon the relatively crude technique of manual titration.

Our experience in Oxford relating pregnancy outcome to maternal anti-D antibody levels was initially reported in 1982 (Bowell et al 1982); the expanded experience, involving more than 1200 Rh(D) sensitized pregnancies between 1978 and 1988 is illustrated in Figure 3.2. With maternal anti-D levels less than 4 i.u./ml, the fetus is likely to be minimally affected with less than 5% requiring neonatal exchange transfusion for hyperbilirubinaemia. Levels between 4–8 i.u./ml may lead to moderate

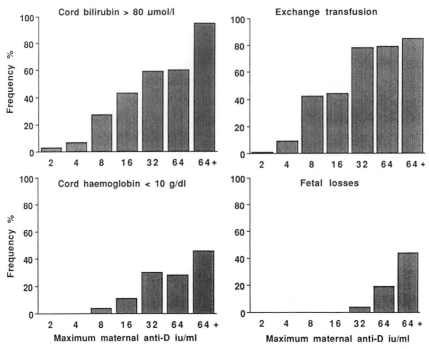

Fig. 3.2   Pregnancy outcome according to maternal anti-D levels in more than 1200 patients during 1978–1988 in the Oxford Health Region.

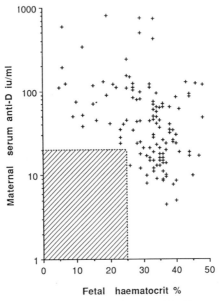

Fig. 3.3   Relationship between maternal anti-D levels and fetal haematocrit during the antenatal period. Results of 130 paired blood samples in 70 untransfused pregnancies with a Rh(D) fetus.

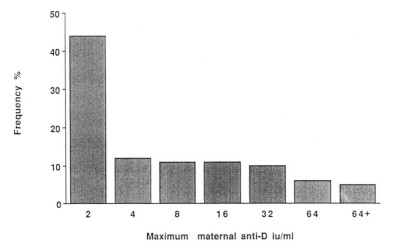

Fig. 3.4   Frequency distribution of maximum maternal anti-D levels in a screened population of over 800 women during the antenatal period.

disease and warrant delivery by 38 weeks gestation. Neonatal exchange transfusion for hyperbilirubinaemia will probably be necessary in 55%; we have seen only two babies with a cord haemoglobin less than 10 g/dl at delivery among more than 800 when the maternal antibody level was < 10 i.u./ml during the 7 days prior to delivery. Anti-D levels above 10 i.u./ml increase the chances of the pregnancy being seriously affected and warrant further investigation, or delivery if at 36 weeks gestation or later. However our growing experience with isoimmunized cases with anti-D quantification values between 10–20 i.u./ml suggests that a higher level than 10 i.u./ml may be set before recommending intra-uterine investigation; as shown in Figure 3.3, we have had no cases where the fetal haematocrit was below 27% when the maternal anti-D was less than 20 i.u./ml. More data are still required before we can be totally confident about changing our threshold. Figure 3.4 illustrates the frequency distribution of cases according to the highest anti-D level recorded during pregnancy in 800 patients: fewer than 20% of patients have anti-D levels greater than 20 i.u./ml, and some achieve these values only late in pregnancy.

Assessment of the identified at risk fetus

In the 1990s, it seems inappropriate to rely on previous obstetric history to decide whether further investigation of the current pregnancy is necessary. The primary decision should be made on the maternal antibody level which is the major factor influencing outcome. This, however, does not precisely predict the degree of fetal anaemia, with a linear regression analysis of maternal anti-D levels and fetal haematocrit giving an R value of 0·39 (Fig.

3.3) suggesting that other factors including fetal genotype, period of antibody contact, IgG subclass, and fetal response may contribute. However if the level is above 10 i.u./ml and delivery is not an option because of fetal immaturity, further investigation is necessary.

A variety of different approaches have been described. The first and most widely used is determining the amniotic fluid optical density at 453 nm ($\hat{}OD^{453}$), based on the observations by Liley (1961). This method has been very useful in managing pregnancies, but since it only assesses amniotic fluid bilirubin concentration, reflecting the degree of fetal haemolysis and not fetal haemopoietic response, it is not always accurate. False predictions were reported by Pridmore et al (1972) and Fairweather et al (1976) and we demonstrated the poor relationship between $\hat{}OD^{453}$ results and fetal haematocrit (MacKenzie & Bowell 1986). Subsequently we reported an 11% under-estimate and 11% over-estimate in the degree of fetal anaemia during both the second and third trimesters (MacKenzie et al 1988): others have also noted similar discrepancies during the second trimester (Nicolaides et al 1986). Analysis of amniotic fluid anti-D concentrations has been studied to determine whether it has greater potential than $\hat{}OD$ measurements in clinical management. Although amniotic fluid and maternal serum anti-D concentrations correlate well, the former has been found to have no added value in predicting the severity of the haemolytic process (Neil & Bowell 1984).

Non-invasive investigations have been proposed during the past 15 years—almost all using ultrasound techniques. Abnormal fetal heart rate patterns have been described in severe rhesus alloimmunization. Sinusoidal and decelerative patterns have been associated with very low cord haemoglobin concentrations at delivery (Visser 1982) and high perinatal death rates (Rochard et al 1976). Although cardiotocography (CTG) will identify the seriously anaemic fetus, significant changes appear as late phenomena and the CTG is insufficiently sensitive to predict mild to moderate anaemia. Measuring fetal cardiac conduction times during the antenatal period has also been suggested with prolonged QRS complexes correlating with anaemia at birth and with stillbirth (Brambati & Pardi 1981). The exact relationship between the length of the QRS complex and decreasing fetal haemoglobin concentrations is not clear enough to make a precise prognosis and organize management: the relationship however warrants further study.

Real time ultrasound examination of the fetus has been used to detect the presence of ascites and other stigmata of hydrops: although reliable in identifying severe disease it appears to be of little benefit in tailoring management before fetal survival is already compromised (Weiner et al 1981). A similar situation applies with fetal movement counting as an effective monitoring method, movements usually declining only when the disease is far advanced (Sadovsky et al 1979, Frigoletto et al 1986). More specific features have been described as pathognomonic of severe disease including the degree of umbilical vein dilatation (DeVore et al 1981), and liver size (Vintzileos et al 1987, Roberts et al 1989). Pulsed Doppler ultrasound observing blood flow in the umbilical vein suggest there is increased blood flow in the anaemic fetus (Kirkinen et al 1983). However, Doppler studies on the umbilical artery and descending fetal aorta do not correlate well with the degree of fetal anaemia (Copel et al 1989a) and misleading results were obtained by some workers in a case developing hydrops (Barss et al 1987). Although Copel et al (1989b) suggest that Doppler assessed fetal cardiac output is higher in anaemic than non-anaemic fetuses, they failed to define anaemia and were unable to correlate output with the degree of anaemia. They concluded that this approach to management was unlikely to be helpful at the present time. It is obviously imperative that a scientific assessment of the value of Doppler in this situation is made before it is used to tailor patient management.

The only direct method of assessing the severity of the disease is measuring fetal haematocrit. This was first suggested in 1983 (MacKenzie 1984). Several techniques have been described for collecting antepartum fetal blood samples: initially a fetoscopic technique was used but most centres now use ultrasound guidance. Whichever method is used, the procedure is invasive and may result in abortion or preterm labour: the incidence of abortion following ultrasound guided fetal blood sampling is quoted at 2% for 606 patients by Daffos et al (1985) and our experience in Oxford has been 3 losses (3%) in 107 patients having 243 samplings performed for rhesus management. In addition each procedure can provoke marked increases in maternal antibody levels although the risk appears to be similar to that following amniocentesis; this can be minimized by ensuring that wherever possible a transamniotic approach is used avoiding the placenta (Bowell et al 1988b). Other complications of fetal blood sampling have been described including exsanguination, fetal bradycardia, failure to obtain a sample, and cord constriction (Berkowitz et al 1987,

Table 3.2   The Oxford guidelines using maternal anti-D levels for the management of Rh(D) sensitized pregnancies

Anti-D level (i.u./ml)	Mat anti-D repeat quant'n	Fetal blood sampling			Intra-peritoneal transfusion	Delivery probably at (weeks)
		First occas'n	Rhesus (D) typing	Hct level		
<0·5	4 weeks	None	No	No	No	40
0·5–4·0	2 weeks	None	No	No	No	40
4·0–10	2 weeks	None	No	No	No	36–38[a]
10–20	2 weeks	28 weeks[b]	Yes	Yes	Prob. no[c]	33–38[a/d]
>20	2 weeks	18 weeks[b]	Yes	Yes	Prob. yes[c]	33–38[a/d]

[a] Precise timing determined from (sometimes computer predicted) Hct values
[b] Thereafter, within 1 week of maternal anti-D first exceeding 10 i.u./ml
[c] If fetal Hct < 25% before 26 weeks gestation; if fetal Hct < 30% after 26 weeks gestation
[d] Objective being to reach at least 34 weeks gestation

Reece et al 1988, Benaceraff et al 1987). In view of the morbidity associated with fetal blood sampling and amniocentesis, they should only be performed when indicated by maternal serum antibody levels rising above the threshold values: our approach to fetal blood sampling is illustrated in Table 3.2.

In cases where the father of the pregnancy is heterozygous for the offending antigen, fetal blood sampling has the advantage of restricting the investigation to a single procedure if the fetus is found to be antigen negative (Philip et al 1978, MacKenzie et al 1983). An alternative to fetal blood sampling for fetal phenotyping is the analysis of red blood cells in samples of trophoblast obtained at first trimester chorion villus sampling. Goto et al (1980) demonstrated that the Rh(D) antigen can be detected by immunofluorescence and this approach has been used in clinical practice (Kanhai et al 1987, Rodesch et al 1987). However the risks of miscarriage and increased sensitization using this technique remain a hazard and it should only be used in cases with appropriately raised antibody levels.

Most of the above methods of fetal assessment have not been assessed scientifically and most, unfortunately, only identify severely affected fetuses rather than those which are becoming anaemic, when corrective management has a good chance of improving outcome. Measuring other constituents of fetal blood including bilirubin, albumin (Rodeck et al 1984, MacKenzie et al 1988), and reticulocytes (Nicolaides et al 1988) have not proved useful in assessing fetal condition or predicting outcome.

ANTENATAL MANAGEMENT

Fetal transfusions

Since 1963, Liley's method of intraperitoneal fetal transfusion has been used world-wide with great success. He used fluoroscopic screening to guide a transfusion needle and catheter to the correct position in the fetal peritoneal cavity, and his technique was used by everyone until the mid 1970s when Hobbins et al (1975) reported the use of ultrasound guidance. With both approaches, the decision to transfuse had been made following the collection of amniotic fluid for $\hat{}OD^{453}$ estimation. Once the $\hat{}OD$ value was in or approaching Liley's zone III (Liley 1961), a transfusion was performed. In many cases the decision was made following the principle of instituting treatment 10 weeks earlier than the previous pregnancy had been lost or fetal hydrops detected (Whitfield 1983). In most units, transfusions were not carried out before 24 weeks gestation since survival figures before that gestation were generally very poor.

The possibility of transfusing directly into the fetal circulation was first explored at the end of the 1970s in patients undergoing termination of pregnancy (MacKenzie et al 1982). The first reports of clinical management appeared in the literature in the early 1980s (Rodeck et al 1981, Bang et al

1982). Initially performed under direct vision by fetoscopy, virtually all units performing intravascular transfusions are now using an ultrasound guided needle technique.

The decision to start transfusing has been made using $\hat{O}D^{453}$ values and in recent years by measuring fetal haematocrit levels, either as an initial assessment or as confirmation of suspected fetal anaemia following amniocentesis. The fetal haematocrit at which transfusion is considered appropriate varies according to the specialist centre and is often unquoted in published reports; haematocrit levels above 40% at any gestation should not require transfusion and a value of 25–30% is probably more realistic. Our practice in Oxford has been to diagnose significant anaemia if the haematocrit is <25% before 26 weeks gestation and <30% after that gestation. We have observed 10 (22%) fetuses among 47 undergoing fetal blood sampling before 30 weeks gestation where the haematocrit was between 30–39% and remained in that range for at least 4 weeks until delivered; the other 37 fetuses were managed by intra-uterine transfusions. Most workers use ORh − ve, CMV − ve, haemolysin negative donor blood cross-matched against maternal serum with an haematocrit of 75–90%; many groups irradiate the blood prior to transfusion to reduce the risk of a graft-versus-host reaction. In most centres maternal premedication is given for maternal and fetal sedation, while some have also given tocolytics and antibiotics to the mother, and diuretics, cardiac stimulants and paralysing agents to the fetus: no prospective studies have been conducted to determine the value of any of these pharmacological additions. Our practice during the last 3 years has been to give betamethasone 6 mg b.d. for 48 hours before transfusions at 28–33 weeks gestation in view of the apparently proven benefit of such therapy to the very preterm neonate (Crowley 1989).

The umbilical cord vessel used for transfusion is frequently stated to be the vein at its junction with the placenta, although this is not universal, and in some instances transfusions have been given into the intrahepatic portion of the vein (Bang et al 1982), the inferior vena cava (Doyle et al 1986) or one of the cardiac ventricles (Vintzileos et al 1987, Westgren et al 1988). There is no convincing evidence that any one site or vessel is better than another for the transfusion technique, since there is apparently minimal change in fetal blood acid-base status during the transfusion (Westgren et al 1989). However transfusion into one of the cord arteries theoretically allows equilibration of blood constituents while passing through the placenta. Rates of transfusion are not always quoted in publications many of which report experience with fewer than 10 cases, but where stated, a rate of 1–3 ml per minute is most frequently used. Most report a technique of direct injection of blood into the fetal circulation, while a few refer to an 'exchange' method which usually involves removing aliquots of blood from the fetal circulation at intervals during the transfusion, but rarely similar volumes removed to those transfused (MacKenzie et al 1982, Grannum et al 1986, Lemery et al 1989).

Volumes transfused are usually determined by checking the fetal haematocrit at intervals during the procedure and stopping the transfusion when the recipient haematocrit has reached 35–45%: transfused volumes are often not stated while in some the volume amounts to only a few millilitres and is thus of dubious value. Formulae have been devised to determine transfusion volumes required according to the initial fetal haematocrit, the donor haematocrit and the ultrasonically estimated fetal weight (Grannum et al 1986, Socol et al 1987, Nicolaides et al 1988). Personal experience using a microcomputer programme indicates it is possible to predict the increase in recipient haematocrit for a given donor volume with less than a 10% error (Selinger et al 1990).

When to give the next transfusion appears to have been determined empirically from many reports and it is generally after an interval of 1–3 weeks. Measurement of the fetal haematocrit and analysis of red blood cell populations immediately prior to the next transfusion provides a check on the success of the previous transfusion and enables a more rational approach to management; there are rarely more than 5% fetal cells remaining in the fetal circulation after two intra-uterine transfusions if the previous transfusions have been successful. A few workers have developed computer programmes to calculate the expected decrease in the fetal haematocrit following a transfusion and again personal experience indicates how helpful this can be; we have found a decline from 40% to 25% takes about 21 days as a general guide, irrespective of gestation.

It is the opinion of many that intravascular transfusions represent a major advance in therapy over intraperitoneal transfusions. However, such claims are not based on scientific evidence. When we initially explored the idea of direct intravascular transfusions in 1980, it was with a view to offering a treatment method for those pregnancies severely compromised before 24 weeks gestation when most workers would not contemplate an intraperitoneal transfusion (MacKenzie et al 1982). It appeared with growing experience and following reports by other groups, that there was also a place for intravascular transfusion at more advanced gestations, since losses had occurred with intraperitoneal transfusion especially if the fetus was hydropic and on occasions due to fetal trauma. Although enthusiastic and extravagant claims have been made for intravascular transfusion, the overall picture during the past 4 years has not supported the initial optimism of its superiority over intraperitoneal transfusions as illustrated in Tables 3.3 and 3.4. Intravascular transfusions are not hazard-free and the specific problems encountered include cord haematoma (Poissonnier et al 1989, Ronkin et al 1989), fetal thrombocytopenia (Harman et al 1988), leukoencephalopathy (Parer 1988), and haemorrhage (Ronkin et al 1989). Fetal bradycardia often without explanation appears the most serious complication, occasionally leading to unexpected death, and has been reported in many series reviewed (Grannum et al 1986, Berkowitz et al 1986, MacKenzie et al 1987, Voto & Margulies 1989, Ronkin et al 1989,

Table 3.3 Intravascular transfusions: results from selected series involving 3 or more patients. *Key*: IUT, intra-uterine transfusion; IVT, intravascular transfusion; exch IVT, exchange intravascular transfusion; IVC, inferior vena cava used for transfusion; i-cardiac, intracardiac transfusion; HV, hepatic vein used for transfusion; N/S, not stated

Reference	Total		Transfusion						Survivors	
	Patients	IUT	Method	Vol.	Rate (ml/min)	Freq.	Pre-transfusion haematocrit[b]	Gestation (wks)	Total	Hydropic
Ronkin et al (1989)	8	31	exch IVT[a]	7–110	3	2 wkly	5–37	21–35	8(100%)	2 of 2
Westgren et al (1988)	6	25	i-cardiac[a]	5–20	1	1–3 wkly	6–24	19–31	4(67%)	2 of 4
Socol et al (1987)	3	12	IVT	30–85	1–3	1–3 wkly	8–32	23–32	3(100%)	3 of 3
Berkowitz et al (1986)	7	18	IVT	12–65	1–2	N/S	2–35	21–31	5(72%)	2 of 4
Doyle et al (1986)	8	35	IVC & HV	N/S	N/S	N/S	11–38	29–34	5(60%)	N/S
Poissonier et al (1989)	107	200	IVT[a]	N/S	N/S	N/S	N/S	N/S	N/S	29 of 47
Rodeck et al (1984)	25	77	IVT[a]	N/S	1–3	1–3 wkly	7–30	19–28	18(72%)	11 of 15
MacKenzie et al (1987)	10	17	exch IVT	3–97	0.5–2	2–3 wkly	6–36	18–30	2(20%)	0 of 5
Grannum et al (1986)	4	9	IVT[a]	10–60	1–3	N/S	6–20	24–31	3(75%)	0 of 1
Lemery et al (1989)	15	30	exch IVT[a]	15–236	N/S	2–8 wkly	11–29	19–34	10(67%)	2 of 4
Voto & Margulies (1989)	33	90	IVT	N/S	N/S	N/S	N/S	N/S	10(30%)	N/S

[a] Intraperitoneal transfusion was necessary in some cases.
[b] Where Hb values are reported, they have been converted to haematocrits by 3 fold multiplication.

Table 3.4 Intraperitoneal transfusions in the 1980s; results from selected series.
Key: IUT, intra-uterine transfusion; N/S, not stated

Reference	Total Patients	IUT	Transfusion Vol	Interval	Gestation (wks)	Survivors Total	Hydropic
Bowman (1987)[a]	75	202	N/S	3–4 wkly	N/S	57 (76%)	18 of 30
Parer (1988)	45	120	N/S	N/S	N/S	35 (78%)	N/S
Bennebroek Gravenhorst et al (1989)	31	66	N/S	1·5–3 wkly	19–32	18 (58%)	8 of 19

[a] Refers to 1980–1986 experience.

Poissonnier et al 1989). In addition, technical difficulties are not uncommon, often related to displacement of the transfusion needle, which in many instances has resulted in abandoning the transfusion or resorting to the intraperitoneal approach (Doyle et al 1986, Grannum et al 1986, Berkowitz et al 1987, Socol et al 1987, Ronkin et al 1989). Although hydrops may resolve following IVT and is considered a major advantage, this is not inevitable (Berkowitz et al 1987, Doyle et al 1986, Voto & Margulies 1989, Poissonnier et al 1989).

Our 6 year experience using intravascular transfusions led us to critically review our intravascular technique and at the beginning of 1988 we abandoned it in favour of a modification of Liley's intraperitoneal method at all gestations from 18 weeks to 33 weeks. Having first confirmed that transfusion is necessary by measuring fetal haematocrit, transfusions are given via a 20 gauge spinal needle guided by ultrasound into either fetal iliac fossa, and donor blood with an haematocrit of 85–90% is injected at 5–10 ml per minute. The transfusion volume required to raise the recipient haematocrit to 40–45% is calculated using a computer program which takes account of the initial fetal haematocrit, donor blood haematocrit, and fetal circulating volume. Confirmation of effective transfusion volume is obtained by measuring the fetal haematocrit before the start of the next transfusion which has been timed to coincide with a fall in fetal haematocrit to the transfusion threshold level previously described. Our results, shown in Table 3.5, of 26 consecutive pregnancies receiving an intravascular or intraperitoneal transfusion indicate that volumes transfused with each method are similar, while transfusion rates at 5–10 ml/min are faster intra-peritoneally even in early gestations in the presence of hydrops; we have had fewer complications with the intraperitoneal route than the intravascular route. It is currently our view that the intravascular route may have a place in the moribund fetus before 20 weeks gestation but even this needs to be objectively demonstrated. In view of the results reported by a number of centres during the latter part of the 1980s, it would seem reasonable to look at the two transfusion techniques objectively, ideally in a multicentre

Table 3.5   Comparison of intravascular and intraperitoneal transfusions in 26 patients managed in Oxford 1987–1989.

	Intravascular transfusions	Intraperitoneal transfusions
n patients	12	14
n transfusions	32	38
Maternal anti-D (i.u./ml) at first transfusion		
Mean	209	86
Range	35–677	14–136
Gestation (wks) at first transfusion		
Mean	26·8	26·3
Range	19–31	18–32
<20	0	5
21–25	5	2
25+	7	7
Fetal haematocrit at first transfusion		
Mean	20·8	18·9
Range	12–33	7–31
Transfusion interval (wk)		
Mean	2·25	2·0
Range	0·5–6	1–5·5
Transfusion vol. (ml)		
Mean	36·4	50·3
Range	20–120	10–85
Fetal bradycardia with transfusion	9 (28%)	0
Immediate delivery by LSCS	4	0
Losses <28 weeks	0	3 (21%)
>27 weeks	3 (25%)	0

prospective randomized trial. However to mount such a trial is likely to prove impossible, since clinicians believing their current technique is the best are unlikely to agree to using the alternative.

Plasmapheresis

Introduced in the late 1960s (Bowman et al 1968), the technique relies on removal of as much antibody as possible from the maternal circulation. The procedure is carried out three to four times a week removing 1–3 litres of plasma on each occasion. Plasmapheresis can reduce the serum antibody level by up to 75% and exponents of the technique report cases treated this way which have ended with a healthy infant when the previous baby died from severe rhesus disease. Bowman (1987), however, observed no obvious benefit in 10 women managed with plasma exchange, all fetuses requiring intra-uterine transfusions. If plasmapheresis is to be used, it would seem prudent before commencing treatment to confirm that the fetus is antigen positive by fetal blood sampling in those cases where the father of the pregnancy is heterozygous for the rhesus factor. At present however, there seems little scope for this strategy since intra-uterine transfusions can be commenced at 18 weeks gestation, the earliest stage that fetal haemolysis from alloimmunization occurs.

Other treatment modalities

Promethazine hydrochloride 25–500 mg daily has been used as an immunosuppressant during pregnancy and claims have been made of a reduced need for neonatal exchange transfusions (Gusdon 1981, Charles & Blumenthal 1982). However, studies looking at the possible benefits of 100–150 mg daily failed to demonstrate any advantage when compared with matched controls (Stenchever 1978, Caudle & Scott 1982).

Oral desensitization with erythrocyte membrane was proposed by Bierme et al (1979), the rationale being the subversion of the maternal immune response from the production of IgG antibody to mainly IgA and IgM, neither of which cross the placenta. Although the French have reported success with treatment, others have not been able to reproduce their results (Gold et al 1983). Prospective randomized trials are required before any genuine value can be discerned from this treatment.

Immunoglobulin therapy, acting possibly by feedback inhibition of antibody synthesis and reticuloendothelial Fc blockade and Fc-mediated antibody transport across the placenta, has been tried in the mangement of severe rhesus disease (Berlin et al 1985, Camara et al 1988). Evidence presented to date, however, is unconvincing of any advantage and as with other treatments objective assessment is necessary before conclusions can be reached.

Transfusion of marrow stem-cell has been tried to effect a marrow graft from a rhesus negative mother to her rhesus positive fetus but it was concluded to have been ineffective (Linch et al 1986). Further basic research should be conducted before human studies are explored with this potentially hazardous approach.

PROPHYLAXIS

Introduced in 1967, there was soon widespread acceptance of the principle which was adopted into routine obstetric management of the mother 'at risk' of Rh(D) sensitization. It has been common practice to give passive immunization at times of recognized risk of feto-maternal transfusion, including threatened, inevitable, and therapeutic abortions, for ectopic pregnancy, during prenatal diagnostic investigations such as chorion villus sampling and amniocentesis, external cephalic version, and at delivery at all gestations; the true risk to pregnancies before 12 weeks gestation remains uncertain but it seems wise to advise prophylaxis on all the above occasions until more information is available. An intramuscular injection of immuno-globulin 250 i.u. should be given within 72 hours of the traumatic insult up to 20 weeks gestation and 500 i.u. after that; injections can be given after that time if prior administration had been overlooked. A Kleihauer test (Kleihauer et al 1957) should be performed to determine whether the dose given is sufficient to remove all the fetal red-cells from the maternal circulation: 250 i.u. should be sufficient to protect against a feto-maternal haemorrhage of 4 ml.

Antibody production following initial sensitization is usually relatively slow and modest, whereas the secondary response to a further inoculum can be dramatic and result in high levels of antibody. The dose of antigen required to initiate primary response is usually many times greater than that for secondary sensitization. Rh sensitization, therefore, tends to occur more frequently at delivery than during pregnancy when any transplacental haemorrhage will be relatively small.

Without recourse to immuno-prophylaxis, about 1% of (Rh)D-negative women would develop anti-D by the end of their first pregnancy, and a further 3 to 5% would have detectable antibodies 6 months post-delivery. About as many women again, however, produce anti-D during a second (Rh)D-positive pregnancy, suggesting that they might have been primarily immunized at their first delivery (Mollison et al 1987).

About 90% of the sensitizations that would otherwise follow pregnancy can be prevented with the administration of anti-D at delivery. Nevertheless we, like many others, have found a significant residual level of (Rh)D-sensitization and about 1·7% of (Rh)D-negative women show evidence of active D-sensitization (Bowell et al 1985).

It is now widely accepted that antenatal administration of anti-D would prevent immunization for virtually all (Mollison et al 1987). However, if the current post-delivery dose of 500 i.u. is given as suggested to (Rh)D-negative women at 28 and again at 34 weeks (Tovey et al 1983), this would require a four-fold increase in production of hyper-immune anti-D, with consequent increased risks for the volunteer donors concerned. A multicentre controlled trial of a lower dose (250 i.u.) therefore, has recently been initiated.

OTHER RED CELL ANTIBODIES AND THEIR MANAGEMENT

Many of the 700 red-cell antibodies can cause haemolytic transfusion reactions in the mother, but few cause severe HDN. Of those that do, the majority cause only mild or moderate HDN occasionally in the third trimester, but more usually following delivery. The factors that determine whether an antibody is clinically significant are immunoglobin class/subclass and the immunogenicity/fetal development of the blood group antigen. For erythroblastosis fetalis to occur during the antenatal period, the antibody must enter the fetal circulation and only those that are IgG in nature are capable of crossing the placenta; of the IgG subclasses, only IgG1 and IgG3 seem to have a role in HDN. The immunogenicity of Rh(D) is high with 80% D-negative volunteers stimulated to produce antibodies when provoked, compared with only 10% Kell negative and 1% of Fya negative volunteers similarly provoked. Additionally, many blood group antigens are only poorly developed on fetal red cells e.g. Lea/Leb, Lua/Lub, P1, I, and A/B (Mollison et al 1987). While many red cell antibodies are clearly 'immune', having been stimulated by pregnancy or transfusion, some are naturally occurring. Most of these are IgM in nature, and are thus of no threat to the fetus.

In consequence few other red cell antibodies need to be considered.

ABO incompatibility

Anti-A and anti-B generally cause relatively mild forms of HDN. Most examples of ABO HDN seem to occur when the mother is group O and her baby is group A or B (15% pregnancies). In spite of this relatively high frequency of incompatibility, very few babies show any evidence of HDN. About 1 in 30 ABO incompatibility pregnancies show mild neonatal jaundice, 1 in 150 mild anaemia, and 1 in 3000 require an exchange transfusion. To our knowledge, no intra-uterine deaths due to ABO incompatibility have been recorded. Unlike Rh(D) HDN, ABO HDN occurs as often in a first pregnancy as in subsequent pregnancies and without a tendency to increasing severity (Mollison 1951). Amniocentesis is therefore never indicated and many serologists take the view that it is generally not necessary to predict ABO HDN. Instead, tests are reserved for those with a history of past ABO HDN or for new cases of unexplained neonatal jaundice.

Anti-Kell, anti-c, and others

Among the non-D antibodies found in pregnancy, anti-c and anti-Kell are probably those most frequently associated with severe HDN. While many other immune antibodies have been cited (Beal 1979, Issit 1985, Mollison et al 1987), these are largely anecdotal reports. Relative to anti-D where 2·9 per 1000 confinements show the antibody, 0·63 show evidence of anti-c and 1·2 per 1000 show anti-Kell alloimmunization. In England and Wales anti-c and anti-Kell jointly cause about 4 fetal losses per year (Clarke et al 1987); yet there are probably more than 1100 confinements annually where anti-c and anti-Kell can be demonstrated. Severe clinical problems due to anti-c and anti-Kell therefore are relatively infrequent.

In a 10 year period in the Oxford Health Region, only 4 babies among 350 000 confinements showed significant HDN due to anti-Kell, resulting in stillbirth in 2. Over a similar period, there were 11 babies requiring exchange transfusions because of HDN due to anti-c, 9 with hyperbili-rubinaemia, 2 with severe anaemia and 1 died in the neonatal period. It appears that all 3 babies that died could have been saved if appropriate attention had been paid to the presence of the antibodies during the antenatal period.

As with anti-D, management depends on monitoring maternal antibody levels. Unlike anti-D, antibody measurement is performed by the manual antibody titration method. Although it has been recognized for some years that the automated method provides much greater precision, its use for anti-c and anti-Kell for the relatively few samples each week for the largest serological laboratories would be inefficient in time, money and effort. We believe titration values at or greater than an IAGT titre of 1/64 indicate further investigation of the pregnancy by fetal blood sampling or delivery if at the appropriate gestation: the place of amniocentesis in non-(Rh)D allo-immunization is even more debatable than it is for (Rh)D sensitized pregnancies. Management of the pregnancy when fetal anaemia has been detected will follow that already outlined for Rh(D) cases, with anticipated similar outcomes.

Occasionally, patients present with either a complex mixture of relatively common antibodies (e.g. Fyb + Jkb) or examples of antibodies to high frequency antigens (e.g. k,Yta,Vel). Although this presents considerable problems in the provision of blood for the mother if a transfusion is necessary, these incompatibilities rarely result in severe HDN. It should, however, be remembered that patients whose pregnancies are transfused may develop further antibodies which could compromise the situation in the future (Pratt et al 1989). This further endorses the view that transfusions should only by given when there is compelling evidence for action.

NEONATAL MANAGEMENT

The principle in management of the neonate delivered following pregnancy complicated by alloimmunization, is the prevention and correction of anaemia and avoidance of hyperbilirubinaemia leading to kernicterus. At delivery, samples of cord blood are collected to assay haemoglobin, ABO and rhesus (D) group, direct Coombs' test and bilirubin concentration. The haemoglobin should not be unexpectedly low if appropriate antenatal care has been provided; in general, if the Hb is below 10 g/dl in the neonate not given an intra-uterine transfusion, an exchange transfusion is required. If more than two intra-uterine transfusions have been given, there is usually less urgency and a top-up transfusion is necessary.

Hyperbilirubinaemia is a more serious threat than anaemia to the neonate. At delivery, the bilirubin concentration is unlikely to be higher than 150 µmol/l, the highest antenatal fetal level we have measured (MacKenzie et al 1988). Serial measurements of bilirubin concentrations are essential at 6 hour intervals for the first 48 hours and a value of more than 340 µmol/l in the term baby and 250 µmol/l in the preterm baby, are indications for exchange transfusion. A double volume exchange transfusion calculating 170 ml blood per kg neonatal weight, exchanged at a rate of 10–20 ml per minute, will replace up to 90% of the baby's circulating blood volume and 30% of the total body indirect bilirubin. The necessity for repeat exchange transfusion is determined by monitoring bilirubin levels and it is rare that more than five are required.

Phototherapy may be used for the less severely affected neonate or as prophylaxis; although of little value on its own in severe disease, it may be helpful as an adjunct to exchange transfusions by delaying the need for the next transfusion. Blue or blue-green light 430–470 nm converts 20% toxic indirect bilirubin into water-soluble, non-toxic isomers which are rapidly excreted in urine and bile thus reducing peak indirect bilirubin levels.

Babies delivered after more than two intra-uterine transfusions are unlikely to develop hyperbilirubinaemia since they have predominantly compatible donor blood circulating. However, prolonged haemopoietic suppression can occur and a chronic hypoplastic anaemia will prevail during the first 4–5 months and top-up transfusions will often be necessary. The anaemia almost always resolves by 6 months of age.

Enhancement of liver enzyme systems has been proposed as a method for reducing the risk of hyperbilirubinaemia. Administration of phenobarbital 10 mg/kg/24 hours to the newborn to mature the glucoronyl transferase enzyme system was found to reduce peak values of bilirubin (Trolle 1968). This approach has not been widely accepted and needs further evidence of its efficacy before it can be recommended for routine management particularly since there is a delay of 2 or 3 days before the enzyme system is stimulated (Queenan 1977).

LONG-TERM FOLLOW-UP

Kernicterus should not occur with modern neonatal care. The consequences of prematurity will vary according to the gestation at delivery. Follow-up of babies managed by intraperitoneal transfusion has been conducted by a number of workers and a review by Hardyment et al (1979) found that 78% were normal, 17% had minor disturbances of neurological function, and 5% suffered severe neurological damage. In a controlled study, White et al (1978) reported that infants treated by intraperitoneal transfusion were similar to the controls when gestation, birthweight and delivery method were taken into account. To date, no large long-term studies of babies managed by intravascular transfusion have been reported. This aspect of assessing the value of this approach to management is essential before widespread advocacy and acceptance.

FUTURE POSSIBILITIES IN RHESUS INVESTIGATION AND MANAGEMENT

Continued promotion of anti-D prophylaxis is essential since cases of omission still occur. The evidence for antenatal prophylaxis appears compelling but reserves of immunoglobulin are limited. The need for a synthetic antibody remains a goal and with the development of the 'new genetics', it is hoped that one will become available before long. At present 28 monoclonal antibodies to the Rh(D) antigen produced primarily by the Epstein-Barr virus have been examined but very few have been found to be adequate. It seems that different isotypes and allo-types of anti-D antibodies mediate removal of the red cell by the effector cells via dissimilar Fc receptor interactions (Kumpel et al 1989). It may be that pools of different cell lines will need deploying before prophylaxis using monoclonals becomes a real possibility.

Investigation of the various antibody subgroups, exploring antigenicity strengths might help determine which sensitized pregnancies are at greater risk of fetal haemolysis. The antibody-dependent cell-mediated cyto-toxicity test (ADCC), by measuring the interaction between sensitized red cells and monocytes, might prove to be an objective indicator of erythro-phagocytosis (Mollison et al 1987) and therefore an adjunct to the quantitation of maternal antibody. However, once sensitization has occurred, improvement in antenatal assessment methods is still required since fetal blood sampling, although precise, is not without hazard. Equally, intra-uterine transfusions, whichever technique is used, are potentially lethal and alternative concepts must be sought.

REFERENCES

Bang J, Bock J E, Trolle D 1982 Ultrasound-guided fetal intravenous transfusion for severe rhesus haemolytic disease. Br Med J 284: 373–374

Barss V A, Doudilet P M, St John-Sutton M et al 1987 Cardiac output in a fetus with erythroblastosis: assessment using pulsed doppler ultrasound. Obstet Gynecol 70: 442–444

Beal R W 1979 Non-Rhesus (D) blood group isoimmunization in obstetrics. Clin Obstet Gynecol 6: 493–508

Benacerraf B R, Barss V A, Saltzman D H, Greene M F, Penso C A, Frigoletto F D 1987 Acute fetal distress associated with percutaneous umbilical blood sampling. Am J Obstet Gynecol 1987: 1218–1220

Bennebroek Gravenhorst J, Kanhai H H H 1989 22 years of intra-uterine intraperitoneal transfusions. Eur J Obstet Gynaecol Reprod Biol 33: 71–77

Berkowitz R L, Chitkara U, Goldberg J D, Wilkins I, Chervenak F A, Lynch L 1986 Intra-uterine intravascular transfusions for severe red blood cell isoimmunization: ultrasound-guided percutaneous approach. Am J Obstet Gynecol 155: 574–581

Berkowitz R L, Chitkara U, Wilkins I, Lynch L, Mehalek K E 1987 Technical aspects of intravascular intrauterine transfusions: lessons learned from 33 procedures. Am J Obstet Gynecol 157: 4–9

Berlin G, Selbing A, Ryden G 1985 Rhesus haemolytic disease treated with high-dose intra-venous immunoglobulin. Lancet i: 1153

Bevis D C A 1952 The antenatal prediction of haemolytic disease of the newborn. Lancet ii: 395–398

Bevis D C A 1956 Blood pigments in haemolytic disease of the newborn. J Obstet Gynaecol Br Commwth 63: 68–75

Bierme S J, Blanc M, Abbal M, Fournie A 1979 Oral Rh treatment for severely immunized mothers. Lancet i: 604–605

Bowell P J, Wainscoat J S, Peto T E A, Gunson H H 1982 Maternal anti-D concentrations and outcome in rhesus haemolytic disease of the newborn. Br Med J 285: 327–329

Bowell P J, MacKenzie I Z, Entwistle C C 1985 Deaths from rhesus D haemolytic disease. Br Med J 291: 1351

Bowell P J, Allen D L, Entwistle C C 1986a Blood group antibody screening tests during pregnancy. Br J Obstet Gynaecol 93: 1038–1043

Bowell P J, Brown S E, Dike A E, Inskip M J 1986b The significance of anti-c alloimmunization in pregnancy. Br J Obstet Gynaecol 93: 1044–1048

Bowell P J, Inskip M J, Jones M N 1988a The significance of anti-C sensitization in pregnancy. Clin Lab Haematol 10: 251–255

Bowell P J, Selinger M, Ferguson J, Giles J, MacKenzie I Z 1988b Antenatal fetal blood sampling for the management of alloimmunized pregnancies: effect on maternal anti-D potency levels. Br J Obstet Gynaecol 95: 759–764

Bowman J M 1987 Haemolytic disease of the newborn. Clin Immunol Allergy 1: 391–425

Bowman J M, Peddle J L, Anderson C 1968 Plasmapheresis in severe Rh iso-immunization. Vox Sang 15: 272–277

Brambati B, Pardi G 1981 The intraventricular conduction time of fetal heart in pregnancies complicated by rhesus haemolytic disease. Br J Obstet Gynaecol 88: 1233–1240

Butler N R, Bonham D G 1963 Perinatal mortality: the first report of the 1958 British perinatal mortality survey. Livingstone, Edinburgh, pp 186–200

Camara C D L, Arrieta R, Gonzalez A, Iglesias E, Omenaca F 1988 High-dose intravenous immunoglobulin as the sole prenatal treatment for severe Rh immunization. N Engl J Med 318: 519–520

Caudle M R, Scott J R 1982 The potential role of immunosuppression plasmapheresis and desensitization as treatment modalities for Rh immunization. Clin Obstet Gynecol 25: 313–319

Charles A G, Blumenthal L S 1982 Promethazine hydrochloride therapy in severely Rh-sensitized pregnancies. Obstet Gynecol 60: 627–630

Clarke C A, Donohoe W T A, McConell R B et al 1963 Further experimental studies on the prevention of Rh haemolytic disease. Br Med J i: 979–984

Clarke C A, Whitfield A G W, Mollison P L 1987 Deaths from Rh haemolytic disease in England and Wales in 1984 and 1985. Br Med J 294: 1001

Copel J A, Grannum P A, Green J J, Belanger K, Hobbins J C 1989a Pulsed doppler flow-velocity waveforms in the prediction of fetal hematocrit of the severely isoimmunized pregnancy. Am J Obstet Gynecol 161: 341–344

Copel J A, Grannum P A, Green J J et al 1989b Fetal cardiac output in the isoimmunized pregnancy: a pulsed doppler-echocardiographic study of patients undergoing intravascular intrauterine transfusion. Am J Obstet Gynecol 161: 361–363

Crowley P 1989 Promoting pulmonary maturity. In: Chalmers I, Enkin M, Keirse M J N C (eds) Effective care in pregnancy and childbirth. Oxford University Press, England, pp 746–764

Daffos F, Capella-Pavlovsky M, Forestier F 1985 Fetal blood sampling during pregnancy with use of a needle guided by ultrasound: a study of 606 consecutive cases. Am J Obstet Gynecol 153: 655–660

Davey M 1979 The prevention of rhesus-isoimmunization. Clin Obstet Gynecol 6: 509–530

DeVore G R, Mayden K, Tortora M, Berkowitz R L, Hobbins J C 1981 Dilation of the fetal umbilical vein in rhesus hemolytic anaemia: a predictor of severe disease. Am J Obstet Gynecol 141: 464–466

Diamond L K 1947 Erythroblastosis foetalis or haemolytic disease of the newborn. Proc R Soc Med 40: 546–550

Doyle L W, Cauchi M, De Crespigny L C et al 1986 Fetal intravascular transfusion of severe erythroblastosis: effects on haematology and survival. Aust N Z J Obstet Gynaecol 26: 192–195

Eklund J 1978 Prevention of Rh immunization in Finland. A national study, 1969–1977. Acta Paediatr Scand Supp. 274, pp 1–57

Fairweather D V I, Whyley G A, Millar M D 1976 Six years experience of the prediction of severity in rhesus haemolytic disease. Br J Obstet Gynaecol 83: 698–706

Frigoletto F D, Greene M F, Benacerraf B R, Barss V A, Saltzman D H 1986 Ultrasonographic fetal surveillance in the management of the isoimmunized pregnancy. N Engl J Med 315: 430–432

Gemke R B R J, Kanhai H H H, Overbeeke M A M et al 1986 ABO and rhesus phenotyping of fetal erythrocytes in the first trimester of pregnancy. Br J Haematol 64: 689–697

Gold W R, Queenan J T, Woody J, Sacher R A 1983 Oral desensitization in Rh disease. Am J Obstet Gynecol 146: 980–981

Goto S, Nishi H, Tomoda Y 1980 Blood group Rh-D factor in human trophoblast determined by immunofluorescent method. Am J Obstet Gynecol 137: 707

Grannum P A, Copel J A, Plaxe S C, Scioscia A L, Hobbins J C 1986 In utero exchange transfusion by direct intravascular injection in severe erythroblastosis fetalis. N Engl J Med 314: 1431–1434

Gusdon J P 1981 The treatment of erythroblastosis with promethazine. J Reprod Med 26: 454–458

Hardyment A F, Salvador H S, Towell M E, Carpenter C W, Jan J E, Tingle A J 1979 Follow-up of intrauterine transfused surviving children. Am J Obstet Gynecol 133: 235–241

Harman C R, Bowman J M, Menticoglou S M, Pollock J M, Manning F A 1988 Profound fetal thrombocytopenia in rhesus disease: serious hazard at intravascular transfusion. Lancet ii: 741–742

Hobbins J C, Davis C D, Webster J 1975 A new technique utilizing ultrasound to aid intra-uterine transfusion. JCU 4: 135–137

Issit P 1985 Applied blood group serology 3rd edn. Montgomery Publications, New York, pp 225–240

Kanhai H H, Bennebroek Gravenhorst J, Gemke R J, Overbeeke M A, Bernini L F, Beverstock G C 1987 Fetal blood group determination in first-trimester pregnancy for the management of severe isoimmunization. Am J Obstet Gynecol 156: 120–123

Kirkinen P, Jouppila P, Eik-nes S 1983 Umbilical vein blood flow in rhesus-isoimmunization. Br J Obstet Gynaecol 90: 640–643

Kleihauer E, Braun H, Betke K 1957 Demonstration of fetal haemoglobin in erythrocytes of a blood smear. Klin Wochenschr 35: 637–638

Kumpel B M, Wiener E, Urbaniak S J, Bradley B A 1989 Human monoclonal anti-D antibodies. Br J Haematol 71: 415–420

Lemery D, Urbain M F, VanLieferinghen P, Micorek J C, Jacquetin B 1989 Intra-uterine exchange transfusion under ultrasound guidance. Eur J Obstet Gynaecol Reprod Biol 33: 161–168

Levine P, Katzin E M, Burnham L 1941 Isoimmunization in pregnancy. Its possible bearing on the etiology of erythroblastosis foetalis. JAMA 116: 825–827

Liley A W 1961 Liquor amnii analysis in management of pregnancy complicated by rhesus sensitization. Am J Obstet Gynecol 82: 1359–1370

Liley A W 1963 Intrauterine transfusion of foetus in haemolytic disease. Br Med J ii: 1107–1109

Linch D C, Rodeck C H, Nicolaides K H, Jones H M, Brent L 1986 Attempted bone-marrow transplantation in a 17-week fetus. Lancet ii: 1453

MacKenzie I Z 1984 Fetoscopy in the management of hemolytic disease of the newborn. Plasma Ther Trans Technol 5: 33–42

MacKenzie I Z, MacLean D A, Fry A, Lloyd-Evans S 1982 Midtrimester exchange transfusion of the fetus. Am J Obstet Gynecol 143: 555–559

MacKenzie I Z, Guest C M, Bowell P J 1983 Fetal blood group studies during midtrimester pregnancy in the management of severe iso-immunization. Prenat Diag 3: 41–46

MacKenzie I Z, Bowell P J 1986 Management of pregnancies complicated by severe Rhesus isoimmunization using repeated fetal blood sampling compared with repeated amnio-centesis. Abstract for 24th British Congress of Obstetrics and Gynaecology. Cardiff 15–18th April 1986, p 170

MacKenzie I Z, Bowell P J, Ferguson J, Castle B M, Entwistle C C 1987 In-utero intravascular transfusion of the fetus for the management of severe rhesus iso-immunization—a reappraisal. Br J Obstet Gynaecol 94: 1068–1073

MacKenzie I Z, Bowell P J, Castle B M, Selinger M, Ferguson J F 1988 Serial fetal blood sampling for the management of pregnancies complicated by severe rhesus (D) isoimmunization. Br J Obstet Gynaecol 95: 753–758

Maclennan Sir H 1967 A gynaecologist looks at the Tudors. Med Hist 11: 66–74

Mollison P L 1951 Blood transfusion in clinical medicine 5th edn, Blackwell Scientific, Oxford, p 391

Mollison P L, Engelfriet C P, Contreras M 1987 Blood transfusion in clinical medicine 8th edn Blackwell Scientific, Oxford, pp 375–378, 649–675

Neil V S, Bowell P J 1984 Amniotic fluid anti-D and the maternal serum: liquor ratio in rhesus haemolytic disease of the newborn. Clin Lab Haematol 6: 39–43

Nicolaides K H, Rodeck C H, Mibashan R S, Kemp J R 1986 Have Liley charts outlived their usefulness? Am J Obstet Gynecol 155: 90–94

Nicolaides K H, Thilaganathan B, Rodeck C H, Mibashan R S 1988 Erythroblastosis and reticulocytosis in anaemic fetuses. Am J Obstet Gynecol 159: 1063–1065

Office of Population, Censuses and Surveys 1985 Abortion statistics—England and Wales 1984. AB No 12 HMSO, London, pp 54–55

Office of Population, Censuses and Surveys 1986 Abortion statistics—England and Wales 1985. AB No 13 HMSO, London, pp 54–55

Parer J T 1988 Severe Rh isoimmunization—current methods of in utero diagnosis and treatment. Am J Obstet Gynecol 158: 1323–1329

Philip J, Brandt N J, Fernandes A, Freiesleben E, Trolle D 1978 ABO and Rh phenotyping of fetal blood obtained by foetoscopy. Clin Genet 14: 324–329

Poissonnier M H, Brossard Y, Demedeiros N et al 1989 200 intrauterine exchange transfusions in severe blood incompatibilities. Am J Obstet Gynecol 161: 709–713

Pratt G A, Bowell P J, MacKenzie I Z, Ferguson J, Selinger M 1989 Production of additional atypical alloantibodies in Rh(D)-sensitized pregnancies managed by intrauterine investigation methods. Clin Lab Haematol 11: 241–248

Pridmore B R, Robertson E G, Walker W 1972 Liquor bilirubin levels and false prediction of severity in rhesus haemolytic disease. Br Med J iii: 136–139

Queenan J T 1977 Modern management of the Rhesus problem, 2nd edn. Harper Row, Hagerstown, p 206

Reece E A, Copel J A, Scioscia A L, Grannum P A T, DeGennaro N, Hobbins J C 1988 Diagnostic fetal umbilical blood sampling in the management of isoimmunization. Am J Obstet Gynecol 159: 1057–1062

Roberts A B, Mitchell J M, Pattison N S 1989 Fetal liver length in normal and isoimmunized pregnancies. Am J Obstet Gynecol 161: 42–46

Rochard F, Schifrin B S, Goupil F, Legrand H, Blottiere J, Sureau C 1976 Nonstressed fetal heart rate monitoring in the antepartum period. Am J Obstet Gynecol 126: 699–706

Rodeck C H, Holman C A, Karnicki J, Kemp J R, Whitmore D N, Austin M A 1981 Direct intravascular fetal blood transfusion by fetoscopy in severe rhesus isoimmunization. Lancet i: 625–627

Rodeck C H, Nicolaides K H, Warsof S L, Fysh W J, Gamsu H R, Kemp J R 1984 The management of severe rhesus in immunization by fetoscopic intravascular transfusion. Am J Obstet Gynecol 150: 769–774

Rodesch F, Lambermont M, Donner C et al 1987 Chorionic biopsy in management of severe Kell alloimmunization. Am J Obstet Gynecol 156: 124–125

Ronkin S, Chayen R, Wapner R J et al 1989 Intravascular exchange and bolus transfusion in the severely isoimmunized fetus. Am J Obstet Gynecol 160: 407–411

Rosenfield R E, Szymanski I O, Kochwa S 1964 Immunochemical studies of the Rh system: quantitation hemagglutination that is relatively independent of source of Rh antigens and antibodies. Cold Spring Harbour Symposium on Quantitative Biology 29: 437

Sadovsky E, Laufer N, Beyth Y 1979 The role of fetal movements assessment in cases of severe Rh immunized patients. Acta Obstet Gynecol Scand 58: 313–315

Scott J R, Branch D W, Kochenour N K, Ward K 1988 Intravenous immunoglobulin treatment of pregnant patients with recurrent pregnancy loss caused by antiphospholipid antibodies and Rh immunization. Am J Obstet Gynecol 159: 1055–1056

Selinger M, Bowell P J, MacKenzie I Z, Ferguson J 1990 Use of microcomputer programmes for in-utero fetal transfusions. Unpublished observations

Socol M L, MacGregor S N, Pielet B W, Tamura R K, Sabbagha R E 1987 Percutaneous umbilical transfusion in severe rhesus isoimmunization: resolution of fetal hydrops. Am J Obstet Gynecol 157: 1369–1375

Stenchever M A 1978 Promethazine hydrochloride: use in patients with Rh isoimmunization. Am J Obstet Gynecol 130: 665–668

Tovey L A D 1988 Anti-D and miscarriages. Br Med J 297: 977–978

Tovey L A D, Taverner J M 1981 A case for the antenatal administration of anti-D immunoglobulin to primigravidae. Lancet i: 878–881

Tovey L A D, Townley A, Stevenson B J, Taverner J 1983 The Yorkshire antenatal anti-D immunoglobulin trial in primigravidae. Lancet ii: 244–246

Trolle D 1968 Decrease of total serum bilirubin concentration in newborn infants after phenobarbitone treatment. Lancet ii: 705

Vintzileos A M, Campbell W A, Deaton J L, Nochimson D J, Erinsum P J 1987 Hydrops fetalis associated with immunologic and nonimmunologic factors. Am J Perinatol 4: 115–120

Visser G H A 1982 Antepartum sinusoidal and decelerative heart rate patterns in Rh disease. Am J Obstet Gynecol 143: 538–544

Voto L S, Margulies M 1989 Frequency and timing of intravascular transfusions reconsidered. Am J Obstet Gynecol 161: 255

Wallerstein H 1946 Treatment of severe erythroblastosis by simultaneous removal and replacement of the blood of the newborn infant. Science 103: 583–584

Weiner S, Bolognese R J, Librizzi R J 1981 Ultrasound in the evaluation and management of the isoimmunized pregnancy. JCU 9: 315–323

Westgren M, Selbing A, Stangenberg M 1988 Fetal intracardiac transfusions in patients with severe rhesus isoimmunization. Br Med J 296: 885–886

Westgren M, Selbing A, Stangenberg M, Phillips R 1989 Acid-base status in fetal heart blood in erythroblastotic fetuses: a study with special reference to the effect of transfusions with adult blood. Am J Obstet Gynecol 160: 1134–1138

White C A, Goplerud C P, Kisker C T, Stehbens J A, Kitchell M, Taylor J C 1978 Intra-uterine fetal transfusion, 1965–1976, with an assessment of the surviving children. Am J Obstet Gynecol 130: 933–939

Whitfield C R 1983 Haemolytic disease of the newborn—a continuing problem. In: Chiswick M L (ed), Recent advances in perinatal medicine, Churchill Livingstone, Edinburgh, pp 95–115

4. Prostaglandins, aspirin and pre-eclampsia

P. McParland   J. M. Pearce

Pregnancy-induced hypertension (PIH) occurs in up to 10% of pregnancies and may cause substantial maternal and fetal mortality and morbidity. The underlying cause remains unknown but most investigators agree that uteroplacental ischaemia plays an important role. Over the past decade substantial evidence has demonstrated a role for prostaglandins in the pathogenesis of PIH. Current knowledge implicates an imbalance between thromboxane and prostacyclin and this appears to play a pivotal role in the clinical and haematological manifestations of PIH. This imbalance may be corrected by low dose aspirin and several studies have demonstrated that low dose aspirin has the capacity to prevent PIH. This review seeks to summarize the role of prostaglandins in PIH and to review the available literature concerning the use of aspirin in pregnancy.

PROSTAGLANDINS

The prostaglandins are a group of 20 carbon unsaturated fatty acids that are similar in structure yet varied in function and have been detected in almost every tissue and body fluid. They produce a multitude of physiological and pharmacological effects that embrace practically every biological function. Interest in prostaglandin production in pregnancy was revived in the late fifties when Bergstrom & Sjovall (1957) isolated the first members of the prostaglandin family, PGE_1 and PGE_2, more than 20 years after Goldblatt (1933) and Von Eular (1937) first postulated the presence of a vasodepressor and smooth muscle stimulating substance in human seminal fluid.

Much of the earlier research on prostaglandins focused on PGE and PGF_2. In the 1970s the successive discoveries of thromboxane A_2 (Hamberg et al 1975, 1976) and prostacyclin (Moncado et al 1976) shifted the focus to these more potent prostanoids which have important regulatory functions on blood pressure and blood flow (Karim & Somers 1972).

The arachidonic acid pathway

Arachidonic acid is a carbon 20 polyunsaturated fatty acid that, in the non-

55

esterified form is the precursor of all prostaglandins. Arachidonic acid is a typical polyunsaturated fatty acid in that it is present in cells predominantly in an esterified form, hence the liberation from glycerophospholipids of arachidonic acid is a key event in the biosynthesis of prostaglandins and is thought to be the rate limiting step in this process (Samuelsson 1978). The release of arachidonic acid is accomplished either directly by the action of phospholipase A_2, or indirectly by the action of phospholipase C.

Liberated arachidonic acid can be metabolized by way of at least 3 major pathways (Fig. 4.1). Attention has been focused on the prostaglandins pathway, though the epoxygenase and leukotriene pathways may have important related functions. The formation of prostaglandins and thromboxanes begins with the action of prostaglandin endoperoxide synthetase (otherwise known as cyclo-oxygenase), on arachidonic acid. There is an inherent peroxidase activity in the holoenzyme, such that PGG_2 is rapidly converted to PGH_2. Although these substances are short-lived intermediates they do possess intrinsic biological activity. It is the formation of these endoperoxide intermediates that is inhibited by non-steroid anti-inflammatory agents such as aspirin (see later). These intermediates are metabolized further to prostaglandins and thromboxanes by the actions of various isomerases.

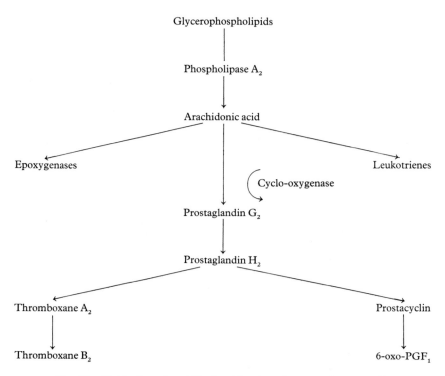

Fig. 4.1   Metabolism of arachidonic acid to thromboxane and prostacyclin.

The first step in the metabolism of prostaglandins is catalysed by 15-hydroxy prostaglandin dehydrogenase (PGDH) which is a cytosolic enzyme. The 15 keto derivatives so formed are biologically inactive and are rapidly converted to the 13, 14-dehydro-15 keto derivatives that are the major circulating forms. Almost all biologically active prostaglandins are metabolized during one passage through the lungs, the major site of metabolism. Such metabolism occurs firstly by uptake into pulmonary cells and secondly by the action of PGDH. Elimination of biologically active prostaglandins is completed by a series of beta and W-oxidations that result in the formation of a wide variety of products that are excreted in the urine. Exceptions do exist, prostacyclin may not be completely metabolized in the lung since it is not a good substrate for the uptake mechanisms that transport prostaglandins into the pulmonary cells for subsequent metabolism.

Prostacyclin

Prostacyclin is a very potent vasodilator and inhibitor of platelet aggregation (Fitzgerald et al 1979, O'Grady et al 1980). It is the most abundant arachidonic acid metabolite, produced in the endothelium of all blood vessels so far studied (Dusting et al 1982) and in the heart and stomach. Prostacyclin is chemically unstable with a half-life of 3 minutes in blood at 37°C (Dusting et al 1978) and therefore its actions are largely limited to the local environment into which it is released. Prostacyclin was at first thought to be a circulating hormone but its presence in the circulation in physiologically significant concentrations has been disputed (Blair et al 1982). This does not of course argue against its role in local vascular haemostasis. The circulatory changes caused by prostacyclin after intravenous infusion into man (vasodilation, tachycardia, hypotension) are reversed within 15 minutes of discontinuing the infusion (O'Grady et al 1980). The platelet effects of inhibition of adenosine diphosphate-induced platelet aggregation, however, persist for up to 105 minutes (O'Grady et al 1980), probably secondary to persistent elevation of platelet cyclic AMP. Prostacyclin has also been shown to inhibit spontaneous motility of isolated normal human myometrium (Omini et al 1979), and to stimulate the renin angiotensin-aldosterone axis (Patrono et al 1982). Prostacyclin activity is determined by measuring its stable metabolite 6-keto-PGF$_{1\alpha}$. In pregnancy the following are known to produce prostacyclin: placenta, umbilical, placental and uterine vessels; ductus arteriosus, amnion, chorion and decidua, and myometrium.

Thromboxane

Thromboxane A$_2$ was discovered in 1975 (Hamberg et al 1975) and in marked contrast to prostacyclin is a potent vasoconstrictor (Svensson et al

1977, Svensson & Fredholm 1977) and platelet aggregator (Hamberg et al 1975, Moncado et al 1979). It is produced primarily by platelets, although other tissues such as lung and spleen are also capable of producing thromboxane A_2. Its biological half-life in blood at 37°C is approximately 30 seconds (Moncado & Vane 1979) and it is therefore usually measured by its stable hydration product, thromboxane B_2 (Granstrom et al 1982).

These two prostaglandins may be seen as powerful biological components which are responsible for vascular tone regulation and the extent to which platelet aggregation and thrombus formation occurs.

PROSTAGLANDINS IN NORMAL PREGNANCY

Prostaglandins have important roles in pregnancy and the mechanisms of parturition in all mammalian species that have been studied. For instance there is overwhelming evidence that prostaglandins are critical in the mechanisms that regulate cervical ripening and uterine contractions. Moreover it is likely that prostaglandins play a significant role in the regulation of uterine and fetoplacental haemodynamics.

Prostaglandins in amniotic fluid

The presence of prostaglandins in amniotic fluid was first demonstrated by Karim in 1966 and shortly thereafter he demonstrated that labour was associated with greatly increased concentrations of amniotic fluid prosta-glandins (Karim 1966, Karim & Devlin 1967). Amniotic fluid has proven to be a popular fluid in which to measure prostaglandins because there is essentially no biosynthesis or metabolism in this fluid. Both 6-keto-$PGF_{1\alpha}$ and thromboxane B_2, the major products of PGI_2 and thromboxane A_2 respectively, have been detected in amniotic fluid (Mitchell et al 1978, 1979). The amniotic fluid concentration of 6-keto-$PGF_{1\alpha}$ level increases with advancing gestational age, and during labour. It originates from various fetoplacental tissues and fetal urine (Ylikorkala & Makila 1985, Ylikorkala et al 1981b). Whether the prostaglandins in amniotic fluid play any part in the mechanisms of the onset and progression of labour in humans is unknown.

Prostaglandins in the maternal circulation

Reliable measurements of prostaglandins in peripheral plasma are difficult to obtain because concentrations of prostaglandins in the peripheral circulation are extremely low due to the high metabolic activity of the lungs. These problems can be overcome to some extent by chronically implanted vascular catheters in the venous drainage of an organ of interest but this is impractical in human pregnancy. Two other methods have therefore been advocated. Firstly the improvement of assay techniques such that peripheral plasma concentrations could be measured accurately and be consistent with levels that have been reported by the use of gas chromotography/mass spectrometry techniques and secondly methods utilizing the measurement of the stable metabolites of prostaglandins.

Despite using adequate anticoagulants and prostaglandin synthesis inhibitors in collecting tubes, minor aggregation of platelets and consequent release of thromboxane B_2 during sampling is unavoidable. Obtaining an index of thromboxane A_2 production by measurements of the degradation product thromboxane B_2 in the peripheral circulation is difficult. Thromboxane A_2 is produced in large amounts by platelets in response to many stimuli. Thromboxane A_2 also combines with plasma proteins in a covalent manner thus making it difficult to draw meaningful conclusions from measurements of thromboxane B_2 in the peripheral circulation. However such measurements that have been made to date suggest little change in thromboxane B_2 levels in plasma throughout normal gestation or labour.

There is also controversy concerning the measurement of the prostacyclin metabolite, 6-keto-$PGF_{1\alpha}$. Initially, measurements using radioimmunoassay techniques and gas chromotography/mass spectrometry provided similar results with peripheral plasma concentrations of approximately 120–150 pg/ml. Subsequently, it has been reported that the circulating concentrations of 6-keto-$PGF_{1\alpha}$ are much closer to those of PGE_2 and PGF_2 i.e. 2–5 pg/ml. Furthermore only 40% of prostacyclin is metabolized to 6-keto-$PGF_{1\alpha}$ (Rosenkranz et al 1980) and so measurement of this metabolite only may not fully reflect prostacyclin metabolism.

The earlier studies measuring maternal plasma 6-oxo-PGF_1 and maternal urinary dinor-6-keto-PGF_1 reported higher levels of prostacyclin in pregnant than in non-pregnant women (Lewis et al 1980, Goodman et al 1982, Mitchell et al 1981). Both groups used combined gas–liquid chromotography-mass spectrometry to measure 6-oxo-PGF_1. These findings have been confirmed by other groups (Barrow et al 1983, Greer et al 1985). On the other hand, no differences between pregnant women and non-pregnant women with respect to plasma 6-oxo-PGF_1 concentrations have been demonstrated (Ylikorkala et al 1981b).

Longitudinal studies in normotensive pregnancies have shown that peak production is achieved by the second trimester, thereafter production appears to be static until term (Lewis et al 1980, Goodman et al 1982). Bolton et al (1981) and Spitz et al (1983) found a peak in the second trimester whilst Greer et al (1985) showed the peak to be achieved by the end of the first trimester followed by a decline until term whilst no changes in plasma levels during pregnancy have been shown by other groups (Ylikorkala et al 1981b, Koullapis et al 1982). The high levels of circulating 6-oxo-PGF_1 that occur during the second trimester may contribute to the physiological mid-trimester fall in blood pressure. The decline after the second trimester may be due to a reduction in prostacyclin synthesis or an increase in its metabolism via an alternative pathway.

The renal excretion of prostacyclin metabolites in normotensive pregnancy is enhanced early in pregnancy and eventually increases to levels 5–10 fold above levels found in non-pregnant women (Goodman et al 1982, Fitzgerald et al 1987). The balance of evidence suggests that prostacyclin production is increased in pregnancy although there have been some conflicting results possibly explained by the different methodology used.

Less information is available about thromboxane A_2 than prostacyclin. Several pregnancy-associated tissues such as amnion, chorion, decidua, and placenta are capable of producing thromboxane B_2 in vitro (Mitchell et al 1978). Plasma thromboxane B_2 levels in normal pregnancy are not known, with studies showing increased (Fitzgerald et al 1987), static (Koullapis et al 1982) or decreasing levels (Greer et al 1985).

The capacity of maternal platelets to synthesize thromboxane A_2 increases during pregnancy (Ylikorkala & Viinikka 1980). Thromboxane B_2 in amniotic fluid appears to increase with advancing gestation (Ylikorkala et al 1981a) and in labour (Makarainen & Ylikorkala 1984).

NORMAL PREGNANCY

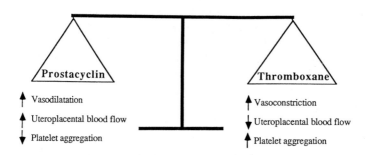

PRE-ECLAMPSIA

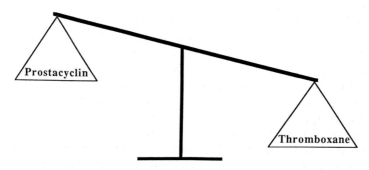

Fig. 4.2   In pre-eclampsia there is an excess of thromboxane when compared to prostacyclin.

PROSTAGLANDINS IN PIH

Numerous studies have attempted to assess prostaglandin production in PIH, but although there is general agreement that the balance is tilted in favour of the actions of thromboxane (Fig. 4.2) there is controversy over the precise details.

The maternal compartment

Several groups have demonstrated a deficiency of prostacyclin production by measuring reduced plasma levels of stable prostacyclin metabolites (Lewis et al 1981, Ylikorkala et al 1981b, Yamaguchi & Mori 1985) and urinary prostacyclin metabolites (Goodman et al 1982, Fitzgerald et al 1987) in PIH. Table 4.1 summarizes the published data on prostacyclin and thromboxane levels in the maternal compartment in pregnancies complicated by pre-eclampsia. Overall it is probable that there is a decrease in prostacyclin production with an increase in thromboxane production.

Table 4.1   Maternal prostacyclin and thromboxane A_2 production in pre-eclampsia versus normal pregnancy. (Adapted from Friedman 1988)

Author	Sample	Method	Prostacyclin	Thromboxane	Prostacyclin/ thromboxane
Ylikorkala et al (1981b)	Venous blood	RIA	Unchanged		
Koullapis et al (1982)	Venous blood	RIA	Increased		
Ylikorkala et al (1986)	Venous blood	RIA	Unchanged	Unchanged	Unchanged
Yamaguchi & Mori (1985)	Venous blood	RIA	Decreased	Increased	Decreased
Bussolini et al (1980)	Subcutaneous vessels	Bioassay	Decreased		
Goodman et al (1982)	Urine	Gas chromo-tography/ mass spectrometry	Decreased		
Fitzgerald et al (1987)	Urine	Gas chromo-tography/ mass spectrometry	Decreased		
Fitzgerald et al (1990)	Urine	Gas chromo-tography/ mass spectrometry		Increased	

The fetal compartment

Other investigators have opted to study prostacyclin and thromboxane production in fetal rather than maternal tissue. The justification for this point of view is that fetal tissues are apparently capable of synthesizing greater amounts of prostacyclin than maternal tissues (Remuzzi et al 1979, Kawano & Mori 1983). The latter group demonstrated that prostacyclin production was very much higher in the umbilical vessels when compared with placental vessels. Various methods have been used including measurement of amniotic fluid levels, fetal blood and plasma levels, in addition to studying the capacity of various vessels (umbilical artery and vein, placental

Table 4.2   Fetoplacental prostacyclin and thromboxane A_2 production in pre-eclampsia versus normal pregnancy. (Adapted from Friedman 1988)

Author	Sample	Method	Prostacyclin	Thromboxane	Prostacyclin/ thromboxane
Bussolino et al (1980)	Placental vein	Bioassay	Decreased		
Remuzzi et al (1980)	Umbilical artery	Bioassay	Decreased		
	Placental vein	Bioassay	Decreased		
Downing et al (1980)	Umbilical artery	Gas chromatography/ mass spectrometry	Decreased		
Bodzenta et al (1980)	Amniotic fluid	Bioassay	Decreased		
Ylikorkala et al (1981a)	Amniotic fluid	RIA	Decreased	Unchanged	Decreased
Carreras et al (1981)	Umbilical artery	RIA	Decreased		
	Placental vein	RIA	Unchanged		
Stuart et al (1981)	Umbilical artery	Thin layer chromatography	Decreased		
Dadak et al (1982)		Bioassay	Decreased		
Mäkilä et al (1984)	Placenta	RIA	Unchanged	Unchanged	Decreased
Walsh et al (1985)	Placenta	RIA	Decreased		
Walsh (1985)	Placenta	RIA	Decreased	Increased	Decreased
Yamaguchi & Mori (1985)	Umbilical venous plasma	RIA	Decreased		
McLaren et al (1987)		Bioassay	Decreased		

vein) and the placenta to synthesize prostacyclin and thromboxane in vitro. The results are more consistent with demonstrating an altered prosta-cyclin/thromboxane ratio than in the maternal compartment and are summarized in Table 4.2.

The source of excess thromboxane production is of some dispute with Walsh et al (1985) suggesting that the placenta is the most likely source. They argue that because prostaglandins are not stored by tissues that the production rate is a better indicator of in vivo situation than simply the tissue level. Fitzgerald et al (1987) have performed an elegant study which suggests that platelets may be the main source, on the basis that the recovery of thromboxane B_2 excretion paralleled the recovery of platelet cyclo-oxygenase following aspirin administration.

A physiological balance between prostacyclin and thromboxane is likely to be of major importance in maintaining the vasodilated state of normal pregnancy and it is probable that the imbalance that exists in PIH is responsible for the generalized vasoconstriction and platelet aggregation (see Fig. 4.2). Vasoconstriction would result in reduced fetoplacental blood flow with subsequent infarction and growth retardation whilst systemic vasoconstriction leads to hypertension. An imbalance favouring thromboxane would increase platelet aggregation and activate the coagulation system leading to thrombocytopenia. It has been suggested on theoretical grounds that low dose aspirin may restore the balance and thus be of use in the prevention and possible treatment of pre-eclampsia.

ASPIRIN

History

In England in the mid 18th century, Reverend Edmund Stone described in a letter to the president of the Royal Society 'an account of the success of the bark of the willow in the cure of agues'. He had accidently tasted the bark of the common white willow (*Salix alba vulgaris*) and the bitterness was to him, strongly reminiscent of Cinchona bark, the source of quinine. He rationalized his finding on the grounds that since the willow grew in damp or wet areas 'where agues drolly abound' it would probably possess curative properties appropriate to that condition.

The active ingredient in the willow bark was a bitter glycoside called salicin first isolated in a pure form in 1829 by Leroux, who also demon-strated its antipyretic effect. On hydrolysis salicin yields glucose and salicylic alcohol. The latter can be converted into salicylic acid either in vivo or by chemical manipulation. Salicylic acid was also prepared from oil of gaultheria (oil of wintergreen) and from extracts of other plants including *Spiraea ulmaria* (a relative of the rose). The synthetic manufacture of this acid from phenol was accomplished by Kolbe and Lautemann. Sodium salicylate was first used for the treatment of rheumatic fever and as an antipyretic in 1875 and the discovery of its uricosuric effects and of its utility in the treatment of gout soon followed. The enormous success of this drug prompted Hoffman, a chemist employed by Bayer, to prepare acetylsalicylic acid. This compound was introduced into medicine in 1899 by Dreser under the name of aspirin—the name probably derived from spiraea.

Mechanism of action

Although the therapeutic effects of aspirin had been appreciated for nearly a century it was not until 1971 that Vane described elaborate experiments in guinea pig lung which suggest that aspirin inhibits synthesis of prostaglandins. Aspirin inhibits the conversion of arachidonic acid to the unstable endoperoxide intermediate PGG_2 (see Fig. 4.1) which is catalysed by cyclo-oxygenase. A few years later this inhibitory effect was shown to result from acetylation of the cyclo-oxygenase enzyme (Roth & Majerus 1975). This effect is irreversible and persists for the lifetime of the enzyme. This is readily demonstrable in the platelet, which has no capacity for protein synthesis (Burch et al 1978). Aspirin acetylates a serine at the active site of the enzyme. In contrast to aspirin, salicylic acid has no acetylating capacity and is almost inactive against cyclo-oxygenase in vitro. Nevertheless it is as active as aspirin in reducing the synthesis of prostaglandins in vivo. The basis of this action is not clearly understood since aspirin is rapidly hydrolyzed to salicylic acid in vivo (half-life in human plasma = 15 min).

The discovery of thromboxane A_2 and prostacyclin as the predominant endoperoxide products in the platelet and in the endothelium, respectively, raised the possibility of a differential inhibitory effect of aspirin on cyclo-oxygenase in the two tissues (Moncado & Vane 1979). According to this hypothesis low doses of aspirin preferentially inhibit platelet thromboxane synthesis leaving endothelial prostacyclin synthesis relatively intact.

In a pharmacological sense, the requirement for such evidence is a statistically significant separation of the close inhibition curves of platelet cyclo-oxygenase and arterial cyclo-oxygenase during short and long term therapy. This has been demonstrated in several studies (Preston et al 1981, Hanley et al 1982, Patrignani et al 1982). The selective mode of action appears to be related to both dosage and kinetics which will be further discussed.

Effect on platelet aggregation

Aspirin inhibits platelet adhesion to collagen under conditions of stasis or low flow but not under normal conditions, that is at physiological rates of shear and haematocrit levels (Ts'ao 1970). Aspirin also inhibits second wave aggregation and the associated release reaction induced by agents such as collagen, ADP and adrenaline.

Aspirin inhibits platelet aggregation by irreversible acetylation as described above; dosages as low as 160 mg inhibit platelet cyclo-oxygenase activity by more than 80% and large doses have little additional effect (Burch et al 1978).

The in vitro effect of aspirin on platelet aggregation is influenced by its concentration, the duration of incubation with platelets, and the aggregating agent (Gordon & McIntyre 1974). The antiplatelet effect of aspirin is maintained over long periods while the subject continues to take aspirin, indicating that aspirin's effect is not overcome by enzyme induction.

Platelets lack nuclei and they are unable to resynthesize cyclo-oxygenase following aspirin administration, and are therefore impaired for the duration of their life span. Nonetheless these platelets can respond to endoperoxides and thromboxanes released from other platelets, and it has been estimated that only a 10% concentration of non-acetylated platelets is needed to restore normal function to the entire platelet population (O'Brien 1968, Cerskus et al 1980).

Effect of coagulation and fibrinolysis

High doses of aspirin prolong the prothrombin time after 2–3 days (Coldwell & Zawidzke 1968). The daily administration of 100 and 300 mg has no effect but doses of 1–2 g/day decrease the level of coagulation factors II, VII, IX and X (Loew & Vinazzer 1976). Sodium salicylate increases the fibrinolytic activity of blood through increased cellular fibrinolysis. Aspirin prolongs the bleeding time (Mielke et al 1970); the degree of prolongation varies between individuals but is usually consistent within an individual and ranges from 1·3 to 3·2 times the control. Prolonged bleeding times have been reported with doses in the range of 300 mg–3·6 g (Mielke & Britten 1970).

PHARMACOKINETICS

Absorption: Orally ingested salicylates are absorbed rapidly partly from the stomach but mostly from the upper small intestine. Appreciable concentrations are found in plasma in less than 30 minutes after a single dose; peak values are reached in about 2 hours and then gradually decline. The rate of absorption is determined by many factors, particularly the disintegration and dissolution rates of tablets, the pH at the mucosal surfaces and gastric emptying.

Absorption occurs by passive diffusion primarily of the non-dissociated lipid soluble molecules across gastrointestinal membranes. The presence of food delays absorption of salicylates.

Distribution: After absorption salicylate is distributed throughout most body tissues e.g. synovial, spinal and peritoneal fluid. Saliva ingested aspirin is mainly absorbed as such but some enters the systemic circulation as salicylic acid, consequent to hydrolysis by esterases in the gastro-intestinal mucosa and the liver. Aspirin can be detected in the plasma only for a short time; for example 30 minutes after a dose of 65 mg, only 27% of the total plasma salicylate is in the acetylated form. As a result of the rapid hydrolysis plasma concentrations of aspirin are always low and rarely exceed 20 mg/ml at ordinary therapeutic doses. At concentrations encountered clinically, 80–90% of the salicylate is bound to plasma protein, especially albumen.

Biotransformation and excretion: The biotransformation of salicylate takes place in many tissues, but particularly in hepatic endoplasmic reticulum and mitochondria. Salicylate is metabolized largely in the liver by four main parallel pathways. Some is excreted in the urine unchanged but predominantly it is excreted after conjugation. The three chief metabolic products are salicyluric acid (the glycine conjugate), the ether glucuronide and the ester glucuronide.

Salicylates are excreted mainly by the kidney. The plasma half-life for aspirin is approximately 15 min; that for salicylate is 2–3 hours in low doses and about 12 hours at normal anti-inflammatory doses.

SAFETY

Any potential benefit from aspirin in pregnancy must be weighed against possible risks of which there are theoretically many including:

Teratogenesis
Altered haemostasis
Prolonged gestation
Effects on fetal circulation
Perinatal mortality
Miscellaneous effects

Teratogenesis

It has generally been recommended that women avoid aspirin in pregnancy especially in the first trimester. Despite this warning, the prevalence of aspirin use during pregnancy is high. Most aspirin ingestion occurs during the first trimester before pregnancy has been recognized. Given such exposure it is important to consider the potential teratogenicity of aspirin.

Animal studies

Numerous reports have shown salicylates to be teratogenic in animals. Warkany & Takacs (1959) found that skeletal defects, particularly craniorhachischisis, could be induced by administering methyl or sodium salicylate in high doses to pregnant female rats from days 9–11 of gestation. Less frequent observed malformations included exencephaly, facial clefts, eye defects, gastroschisis and irregularities of the vertebrae and ribs. Similar findings were reported by Larsson et al (1963), Trasler (1965) and Kimmel et al (1971). The teratogenic effects in the rodents are associated with doses of salicylate considerably greater than usual therapeutic doses in human (e.g. 500 mg/kg/day in Trasler's study). Studies by Wilson (1973) disclosed that doses of aspirin five to six times higher than those used in rodents produced malformations in rhesus monkeys.

The results of these animal experiments however cannot be extrapolated to human studies as there is considerable individual variation and the doses used were considerably higher than those used therapeutically in man.

Human studies

The obvious difficulties in performing controlled human studies means that information on teratogenicity is mainly derived from retrospective case control studies and case reports. McNeil (1973) described 8 cases suggesting that ingestion of aspirin in dosages of 650 mg q.d.s. by women during a critical period of early gestation may result in a variety of congenital defects. Several case control studies using specific and mixed abnormalities have been reported. The usual methodology was to identify

Table 4.3 Studies on aspirin and teratogenesis

Author	Number and type of abnormality	Aspirin usage (%)	Controls (%)	Significance (P value)	Odds ratio	Type of study
Richards (1969)	833 mixed	22·3	14·4	<0·01		Case control
Nelson & Forfar (1971)	458 mixed	62·2	54·3	<0·01		Case control
Saxan (1975)	599 oral clefts	14·9	5·6	<0·001		Case control
Slone et al (1976)	3248 mixed	6·7	6·3	NS		Cohort
Zierler & Rothman (1985)	298 cardiac abnormalities	12·1	9		1·4 (90% CI 0·95–2·0)	Case control
Werler et al (1989)	1381 cardiac abnormalities	25–33	27	NS		Case control
		Incidence of congenital abnormality				
		(%)	(%)			
Turner & Collins (1975)	144 aspirin users	4·2	2·4	NS		Comparative

an abnormal group and compare with a selected control group. Mothers were then interviewed and a detailed drug history taken. This type of study is open to bias in that truly exposed cases recall a positive exposure history more readily than truly exposed controls. Table 4.3 summarizes these studies which are divided on whether aspirin is teratogenic or not. The largest study was a prospective cohort study of 50 282 mother–child pairs which controlled for potential confounding factors using multivariate analysis and concluded that aspirin was not teratogenic.

In summary the balance of evidence suggests that large doses of aspirin during organogenesis may slightly increase the risk of malformation. It is however possible that the symptoms or disease requiring analgesia in the form of salicylates may be in themselves contributory. There is as yet no evidence that low dose aspirin (< 150 mg/day) is teratogenic.

Altered haemostasis

Aspirin is known to inhibit platelet function. Dosages in the range of 50–100 mg of aspirin inhibits platelet function for 5–10 days after ingestion. Thus it is not surprising that there have been several reports on adverse haemostatic effects.

Maternal haemostasis

Lewis & Schulman (1973) demonstrated that the average blood loss at delivery in patients with heavy aspirin ingestion in the last 6 months of pregnancy was significantly increased (340 ml vs 240 ml $P < 0.025$). Collins & Turner (1975) reported a higher incidence of antepartum and postpartum haemorrhage as well as the need for transfusion at delivery in mothers who chronically ingested large amounts of salicylates. There was an excess of maternal bleeding in the form of an abnormal fall in haemoglobin levels postpartum in mothers who ingested 5–15 g of aspirin within 5 days of delivery (Stuart et al 1982) when compared with a control group. Very prolonged maternal bleeding times (up to 25 min) with doses of aspirin 50 mg/day have recently been reported (Uzan et al 1989).

Fetal haemostasis

In 1971 Corby & Schulman suggested that aspirin taken shortly before delivery might cause a decrease in platelet function in the newborn infant. This report was followed by several case reports of minor bleeding tendencies (purpura, petechiae and cephalohaematoma) in infants whose mothers had ingested aspirin prior to delivery (Bleyar & Breckenridge 1970, Haslan et al 1974). In a prospective study of 108 infants born at 34 weeks gestation or earlier and weighing 1500 g or less, the incidence of intracranial haemorrhage in the infants whose mothers had ingested aspirin was significantly greater ($P < 0.05$) (Rumack et al 1981). Increased bleeding tendencies were demonstrated in a case control study of 34 maternal-neonatal pairs (Stuart et al 1982) where aspirin had been ingested within 5 days of delivery. These findings are obviously of clinical relevance especially during difficult traumatic deliveries. A study by Ylikorkala et al (1986) demonstrates the importance of dosage with regard to its effects of fetal vascular synthesis of vasodilator prostaglandins. They determined prostacyclin and thromboxane production by umbilical arteries. Fetal and neonatal prostacyclin was significantly reduced following 500 mg of aspirin, but it was unchanged in infants of mothers receiving 100 mg of aspirin. Fetal thromboxane synthesis was reduced after 100 mg as well as after 500 mg of aspirin ingested by the mother. On the other hand a recent randomized placebo controlled study using 60 mg of aspirin demonstrated neonatal sparing with regard to platelet reactivity (Louden et al 1988). Maternal prostacyclin metabolites were not affected by 20, 60 or 80 mg/day whereas thromboxane B_2 was decreased significantly by 60 and 80 mg (Sibai et al 1989). In this study neonatal serum levels of 6-keto-PGF and thromboxane in addition to platelet aggregation were not affected by 20–80 mg of aspirin. In the prospective studies using low dose aspirin (< 150 mg/day) there have been no bleeding complications.

Length of gestation and labour

As aspirin inhibits prostaglandin synthesis it may be anticipated that uterine contractions might be inhibited and aspirin would therefore delay the onset and increase the length of labour. Tuchmann-Duplessis et al (1975) showed that administration of aspirin 200 mg/kg/day to rats during the last 6 days of gestation causing prolonged duration of pregnancy and appearance of dystocia in some animals. This study has been confirmed by others (Aiken 1972, Chester et al 1972, Waltman et al 1973).

Lewis & Schulman (1973) reported a 20 year retrospective study of 103 patients with rheumatic diseases who had taken doses of aspirin (> 325 mg/day) during the last 6 months of their pregnancy and compared them with two separate control groups. They showed that there was a highly significant increase in length of gestation (286·1 days versus 275·2 days $P < 0.05$) and an increase in the mean duration of labour (12·1 hours versus 7 hours $P < 0.05$).

Collins & Turner (1975) in their study of Australian women who dramatically had taken large doses of salicylates throughout pregnancy also found prolonged gestation and an increase in complicated deliveries. Once again all the above reports relate to much higher dosages than being currently advocated as having a beneficial effect in pregnancy.

Effects on fetal circulation

Administration of indomethacin or sodium salicylate to pregnant rats or rabbits resulted in closure or marked constriction of the ductus arteriosus of their fetuses (Sharpe et al 1974, 1975). This effect was confirmed in fetal lambs (Heymann and Rudolph 1976)—the instillation of aspirin (50–90 mg/kg) resulted in a significant increase ($P < 0.005$) in pulmonary arterial pressure related to constriction of the ductus arteriosus. Doppler echocardiographic studies showed that low doses of aspirin (20–80 mg) in 30 patients did not close the ductus arteriosus and pulmonary pressures were not elevated (Sibai et al 1989). There are no human reports linking aspirin and persistent pulmonary hypertension.

Perinatal mortality

Collins & Turner (1975) found on very limited data significantly decreased birthweights, increased fetal wastage and increased perinatal mortality in infants of mothers who chronically ingested salicylates throughout pregnancy. Conversely Shapiro et al (1976) using the collaborative perinatal project previously described by Slone et al (1976) could find no evidence that prenatal aspirin is a cause of stillbirth, neonatal death or reduced birthweight.

Miscellaneous effects

Usually Reyes syndrome occurs at a median age of 14 months in children who have been taking more than 10 mg/kg of aspirin daily for a febrile illness. Neonates do not appear to be at risk of developing Reyes syndrome nor has there been any association with maternal use of aspirin (Collins & Turner 1975).

Studies in non-pregnant subjects on optimal dosage

The discovery of thromboxane A_2 and prostacyclin as the predominant endoperoxide products in the platelet and the endothelium, respectively, raises the possibility of a differential inhibiting effect of aspirin on cyclo-oxygenase in the two tissues. A number of studies have been performed to determine the doses of aspirin required to preferentially inhibit platelet thromboxane synthesis leaving endothelial prostacyclin relatively intact. Clinical studies addressing this hypothesis of a selective dose of aspirin have reached varying conclusions depending on the trial design and analytic method used. A daily dose of 20 mg aspirin was shown to result in approx 50% enzyme inactivation, with a dose of 650 mg resulting in more than 95% inactivation (Burch et al 1978). The same group looked at enzyme recovery after a single dose (325 mg or 650 mg) and showed that no new platelet enzyme appeared in the circulation for 2 days. Thereafter unacetylated enzyme returned with a time course consistent with platelet turnover.

Jaffe & Weksler (1979) studied the effect of aspirin on endothelial cell production of prostacyclin. They showed that whilst doses of aspirin did inhibit production of prostacyclin, recovery of production occurs within a few hours with the ability of endothelial cells to return to normal levels of production by 35 hours. This suggested that aspirin as an antithrombotic drug should be given no more often than on a daily basis. Masotti et al (1979) compared the effects of different dosages of aspirin on platelet aggregation and prostacyclin production by vessel wall after ischaemia was induced for 3 min in 25 healthy volunteers. Dosages ranged from 2–10 mg/kg. Aspirin inhibited platelet aggregation proportionally in the ranges 2–5 mg/kg but not for larger doses. In this study vessel wall cyclo-oxygenase activity usually returned to normal 24 hours after aspirin administration whereas platelet cyclo-oxygenase was still inhibited 72 hours after aspirin administration which was consistent with studies by Roth et al (1975) and Moncado & Korbut (1975). Masotti et al (1979) concluded that doses of 3·5 mg/kg of aspirin given at 3 day intervals, appear to be able to induce maximum in vivo inhibition of platelet aggregation without significantly affecting prostacyclin production by the vessel wall. Higher doses significantly inhibit prostacyclin production but only slightly increase inhibition of platelet aggregation. This study has been criticized because PGI_2 was measured by an indirect method after the somewhat unphysiological stimulus of 3 min of ischaemia in the forearm.

Preston et al (1981) demonstrated in five healthy adult volunteers given either 150 mg or 300 mg aspirin that prostacyclin production was markedly inhibited much more so than previously reported by Masotti. They confirmed the effects on platelet aggregation and platelet prostaglandin biosynthesis in that thromboxane production by platelets was completely inhibited within 4 hours and persisted for 48 hours after 300 mg and 24 hours after 150 mg. Thereafter there was progressive recovery of prosta-glandin biosynthesis. Recovery of prostacyclin production was demon-strable 6 hours after 300 mg aspirin. Thus they agreed that the effect of aspirin on thromboxane synthesis by platelets is of much longer duration than its inhibitory effect on prostacyclin synthesis by the vessel wall.

A study designed to determine the dose dependance, the cumulative nature and selectivity of aspirin effects on platelet thromboxane and prosta-cyclin production was reported by Patrignani et al (1982). Single doses of 6–100 mg aspirin resulted in a linear ($r = 0·92$, $P < 0·01$) inhibition of platelet production ranging from 12–95% after 24 hours. A daily dose of 0·45 mg/kg given for 7 days produced a cumulative and virtually complete inhibition ($>95\%$) of platelet thromboxane without significantly reducing the urinary excretion of prostacyclin metabolite in both healthy men and women. A further study showed similar results with 40 mg aspirin given every 48 hours (Hanley et al 1982).

In summary none of the studies published so far has presented conclusive evidence for a particular dose of aspirin but the most convincing studies suggest that dosages of less than 100 mg on a daily basis are the optimal dosage schedule.

Studies in pregnancy

The benefits of restoring the balance between prostacyclin to thromboxane have become obvious after several reports over the past decade which suggested that pre-eclampsia was associated with excessive thromboxane production compared with prostacyclin (see above). There are now several studies in the literature addressing the effect of aspirin on thromboxane and prostacyclin production in pregnancy. Makila et al (1983) studied thromboxane and prostacyclin production in umbilical arteries in vitro after the addition of various concentrations of prostaglandin synthetase inhibitors including aspirin. All prostaglandin synthetase inhibitors inhibited platelet cyclo-oxygenase more potently (4–44 times) than vascular wall cyclo-oxygenase, lending support to the above hypothesis. Low dose aspirin significantly decreased production of thromboxane but not prostacyclin in isolated human placental arteries (Thorp et al 1988). As discussed earlier, in an attempt to study the effects in vivo of different dosages healthy pregnant women ingested either 100 mg or 500 mg during labour at term (Ylikorkala et al 1986). Fetal prostacyclin synthesis was reduced in infants of mothers receiving 500 mg of aspirin, but was unchanged in infants with mothers taking 100 mg. The fetal platelet thromboxane synthesis was inhibited by both dosages whilst prostacyclin production was unaffected by the 100 mg dose. This study confirms that aspirin crosses the placenta in appreciable amounts and in such doses so as to have significant action. A dose of 60 mg aspirin resulted in a greater than 90% inhibition of adult thromboxane production with no reduction in prostacyclin production (Benigni et al 1989). Furthermore the same dosage reduced neonatal serum thromboxane by 63% but this increment is thought not to affect fetal haemostasis. Schiff used a dosage of 100 mg/day for 3 weeks in a controlled study and demonstrated a selective reduction in thromboxane production when compared with prostacyclin production.

The refractoriness to angiotensin II in normal pregnancy may be mediated by prostaglandins (Everett et al 1978). Thus low dose aspirin may be expected to alter the sensitivity to angiotensin II. Sanchez-Ramos et al (1987) performed angiotensin II studies before and 2 hours after 80 mg of aspirin was administered to 13 primigravidae between 28 and 34 weeks gestation. Aspirin resulted in a significant decrease in all patients in angiotensin pressor responsiveness (i.e. increased refractoriness). This lends support to the hypothesis that alterations in the production of prostaglandins plays an important role in the pathogenesis of PIH. Low dose aspirin may affect prostaglandin imbalances and thus contribute to the reduction of the sensitivity to vasoactive substances characteristic of pre-eclampsia.

A similar study was performed by Spitz et al (1988) with the angiotensin II test repeated after 81 mg/daily for a week. Low dose aspirin increased the effective pressor dose of angiotensin II when the results of 17 patients were averaged, but on an individual basis only 9 out of 17 (53%) increased their pressor responses. The same group demonstrated optimal selective inhibition of thromboxane production (65%) with no decrease in prostacyclin production. There was an 80% overall reduction in the 7 women whose pressor dose remained below 7 mg/kg/min but with a 25% reduction in prostacyclin production. These differences could not be explained by differences in weight, race or age. However they are consistent with the hypothesis that PIH represents a heterogenous disease with two or three subgroups. It is of interest that of the 6 women sensitive to AII who became refractory after aspirin therapy, only 1 developed non-proteinuric PIH. Conversely of the subgroup that did not respond to aspirin all 7 developed PIH, 6 of them had proteinurea.

CLINICAL STUDIES

After the discovery that prostaglandin production was reduced in pre-eclampsia some groups attempted to treat the disorder by administering prostacyclin to the mother. Because of the short half-life prostacyclin needs to be given as a continuous intravenous infusion. Nine pregnancies complicated by either severe hypertension or IUGR reported in 4 different studies have been treated with prostacyclin after failure of conventional medication (Fidler et al 1980, Lewis et al 1981, Belch et al 1985, Steel & Pearce 1988). In all cases, blood pressure was reduced. Side effects were common and included nausea, vomiting, facial flushing and headache. Fetal bradycardia was observed in two of the pregnancies and only 4 babies survived. Two of the babies died inexplicably during prostacyclin infusion. There are several possible reasons for its lack of effectiveness. Firstly all treated patients were severely hypertensive and were probably end stage. It is also possible that when a systemic vasodilator such as prostacyclin is administered, blood flow will take the path of least resistance to increase flow to other vascular beds rather than the placenta with a resulting decrease in uteroplacental blood flow. Support for this hypothesis is provided by experimental studies in which prostacyclin was infused into the ovine fetus (Parisi & Walsh 1989, Rankin et al 1979). Thus recently attention has focused on correcting the thromboxane/prostacyclin imbalance with low dose aspirin.

Goodlin et al (1978) were one of the first groups to report a beneficial effect of aspirin in pregnancy. Aspirin 1800 mg/day from 22 weeks resulted in correction of thrombocytopenia in a patient with recurrent pre-eclampsia and resulted in a successful pregnancy. This prompted a group in

Table 4.4   Summary of randomized studies of low dose aspirin in the prevention of PIH

	Method to identify risk group	Treatment	Control	Significance
Beaufils et al (1985)	Obstetric Hx.			
Aspirin 150 mg/ dipyridamole (*n* = 102)				
Uncomplicated PIH		19	22	NS
Proteinuric PIH		0	6	<0·01
Severe IUGR		0	4	<0·05
Perinatal deaths		0	5	<0·02
Wallenburg et al (1986)	Angiotensin 11 test			
Aspirin 60 mg (*n* = 46)				
Mild PIH		2	1	NS
Severe PIH		0	3	NS
Proteinuric PET		0	7	<0·01
Schiff et al (1989)	Roll over test			
Aspirin 100 mg (*n* = 65)				
PIH		4	11	=0·024
Non-proteinuric PIH		3	4	NS
Proteinuric PIH		1	7	=0·019
Benigni et al (1989)	Obstetric history			
Aspirin 60 mg (*n* = 33)				
Gestation at delivery (wk)		39	35	<0·01
Birthweight (g)		2922	2264	<0·05
PIH		0	3	NS

Leeds to study retrospectively the incidence of pre-eclampsia in primi-gravida patients taking part in a drug consumption study. The incidence in aspirin users (i.e. >2 aspirin/week) was 4% compared with 16% (*P* = 0·027) in the non-aspirin users (Crandon & Isherwood 1979). Limited conclusions could be drawn from this study due to its retrospective nature, the lack of information on whether groups were well matched and dosage of aspirin ingested. This however did stimulate prospective studies which are summarized in Table 4.4.

The first prospective trial comprised 102 multiparae at risk of developing pre-eclampsia on the basis of their previous obstetric history (Beaufils et al 1985). A combination of aspirin 150 mg/day and dipyridamole 300 mg/day was randomly assigned to half the group with the remainder assigned to routine care. Uncomplicated PIH occurred in approximately 45% in both groups. There were no cases of pre-eclampsia, fetal and neonatal loss of severe growth retardation in the treated group compared with 6, 5 and 4 respectively in the untreated group. This study has been largely criticized because of its lack of placebo control, a higher incidence of chronic hypertension in the control group (38% vs 29%) and a higher incidence of complications in the control group than might be expected even given the previous obstetric history. In addition all patients were multiparous.

A more convincing study was published the following year. Wallenberg et al (1986) identified a group at high risk on the basis of an angiotensin II infusion test at 28 weeks gestation. They performed 207 infusions to identify 46 primigravid women who entered a double blind prospective study (Aspirin 60 mg versus placebo). Only 2 of 23 women assigned to aspirin developed mild PIH whereas 12 of the 23 women treated with placebo developed pre-eclampsia or eclampsia.

Schiff et al (1989) used the roll-over test to identify their at risk population. A total of 791 high risk women were screened with use of the roll-over test between 28 and 29 weeks. Women with abnormal results were assigned to either aspirin 100 mg ($n = 34$) or placebo ($n = 31$). The incidence of pre-eclampsia was reduced to 2·9% from 22·6 ($P = 0·019$) in the aspirin group. The group was able to demonstrate an increased ratio of serum 6-keto prostaglandin F_1 levels to serum thromboxane B_2 levels after 3 weeks treatment with aspirin. These findings support the contention that aspirin mediated correction of prostaglandin imbalance may interfere with the mechanism leading to pre-eclampsia. Similar favourable effects on the prostacyclin/thromboxane ratio were reported by Benigni et al (1989) in a further randomized study of 33 patients. Low doses of aspirin 60 mg were associated with a longer pregnancy and increased birthweight. These studies are summarized in Table 4.4.

A further prospective study designed to assess whether 75 mg reduced the incidence of proteinuric PIH has recently been reported. Doppler studies of the uteroplacental circulation have recently been reported to be

Table 4.5 Pregnancy outcome. (From McParland et al 1990.)

Outcome measure	Placebo group	Aspirin group	Significance
Pregnancy induced hypertension (%)	13 (25)	6 (13)	NS
Proteinuric hypertension (%)	10 (19)	1 (2)	<0·02
Onset of hypertension before 37 weeks (%)	9 (17)	0	<0·01
Gestation at delivery (wks) (s.d.)	38·7 (3·9)	39·5 (2·1)	NS
Birthweight (g) (s.d.)	2954 (852)	3068 (555)	NS
No. of infants (%)			
Less than 2500 g	13 (25)	7 (15)	NS
Less than 1500 g	4 (8)	0	NS
Less than 5th	7 (14)	7 (14)	NS
Blood loss at delivery (ml) (s.d.)	358 (228)	289 (188)	NS
Perinatal deaths	3	1	NS

sensitive in the prediction of the severest forms of hypertension associated with pregnancy (Steel et al 1990). From Doppler studies on 1226 nulliparous patients we identified 106 at risk pregnancies. These patients were randomized to 75 mg aspirin or placebo. Table 4.5 illustrates the outcome and like the studies from Wallenburg et al (1986) demonstrates a significant reduction in the incidence of proteinuric hypertension and of early onset (< 37 weeks) hypertension (McParland et al 1990). There were no deaths associated with hypertension in the aspirin treated group whilst 3 such deaths occurred in the placebo group. These deaths were all in preterm infants with birthweights of less than 1000 g and the pregnancies were complicated by severe proteinuric hypertension.

In addition to a beneficial effect on the incidence and severity of PIH there is some evidence to suggest that low dose aspirin may promote or enhance fetal growth. In a controlled but non-randomized study a treatment group of 24 multigravid women with a history of at least 2 previous pregnancies complicated by growth retardation and placental infarction were treated with 1–1·6 mg/kg aspirin and 225 mg dipyridamole daily from 16 to 34 weeks gestation in a total of 30 pregnancies. Fetal growth retardation occurred in 61% of the control pregnancies and in only 13% of treated pregnancies. Severe fetal growth retardation was not observed in treated pregnancies (Wallenburg & Rotmans 1987). Aspirin treatment (150 mg/day) was associated with an increase of over 500 g when given from 28 weeks to a group of pregnancies with abnormal umbilical artery flow velocity waveforms (Trudinger et al 1988) when compared with a placebo group. A retrospective study analysing the outcome of 38 pregnancies treated with 75 mg aspirin because of a poor obstetric history (only 8 of 84 previous pregnancies resulting in live births) showed that 88% had successful pregnancies (Elder et al 1988).

All of the above studies, though relatively small in terms of patient numbers, demonstrate a consistent beneficial effect of aspirin in high-risk pregnancies particularly in reducing the incidence and severity of PIH and in addition enhancing fetal growth. There are currently many worldwide trials underway including the CLASP study (collaborative low dose aspirin in pregnancy) which should be reported in 1991–1992. Many questions still need to be answered: what is the optimum dosage schedule, when should aspirin be started, if proven to be effective in large studies who should be treated—how do we decide who is high risk or do we treat all primi-gravidae?; is there a role for aspirin in the treatment as well as prophylaxis of pre-eclampsia? The issue of whether low dose aspirin should be used alone or whether it should be combined with dipyridamole is being assessed in several European studies. The role of specific thromboxane synthetic inhibitors (dazoxiben, desmegrel) and thromboxane receptor antagonists needs to be evaluated.

It seems likely that low dose aspirin will prove to be of benefit in some pregnancies but it may be naive to expect that aspirin will be a panacea for a multitude of possibly heterogeneous disorders. We look forward to a wealth of literature which should answer these questions and firmly establish the role of aspirin in pregnancy.

REFERENCES

Aiken J W 1972 Aspirin and indomethacin prolong parturition in rats: evidence that prostaglandins contribute to expulsion of fetus. Nature 240: 21–25

Barrow S E, Blair J A, Waddell K A et al 1983 Prostacyclin in late pregnancy: analysis of 6-oxo-prostaglandin-F_1 alpha in maternal plasma. In: Lewis P J, Moncado S, O'Grady J (eds) Prostacyclin in pregnancy, New York, Raven Press, pp 79–85

Beaufils M, Uzan S, Donsimoni R et al 1985 Prevention of pre-eclampsia by early antiplatelet therapy. Lancet i: 840–842

Belch J J F, Thorburn J, Greer I A et al 1985 Intravenous prostacyclin in the management of pregnancies complicated by severe hypertension. Clin Exp Hypertens in Pregnancy B4: 75–86

Benigni A, Gregorini G, Frusca T et al 1989 Effect of low-dose aspirin on fetal and maternal generation of thromboxane by platelets in women at risk for pregnancy induced hypertension. N Engl J Med 321: 357–362

Bergstrom S, Sjovall 1957 The isolation of prostaglandin. Acta Chem Scand 11: 1086

Blair I A, Barrow S E, Waddell K A et al 1982 Prostacyclin is not a circulating hormone in man. Prostaglandins 23: 579–589

Bleyer W A, Breckenridge R T (1970) Studies in the detection of adverse drug reaction in the newborn: II The effects of prenatal aspirin on newborn hemostasis. JAMA 213: 2049–2053

Bodzenta A, Thomson J M, Poller L 1980 Prostacyclin activity in amniotic fluid in pre-eclampsia. Lancet ii: 650

Bolton P J, Jogee M, Myatt L et al 1981 Maternal plasma 6-oxo-prostaglandin F_1 levels throughout pregnancy: a longitudinal study. Br J Obstet Gynaecol 88: 1101–1103

Burch J W, Stanford P W, Majerus P W 1978 Inhibition of platelet prostaglandin synthetase by oral aspirin. J Clin Invest 61: 314–319

Bussolini F, Benedetto C, Massobrio M, Camussi G 1980 Maternal vascular activity in pre-eclampsia. Lancet ii: 702

Carreras L O, Defreyn G, Van Houtte E, Vermylen J, Van Assche A 1981 Prostacyclin and preeclampsia. Lancet i: 442

Cerskus A L, Ali M, Davies B J, McDonald J N D 1980 Possible significance of small numbers of functional platelets in a population of aspirin treated platelets in vitro and in vivo. Thromb Res 18: 389–397

Chester R, Dukes M, Slater S R et al 1972 Delay of parturition in the rat by anti-inflammatory agents which inhibit the biosynthesis of prostaglandins. Nature 240: 37–38

Coldwell B B, Zawidzke 1968 Effect of acute administration of acetylsalicylic acid on the prothrombin activity of bis-hydroxy-coumarin-treated rats. Blood 32: 945–949

Collins E, Turner G 1975 Maternal effects of regular salicylate ingestion in pregnancy. Lancet ii: 335–337

Corby D G, Schulman I 1971 The effects of antenatal drug administration on aggregation of platelets of newborn infants. J Pediatr 79: 307–313

Crandon A J, Isherwood D M 1979 Effect of aspirin on incidence of pre-eclampsia. Lancet i: 356

Dadak C, Kefalides A, Sinzinger H et al 1982 Reduced umbilical artery prostacyclin formation in complicated pregnancies. Am J Obstet Gynecol 144: 792–795

Downing I, Shepherd G L, Lewis P J 1980 Reduced prostacyclin production in pre-eclampsia. Lancet ii: 1374

Dusting G J, Moncado S, Vane J R 1978 Recirculation of prostacyclin (PGI_2) in the dog. Br J Pharmacol 64: 315

Dusting G J, Moncado S, Vane J R 1982 Prostacyclin: its biosynthesis, actions, and clinical potential. Adv Prostaglandin, Thromboxane and Leukotriene Res 10: 59

Elder M G, de Swiet M, Robertson A et al 1988 Low-dose aspirin in pregnancy. Lancet i: 410

Everett R B, Worley R J, MacDonald P C et al 1978 Effect of prostaglandin synthetase inhibitors on pressor response to angiotensin II in human pregnancy. J Clin Endocrinol Metab 46: 1007

Fidler J, Bennett M J, de Swiet M et al 1980 Treatment of pregnancy hypertension with prostacyclin. Lancet ii: 31

Fitzgerald G A, Friedman L A, Miyamori I et al 1979 A double blind placebo controlled crossover study of prostacyclin in man. Life Sci 25: 665

Fitzgerald D J, Entman S S, Mulloy K et al 1987 Decreased prostacyclin biosynthesis preceding the clinical manifestation of pregnancy-induced hypertension. Pathophysiology and natural history. Circulation 75: 956–963

Fitzgerald D J, Rocki W, Murray R et al 1990 Thromboxane A_2 synthesis in pregnancy-induced hypertension. Lancet 335: 751–754

Goldblatt M W 1933 A depressor substance in seminal fluid. J Soc Chem Ind 52: 1056

Goodlin R 1980 Treatment of pregnancy hypertension with prostacyclin. Lancet ii: 310

Goodlin R C, Haesslein H O, Fleming J 1978 Aspirin for the treatment of recurrent toxaemia. Lancet ii: 51

Goodman R P, Killam A P, Brash A R et al 1982 Prostacyclin production during pregnancy: comparison of production during normal pregnancy and pregnancy complicated by hypertension. Am J Obstet Gynecol 142: 817–822

Gordon J L, McIntyre D E 1974 Inhibition of collagen-induced platelet aggregation by aspirin. Br J Pharmacol 50: 469

Granstrom E, Diczfalusy U, Hamberg et al 1982 Thromboxane A_2: biosynthesis and effects on platelets. Adv Prostaglandin, Thromboxane and Leukotriene Res 10: 15

Greer I A, Walker J J, McLaren M et al 1985 Immunoreactive prostacyclin and thromboxane metabolites in normal pregnancy and the puerperium. Br J Obstet Gynaecol 92: 581–585

Hamberg M, Svensson J, Samuelsson B 1975 Novel transformation of prostaglandin endoperoxides. Formation of thromboxanes. Adv Prostaglandin Thromboxane Res 1: 19

Hamberg M, Svensson J, Samuelsson B 1976 Thromboxanes: a new group of biologically active compounds derived from prostaglandin endoperoxides. Proc Nat Acad Sci USA 72: 2994–2998

Hanley S P, Bevan J, Cockbill S R et al 1982 A regimen for low-dose aspirin? Br Med J 285: 1299–1302

Haslan R R, Ekert H, Gilla G L 1974 Haemorrhage in a neonate possibly due to maternal ingestion of salicylate. J Pediatr 84: 556

Heymann M A, Rudolph A M 1976 Effects of acetylsalicylic acid on the ductus arteriosus and circulation of fetal lambs in utero. Circ Res 38: 418–422

Jaffe E A, Weksler B B 1979 Recovery of endothelial cell prostacyclin production after inhibition by low doses of aspirin. J Clin Invest 63: 532–535

Karim S M M 1966 Identification of prostaglandins in human amniotic fluid. J Obstet Gynaecol Br Commonwealth 73: 903–908

Karim S M M, Devlin J 1967 Prostaglandin content of amniotic fluid during pregnancy and labour. J Obstet Gynaecol Br Commonwealth 74: 230–234

Karim S M, Somers K 1972 Cardiovascular and renal actions of prostaglandins. In: Karim S M (ed) The prostaglandins: progress in research. Asia Publishing House, Bombay, p 165

Kawano M, Mori N 1983 Prostacyclin in producing activity of human umbilical, placental and uterine vessels. Prostaglandins 26: 645–662

Kimmel C A, Wilson J G, Schumacher J H 1971 Studies on metabolism and identification of the causative agent in aspirin teratogenesis in rats. Teratology 4: 15–24

Koullapis E N, Nicolaides K H, Collins W P et al 1982 Plasma prostanoids in pregnancy-induced hypertension. Br J Obstet Gynaecol 89: 617–621

Larsson K S, Bostrom H, Ericson B 1963 Salicylate-induced malformations in mouse embryos. Acta Paediatr Scand 52: 36–40

Lewis R B, Schulman J D 1973 Influence of acetylsalicylic acid, an inhibitor of prostaglandin synthesis on the duration of human gestation and labour. Lancet ii: 159

Lewis P J, Boylan P, Friedman L A et al 1980 Prostacyclin in pregnancy. Br Med J i: 1581–1582

Lewis P J, Shepherd G L, Ritter J et al 1981 Prostacyclin and pre-eclampsia. Lancet i: 559

Loew D, Vinazzer H 1976 Dose dependent influence of acetylsalicylic acid on platelet functions and plasmatic coagulation factors. Haemostasis 5: 239–249

Louden K A, Broughton-Pipkin F, Heptinstall S, Mitchell J R A, Symonds E M 1988 Studies of the effect of low dose aspirin on thromboxane production and platelet reactivity in normal pregnancy, PIH, and neonates. Paper presented at 1st European Congress on Prostaglandins in Reproduction, July 6–9 1988, Vienna (Abstract No 30)

McLaren M, Greer I A, Walker J J et al 1987 Reduced prostacyclin production by umbilical arteries from pregnancy complicated by severe pregnancy induced hypertension. Clin Exp Hypertens in Pregnancy B6 (2): 365–374

McNeil J R 1973 The possible teratogenic effect of salicylates on the developing fetus: brief summaries of 8 suggestive cases. Clin Paediatr 12: 347–350

McParland P, Pearce J M, Chamberlain G V P 1990 Low dose aspirin in nulliparous patients with abnormal doppler uteroplacental flow velocity waveforms—a placebo controlled double blind randomized study. Lancet 335: 1552–1555

Makarainen L, Ylikorkala O 1984 Amniotic fluid 6-keto-prostaglandin F_1 and thromboxane B_2 during labor. Am J Obstet Gynecol 150: 765–768

Makila U M, Kokkonen E, Viinikka L et al 1983 Differential inhibition of fetal vascular prostacyclin and platelet thromboxane synthesis by nonsteroidal anti-inflammatory drugs in humans. Prostaglandins 25: 39–47

Makila U M, Viinikka L, Ylikorkala O 1984a Increased thromboxane A_2 production but normal prostacyclin by the placenta in hypertensive pregnancies. Prostaglandins 27: 87–95

Makila U M, Viinikka L, Ylikorkala O 1984b Evidence that prostacyclin deficiency is a specific feature in preeclampsia. Am J Obstet Gynecol 148: 772–774

Masotti G, Galanti G, Poggesi L et al 1979 Differential inhibition of prostacyclin production and platelet aggregation by aspirin. Lancet i: 1213–1216

Mielke C H, Britten A F H 1970 Aspirin as an antithrombotic agent: template bleeding time—test of antithrombotic effect. Blood 36: 855

Mielke C H, Kaneshiro M M, Maher I A et al 1970 The standardized normal Ivy time and its prolongation by aspirin. Blood 34: 204–215

Mitchell M D 1981 Prostaglandins during pregnancy and the perinatal period. J Reprod Fertil 62: 305–308

Mitchell M D, Keirse M J N C, Anderson A B M et al 1978 Thromboxane B_2 in amniotic fluid before and during labour. Br J Obstet Gynaecol 85: 442–445

Mitchell M D, Keirse M J N C, Brunt J D et al 1979 Concentrations of the prostacyclin metabolite, 6-keto-prostacyclin F1α in amniotic fluid during late pregnancy and labour. Br J Obstet Gynaecol 86: 350–353

Moncada S, Korbut R 1975 Dipyridamole and other phosphodiesterase inhibitors act as antithrombotic agents by potentiating endogenous prostacyclin. Lancet i: 1286–1289

Moncada S, Vane J R 1979 Arachidonic acid metabolites and the interactions between platelets and blood-vessel walls. Physiol Med 300: 1142–1147

Nelson M M, Forfar J O 1971 Associations between drugs administered during pregnancy and congenital abnormalities of the fetus. Br Med J 1: 523–527

O'Brien J R 1968 Effects of salicylates on human platelet. Lancet i: 779–783

O'Grady J, Warrington S, Moti M J et al 1980 Effects of intravenous infusion of prostacyclin (PGI_2) in man. Prostaglandins 19: 319–327

Omini C, Folco G C, Pasargiklian R et al 1979 Prostacyclin (PGI_2) in pregnant human uterus. Prostaglandins 17: 113–120

Parisi V M, Walsh S W 1989 Fetoplacental vascular responses to prostacyclin after thromboxane induced vasoconstriction. Am J Obstet Gynecol 160: 502–507

Patrignani P, Filabozzi P, Patrono C 1982 Selective cumulative inhibition of platelet thromboxane production by low-dose aspirin in healthy subjects. J Clin Invest 69: 1366–1372

Patrono C, Pugliese F, Ciabattoni G et al 1982 Evidence for a direct stimulatory effect of prostacyclin on renin release in man. J Clin Invest 69: 231

Preston F E, Whipps S, Jackson C A et al 1981 Inhibition of prostacyclin and platelet thromboxane A_2 after low-dose aspirin. N Engl J Med 304: 76–79

Rankin J H G, Phernetton T M, Anderson D F 1979 Effect of prostaglandin I_2 on ovine placental vasculature. J Dev Physiol 1: 151–160

Remuzzi G, Misiani R, Muratore D et al 1979 Prostacyclin and human foetal circulation. Prostaglandins 18: 341–348

Remuzzi G, Marchesi D, Zoja C et al 1980 Reduced umbilical and placental vascular prostacyclin in severe pre-eclampsia. Prostaglandins 20: 105–110

Richards I D 1969 Congenital malformations and environmental influences in pregnancy. Br J Preventive and Social Med 23: 218–225

Rosenkranz B, Fischer C, Weimer K E, Frolich J C 1980 Metabolism of prostacyclin and 6-keto-prostaglandin F_1 alpha in man. J Biol Chem 255: 1094–1098

Roth G J, Majerus P W 1975 The mechanism of aspirin on human platelets I acetylation of a particulate fraction protein. J Clin Invest 56: 624–632

Roth G J, Stanford N, Majarus P W 1975 Acetylation of prostaglandin synthetase by aspirin. Proc Natl Acad Sci USA 72: 3073–3076

Rumack C M, Guggenheim M A, Rumack B H et al 1981 Neonatal intracranial hemorrhage and maternal use of aspirin. Obstet Gynecol 58: 52S–56S

Samuelsson B 1978 Prostaglandins and thromboxanes. Recent Prog Horm Res 34: 239

Sanchez-Ramos L, O'Sullivan M J, Garrido-Calderon J 1987 Effect of low-dose aspirin on angiotensin II pressor response in human pregnancy. Am J Obstet Gynecol 156: 193–194

Saxan I 1975 Association between oral clefts and drugs during pregnancy. Int J Epidemol 4: 37–43

Schiff E, Peleg E, Goldenberg M et al 1989 The use of aspirin to prevent pregnancy-induced hypertension and lower the ratio of thromboxane A_2 to prostacyclin in relatively high risk pregnancies. N Engl J Med 321: 351–356

Shapiro S, Monson R R, Kaufman D W et al 1976 Perinatal mortality and birth-weight in relation to aspirin taken during pregnancy. Lancet i: 1375–1377

Sharpe G L, Thalme B, Larsson K S 1974 Studies on closure of the ductus arteriosus:XI. Ductal closure in utero by a prostaglandin synthetase inhibitor. Prostaglandins 8: 363–368

Sharpe G L, Larsson K S, Thalme B 1975 Studies on closure of the ductus arteriosus:XII. In utero effect of indomethacin and sodium salicylate in rats and rabbits. Prostaglandins 9: 585–596

Sibai B M, Mirro R, Chesney C M et al 1989 Low-dose aspirin in pregnancy. Obstet Gynecol 74: 551–556

Slone D, Sisking V, Heinonen O P et al 1976 Aspirin and congenital malformations. Lancet ii: 1373–1375

Spitz B, Deckmyn H, van Assche F A et al 1983 Prostacyclin production in whole blood throughout normal pregnancy. Clin Exp Hypertens in Pregnancy B2: 191–202

Spitz B, Magness R R, Cox S M et al 1988 Low-dose aspirin 1. Effect on angiotensin II pressor responses and blood prostaglandin concentrations in pregnant women sensitive to angiotensin II. Am J Obstet Gynecol 159: 1035–1043

Steel S A, Pearce J M F 1988 Specific therapy in severe intrauterine growth retardation: failure of prostacyclin. J Roy Soc Med 81: 214–216

Steel S A, Pearce J M F, McParland P, Chamberlain G V P 1990 Early ultrasound screening in the prediction of hypertensive disease of pregnancy. Lancet 335: 1548–1551

Stuart M J, Clark D A, Sunderji S G et al 1981 Decreased prostacyclin production: a characteristic of chronic placental insufficiency syndromes. Lancet: 1126–1128

Stuart M J, Gross S J, Elgard H et al 1982 Effects of acetylsalicylic-acid ingestion on maternal and neonatal hemostasis. N Engl J Med 307: 909–912

Svensson J, Fredholm B B 1977 Vasoconstrictor effect of thromboxane A_2. Acta Physiol Scand 101: 366–368

Svensson J, Strandberg K, Tuvemo T et al 1977 Thromboxane A_2: effects on airway and vascular smooth muscle. Prostaglandins 14: 425–436

Thorp J A, Walsh S W, Brath P C 1988 Low-dose aspirin inhibits thromboxane, but not prostacyclin, production by human placental arteries. Am J Obstet Gynecol 159: 1381–1384

Trasler D G 1965 Aspirin-induced cleft lip and other malformation in mice. Lancet i: 606–607

Trudinger B J, Cook C M, Thompson R S et al 1988 Low-dose aspirin therapy improves fetal weight in umbilical placental insufficiency. Am J Obstet Gynecol 159: 681–685

Ts'ao C 1970 Ultrastructural study of the effect of aspirin on in vitro platelet–collagen interaction and platelet adhesion to intima in the rabbit. Am J Pathol 59: 327–332

Tuchman-Duplessis H, Hiss D, Mottot G et al 1975 Effects of prenatal administration of acetylsalicylic acid in rats. Toxicology 3: 207

Turner G, Collins E 1975 Fetal effects of regular salicylate ingestion in pregnancy. Lancet ii: 338–339

Uzan S, Beaufils M, Bazin B et al 1989 Idiopathic recurrent fetal growth retardation and aspirin-dipyridamole therapy. Correspondence. Am J Obstet Gynecol 157: 763

Von Eular U S 1937 On the specific vasodilating and plain muscle stimulating substances from accessory genital glands in man and certain animals (prostaglandin and vasiglandin). J Physiol 88: 213

Wallenburg H C S, Rotmans N 1987 Prevention of recurrent idiopathic fetal growth retardation by low-dose aspirin and dipyridamole. Am J Obstet Gynecol 157: 1230–1235

Wallenburg H C S, Dekker G A, Makovitz J W et al 1986 Low-dose aspirin prevents pregnancy-induced hypertension and pre-eclampsia in angiotensin-sensitive primigravidae. Lancet i: 1–3

Walsh S W 1985 Preeclampsia: an imbalance in placental prostacyclin and thromboxane production. Am J Obstet Gynecol 152: 335–340

Walsh S W, Behr M J, Allen N H 1985 Placental prostacyclin production in normal and toxemic pregnancies. Am J Obstet Gynecol 151: 110–115

Waltman R, Tricomi V, Shabanah E H et al 1973 The effect of anti-inflammatory drugs on parturition parameters in the rat. Prostaglandins 4: 93–106

Warkany J, Takacs E 1959 Experimental production of congenital malformations in rats by salicylate poisoning. Am J Pathol 35: 315–331

Werler M M, Mitchell A A, Shapiro S 1989 The relation of aspirin use during the first trimester of pregnancy to congenital cardiac defects. N Engl J Med 321: 1639–1642

Wilson J G 1973 Causes of developmental defects in man. In: Environment and birth defects. Academic Press, New York, p 48

Yamaguchi M, Mori N 1985 6-Keto prostaglandin F_1, thromboxane B_2, and 13, 14-dihydro-15-keto prostaglandin F concentrations of normotensive and preeclamptic patients during pregnancy, delivery, and the postpartum period. Am J Obstet Gynecol 151: 121–127

Ylikorkala O, Makila U M 1985 Prostacyclin and thromboxane in gynecology and obstetrics. Am J Obstet Gynecol 152: 318–329

Ylikorkala O, Viinikka L 1980 Thromboxane A_2 in pregnancy and puerperium. Br Med J 281: 1601–1602

Ylikorkala O, Makila U M, Viinikka L 1981a Amniotic fluid prostacyclin and thromboxane in normal, preeclamptic, and some other complicated pregnancies. Am J Obstet Gynecol 141: 487–490

Ylikorkala O, Kirkinen P, Viinikka L 1981b Maternal plasma prostacyclin concentration in pre-eclampsia and other pregnancy complications. Br J Obstet Gynaecol 88: 968–972

Ylikorkala O, Makila U M, Kaapa P et al 1986 Maternal ingestion of acetylsalicylic acid inhibits fetal and neonatal prostacyclin and thromboxane in humans. Am J Obstet Gynecol 155: 345–349

Zierler S, Rothman K J 1985 Congenital heart disease in relation to maternal use of Bendectin and other drugs in early pregnancy. N Engl J Med 313: 347–352

5. Drugs, hypertension and pregnancy

C. W. G. Redman

Medical treatment of the hypertensive conditions of pregnancy is becoming better rationalized. Three classes of drugs—antihypertensive, anti-convulsant and antiplatelet—are now relevant. Other types of management, such as plasma volume expansion for the treatment of severe pre-eclampsia (Belfort et al 1989) or calcium supplementation for its prevention (Lopez-Jaramillo et al 1989), are not reviewed, simply because they do not involve the use of drugs, not because they are unimportant.

ANTIHYPERTENSIVE DRUGS

It is taken for granted that severe hypertension in pregnancy should be treated. The principle has never been formally tested, but is based on circumstantial reasoning. It is consistent with the management of non-pregnant hypertensive individuals (Breckenridge et al 1970), has some validity derived from animal experiments (Byrom 1954) and takes account of the well known fact that when women die of pre-eclampsia/eclampsia it is more commonly of cerebral haemorrhage (Department of Health and Social Security 1989) thought to be caused by severe hypertension. Severe hypertension usually means blood pressures at or above 170/110 mmHg. In our practice, if the systolic *or* diastolic readings repeatedly reach or exceed these limits, the threshold of severe hypertension has been crossed, although average or baseline readings are lower. This definition is arbitrary and its implications have not been rigorously defined. The reader should be aware that what is propounded with the authority of consensus, is based on a relatively weak framework of which the validity has not been properly tested.

These uncertainties are magnified when the issue of treating mild to moderate hypertension is considered. In general medical practice an initial enthusiasm has moderated as the results of large controlled trials have become available (Swales et al 1989). In obstetric practice the issue is totally unresolved. On the one hand mild to moderate hypertension (140/90 to 169/109) is associated with (but does not necessarily cause) increased perinatal morbidity. On the other hand this degree of hypertension is common (about 1 in 5 of all women in Oxford, Redman 1989), the effects of fetal drug exposure are a cause for concern, and the pathology which the treatment is intended to prevent—the 'damage' caused by modest hypertension—is undefined. The problem is complicated by the heterogeneity of causes for the hypertension—pre-eclampsia, chronic hypertension, or combinations of both conditions—and confusion about whether antecedent or chronic hypertension is, of itself, a disability in pregnancy. It is well known that it predisposes to superimposed pre-eclampsia (Redman 1984). But the majority of chronically hypertensive women who do not get pre-eclampsia, particularly multiparae, have normal outcomes. Therefore mild chronic hypertension of itself is not harmful and, in consequence, its treatment is unlikely to be beneficial. With respect to early pre-eclampsia the question arises whether treatment of the raised pressure can halt or retard progression of the disease. All the evidence and everyday clinical experience suggest that it cannot (Redman 1984).

The question is more complicated than it seems. First, pre-eclamptic hypertension is clearly secondary to intra-uterine disturbances: when the pregnancy ends the problem resolves. Its medical treatment may be palliative but cannot be expected to cure the condition. Then there is no defined mechanism to explain why the mild hypertension should cause or aggravate the problem. Many of the features of pre-eclampsia could arise from focal or generalized maternal endothelial cell injury, mediated by substances released by the placenta (Roberts et al 1989). It is possible, although not probable, that mild to moderate hypertension enhances endothelial damage or its consequences. In addition, antihypertensive drugs do not only lower the blood pressure, but have other actions which may be potentially more beneficial: for example calcium channel and beta adrenergic blocking agents inhibit platelet function (Nyrop & Zweifler 1988). Therefore apparent benefit may derive from actions other than their antihypertensive action. Although there is evidence that some agents do not reduce uteroplacental blood flow (Jouppila et al 1986) it is sometimes believed that antihypertensive drugs may confer benefit by enhancing flow after relaxing the uteroplacental arteries. If this were true, then the agents would be used for their vasodilating effects: antihypertensive actions would be incidental. Finally, blood pressure readings are a cue for obstetric intervention which although well intended may, in fact, have deleterious consequences. Treatment that hides the cue may benefit the patient by protecting her from her obstetrician. Better insight into the problems of hypertension in pregnancy and how to deal with them should resolve this difficulty. It should not be addressed by the prescription of drugs. However, in this context treatment of *severe* hypertension may be genuinely beneficial by delaying the valid need to expedite immediate delivery.

With these complexities in mind, the reader should know of a recent placebo-controlled trial of the treatment of moderate hypertension (Plouin et al 1990). Active treatment comprised oxprenolol with or without hydralazine. Treatment did not influence the consequences of pre-eclampsia, including the evolution of proteinuria or its appearance de novo, the degree of hyperuricaemia, perinatal survival, birthweight or weight for gestational age, but it did affect indices of intervention such as induction and Caesarean sections during labour. Treatment was also associated with significantly shorter duration of special care for those neonates who needed it. Were the benefits because the treatment ameliorated a basic pathological process, or because the patterns of intervention were altered? In contrast, a double blind trial of labetolol compared with placebo showed no definite benefits (Pickles et al 1989).

Methyldopa or adrenergic beta blocking agents?

Methyldopa is the oldest and best characterized antihypertensive drug for use in pregnancy (Redman et al 1976, 1977). It is effective and safe for both mother and fetus. Drug exposure in utero does not affect later growth and development (Cockburn et al 1986). Its major side effect of lethargy is less important if its use is restricted to the treatment of severe hypertension. Many have preferred to use adrenergic beta blocking agents after encouraging reports of their effectiveness (Rubin et al 1983, Gallery et al 1985). Atenolol has a long half-life and flat dose response curve, desirable for prolonged ingestion by non-pregnant chronically hypertensive individuals, but less suitable for the management of hypertension in pregnancy where the problem is unstable and demands fast acting therapies. Neither labetolol nor oxprenolol suffer from this drawback and both appear to be suitable alternatives to methyldopa. Early fears that beta adrenergic blockade might alter the fetal heartrate pattern or be deleterious for the neonate have not been substantiated (Rubin et al 1983, 1984, Reynolds et al 1984, McPherson et al 1986, Pickles et al 1989).

A report that oxprenolol may promote fetal growth (Gallery et al 1985) has not been confirmed (Fidler et al 1983). On the contrary, there is now good evidence that atenolol given from early in the second trimester powerfully retards fetal growth (Rubin et al 1990). This may be related to inhibition of the secretion of placental lactogen, previously reported (Rubin et al 1984). These observations are extremely important and show that beta adrenergic blocking agents should not be used in pregnancy, except perhaps as a short-term expedient shortly before delivery. Thus if a woman conceives whilst taking beta blocking agents, her regimen should be reviewed at a gestational age of around 3 months. In many, the fall in blood pressure induced by normal pregnancy is such that all treatment can be stopped; in which case it will probably need to be re-introduced during the third trimester. If not, it should be changed to methyldopa.

Calcium channel blockers

Calcium channel blocking agents are potent vasodilators and for this reason are increasingly being used for the treatment of medical and obstetric hypertension. Calcium ions are essential for the full depolarization and activation of contractile cells. Depolarization initially depends on Na^+ entry through 'fast channels' and is subsequently sustained because slow voltage dependent calcium channels are opened (Braunwald 1982). An increase of intracellular ions activates vascular smooth muscle and prevents vasoconstriction. Calcium channel blockers selectively block the latter process. Arterioles are more sensitive than venules so that nifedipine and related drugs are antihypertensive because they dilate arteriolar beds and decrease peripheral resistance (Braunwald 1982).

Two oral preparations of nifedipine are available which act rapidly: nifedipine capsules within 10 to 15 minutes, and nifedipine slow release tablets within 45 to 60 minutes, with a more prolonged effect. The higher the starting pressure the greater is the hypotensive action. This attribute, combined with its rapid action and ability to maintain or enhance cerebral blood flow (Edvinsson et al 1979) makes nifedipine a useful drug for hypertensive emergencies (Bertel et al 1983). Its introduction into obstetric practice has been appropriately cautious. It appears to be at least as safe as hydralazine, more convenient to use and have actions that are particularly desirable in the context of pre-eclampsia. The last include inhibition of platelet function in vitro (Hann et al 1983) and in vivo (Dale et al 1983) and a possible anticonvulsant action (Larkin et al 1988). Unfortunately formal case-control comparisons of its use have not been reported. They are difficult to do well and the pharmaceutical industry has been reluctant to be involved with extensions of drug use in pregnancy. An initial report (of the use of nifedipine) was encouraging (Walters & Redman 1984) as was a small study of nitrendipine (Allen et al 1987). The slow release formulation of nifedipine is useful as a second line drug for chronic administration during pregnancy (Constantine et al 1987). An apparently beneficial effect on the platelet counts of pre-eclamptic women has been reported (Rubin et al 1988). Because nifedipine is tocolytic, indeed has been used to treat preterm labour (Ulmsten 1984), it is possible that it would predispose to postpartum haemorrhages, particularly if platelet function is also impaired. This problem has not been reported but it has yet to be addressed definitively.

The main concern is the possibility of fetal problems either directly, owing to impaired fetal or neonatal vascular responses, or indirectly by reduced uteroplacental blood flow. Acute experiments in sheep have suggested adverse effects including reduced uteroplacental blood flow and fetal oxygenation (Harake et al 1987) or reduced fetoplacental blood flow, fetal acidaemia and death (Parisi et al 1989). These have been pharmacological experiments that do not emulate the way in which calcium channel blockers are used clinically, so it is reassuring that nifedipine given to pregnant women does not reduce uteroplacental blood flow (Lindow et al 1988), nor alter the Doppler ultrasound flow velocity waveforms of the uteroplacental or umbilical arteries (Hanretty et al 1989).

The most common side effect is a headache, often severe, that can raise concern about impending eclampsia. Magnesium may potentiate the hypotensive actions of nifedipine (Waisman et al 1988), an important consideration if magnesium sulphate is used as anticonvulsant therapy. Nifedipine has a negative inotropic action on the myocardium and in combination with beta adrenergic blockade, can precipitate heart failure (Robson & Vishwanath 1982); this should be borne in mind if it is used to supplement the action of beta adrenergic blocking agents.

Angiotensin converting enzyme (ACE) inhibitors

ACE inhibitors such as captopril and enalapril belong to a relatively new class of antihypertensive drugs, which inhibit the formation of angiotensin II from its inactive precursor angiotensin I. They are particularly useful where the hypertension is renal in origin although they are also effective in individuals with essential and other forms of hypertension. Side effects include rashes, loss of taste, hypotension and renal failure, the last most commonly in individuals with renal vascular problems.

Early experimental work indicated that in pregnancy ACE inhibitors might not be safe for the fetus (Broughton Pipkin et al 1980, 1982). The first case in which their use in human pregnancy was reported (Guignard et al 1981) was complicated by neonatal anuria. Since then, 13 more cases have been reported (Rosa et al 1989) which confirm that this is a dangerous side effect of ACE inhibitors. The neonatal renal failure is often preceded by oligohydramnios, is associated with neonatal hypotension, is irreversible and frequently fatal. Nevertheless, ACE inhibitors can be used in some pregnant women, even from conception, without problems (Kreft-Jais et al 1988), but it is clear that these drugs should not be used routinely in pregnancy although they might have a role for the treatment of puerperal hypertension. In this regard it is relevant that enalapril does not enter breast milk in significant amounts (Redman et al 1990).

ANTIPLATELET AGENTS

The hypertension of pre-eclampsia is secondary; therefore its treatment is at best palliative and, it is to be hoped, will be supplanted by better strategies that can prevent the disease. Of these the most promising is the use of prophylactic low-dose aspirin as antiplatelet therapy. The increasing evidence that platelet disturbances could be an early event in the time course of pre-eclampsia (Redman et al 1978) gave the rationale; reinforced by measurements showing an imbalance between production of prostacyclin and thromboxane (Walsh 1985, Yamaguchi & Mori 1985, Fitzgerald et al 1987) with opposing actions on platelets, antiaggregatory and aggregatory respectively.

Low-dose aspirin is thought to act by acetylating cyclo-oxygenase, necessary for the synthesis of both prostacyclin and thromboxane. Platelets mainly synthesize thromboxane and, as anucleate cells, cannot recover from the effects of aspirin; whereas endothelial cells synthesize mainly prostacyclin and can replace inactivated cyclo-oxygenase quickly. The dosage of aspirin is chosen to maximize this differential effect, which is achieved at about 20 mg per day, although higher doses are needed to inhibit platelet function maximally (Fitzgerald et al 1983). In addition, aspirin at higher doses has a mild anticoagulant effect and enhances fibrinolysis (Editorial 1986). Much of this knowledge has been derived from studies of non-pregnant individuals in relation to the use of aspirin to prevent coronary or cerebral artery thromboses. However, 60 mg of aspirin per day has now been shown to inhibit the generation of thromboxane B_2 as maternal blood clots, the production of thromboxane B_2 from maternal platelets stimulated by collagen or adenosine diphosphate, but not to alter serum levels of the prostacyclin metabolite 6-keto-prostaglandin-F1$_a$ (Sibai et al 1989). These results have been confirmed in pregnant women and extended by measuring a differential effect on the excretion or urinary metabolites of prostaglandins derived from platelets or circulating prostacyclin (Benigni et al 1989) and demonstrating the expected reduction in the ratio between serum metabolites of thromboxane A_2 and prostacyclin (Schiff et al 1989, Spitz et al 1988).

Anecdotal reports of the effectiveness of aspirin in preventing pre-eclampsia (Goodlin et al 1978) were followed by controlled trials (Beaufils et al 1985, Wallenberg et al 1986) of differing designs, using aspirin with or without dipyridamole. The results were promising and have been confirmed by further small trials (Schiff et al 1989, McParland et al 1990, Breart et al unpublished observation, 1990), so that, increasingly low dose aspirin seems to be the first effective medical treatment for preventing pre-eclampsia, or even treating its earliest signs (Cunningham & Gant 1989). An increased sensitivity to the pressor action of infused angiotensin II is one of the earliest prodromal signs of pre-eclampsia (Gant et al 1973). Low-dose aspirin (80 mg) diminishes this pressor response in normal women (Sanchez-Ramos et al 1987), and in those abnormally sensitive to infused angiotensin II although a normal response cannot be restored (Spitz et al 1988). There are numerous unanswered questions about the possible use of low dose aspirin in obstetric practice. What is the most effective regimen? If it works to prevent the onset of the disease can it also ameliorate the progression once pre-eclampsia is established? If so, is there no stage at which aspirin ceases to have some effect? But most important of all—what are the side effects, particularly on the fetus and neonate?

The main concern centres on the intended action of low-dose aspirin which is to inhibit part of the mechanism of haemostasis. It is unlikely that this can be achieved without altering the risks of maternal, fetal or neonatal bleeding. Many reports relate to maternal ingestion of high dose aspirin. Uncontrolled observations suggest an increased risk of antepartum and postpartum haemorrhages (Collins & Turner 1975), and of neonatal intra-cranial haemorrhage (Rumack et al 1981). A controlled study has confirmed an increased liability to neonatal haemorrhagic problems (Stuart et al 1982). It is to be expected that low-dose aspirin will share at least some of these undesirable attributes, particularly as maternal exposure alters the production of thromboxane from neonatal platelets (Ylikorkala et al 1986, Benigni et al 1989).

The risk of teratogenesis is largely confined to the first trimester of pregnancy when it has not been necessary to use low dose aspirin. Exposure to high dose aspirin at this time has been associated with an increased risk of congenital heart disease (Zierler & Rothman 1985), an observation refuted in a more recent study (Werler et al 1989). Problems attributable to the actions of prostaglandins synthetase inhibition, including prolongation of labour or premature closure of the ductus arteriosus are probably not relevant. Of more concern has been the report that intra-uterine exposure to aspirin may marginally impair later neonatal development (Streissguth et al 1987) although this has not been confirmed in a later study (Klebanoff and Berendes 1988).

Although low dose aspirin is the first medical treatment to prevent or retard effectively the development of pre-eclampsia, its safety in pregnancy has yet to be defined. The potential number of recipients is large so this issue should not be ignored. For these reasons the results of large randomized controlled trials now in progress should be awaited before low dose aspirin is used routinely. One such trial in the United Kingdom (CLASP) is the largest multi-centre collaborative trial of obstetric manage-ment so far to be implemented. It is to be hoped that it proves to be a model for testing rigorously the other aspects of the management of the hyper-tensive diseases of pregnancy.

ANTICONVULSANTS AND ECLAMPSIA

It is not known what causes eclamptic convulsions (Redman 1988), but it is clear that although hypertension may contribute to the problem it is not the prime cause. Most women with extreme pre-eclamptic hypertension do not have fits; conversely many episodes of eclampsia occur when the blood pressure is relatively low or even, at times, normal. Thus eclampsia is not prevented simply by adequate blood pressure control, although it is probable, but by no means proven, that the risks are ameliorated. Inevitably, anticonvulsants must be used in appropriate cases: there is considerable uncertainty about what preparation is to be preferred and the problem that few obstetricians in the United Kingdom see enough cases of severe pre-eclampsia or eclampsia to acquire skill in the use of anti-convulsants. This fact alone is a compelling reason for establishing the Regional Centres recommended by the Committee conducting the triennial confidential enquiries into maternal deaths in England and Wales

(Department of Health and Social Security 1986), which the profession have been too slow in implementing. Two therapeutic preparations need to be considered—magnesium sulphate and phenytoin.

Magnesium sulphate remains the standard treatment for severe pre-eclampsia and eclampsia in North America but is little used in Britain. The reasons for these differences in practice seem arbitrary; there continues to be controversy about what is its mode of action (Donaldson 1986) and whether it should be adopted more widely, or conversely if it should be used at all (Dinsdale 1988, Kaplan et al 1988).

It is given to prevent rather than terminate seizures, diazepam being the drug of choice for the latter indication. The issue that worries many clinicians is whether magnesium has anticonvulsant properties (Sibai et al 1984, Koontz & Reid 1985) or indeed whether, when given clinically, it even reaches the central nervous system (Hilmy & Somjen 1968), although it certainly can reach the cerebrospinal fluid where concentrations correlate significantly with those in plasma (Thurnau et al 1987). Because the central nervous system is sensitive to magnesium when it is directly administered in experimental animals, the advantage of magnesium over other preparations, namely the absence of any sedative effect (Mordes & Wacker 1978) for mother or neonate, is in a way evidence that it does not reach the brain.

Magnesium sulphate has some effects on vascular smooth muscle and hence on the cardiovascular system. Reduced magnesium concentrations potentiate the actions of angiotensin II, catecholamines and serotonin in vitro (Altura & Altura 1981). Conversely a high extracellular magnesium concentration reduces the excitability of smooth muscle (Altura & Altura 1981), possibly by inhibiting entry of calcium ions into the cell (Altura et al 1983). It has been suggested that magnesium functions as a physiological calcium channel blocker (Iseri & French 1984); the effects of a magnesium infusion on intracellular free calcium are the same as calcium antagonists (Lenz et al 1987). Hence its use may interact with and potentiate the action of nifedipine or other calcium channel blockers used for the control of hypertension (Waisman et al 1988). In vivo, the effect of magnesium administration, on its own, on pre-eclamptic hypertension is transient (Pritchard 1955, Mroczek et al 1977, Cotton et al 1984). However the use of magnesium attenuates the pressor response to intubation in hypertensive pregnant patients (Cork & James 1985) which is a desirable attribute. Furthermore, magnesium ions inhibit catecholamine release from the adrenal gland and peripheral sympathetic nerve ends and reduce sensitivity of the alpha adrenergic receptors (von Euler et al 1973) that make vascular smooth muscle sensitive to catecholamines. Intravenous magnesium sulphate can thus stabilize the blood pressure where there is major autonomic dysfunction as, for example, with severe tetanus (Lipman et al 1987). Extreme hypermagnesaemia has been associated with refractory hypotension in a non-gravid patient (Mordes et al 1975) and in preeclamptic patients with therapeutic plasma concentrations (Bourgeois et al 1986). Magnesium acts on endothelium to stimulate release of prostacyclin (Watson et al 1986) which would be a desirable action in pre-eclampsia. Cardiac and uterine muscle contractility are also impaired.

Although in skilled hands it is a safe preparation its side effects include failure to control fits (Pritchard & Stone 1967, Sibai et al 1981), maternal death from overdosage (Hibbard 1973, Pritchard et al 1984), hypocalcaemic tetany (Eisenbud & Lobue 1976) and hypersensitivity reactions (Thorp et al 1989). The side effect of an overdose is cardiac arrest (McCubbin et al 1981). At high blood concentrations it also causes a relative blockade of the neuromuscular junction (Ramanathan et al 1988) which can lead to a loss of deep tendon reflexes, respiratory depression or respiratory arrest (Pritchard & Stone 1967, Pritchard et al 1984) and augments the action of depolarizing and non-depolarizing muscle relaxants used for anaesthesia (Ghoneim & Long 1970, Sinatra et al 1985). Neonatal hypermagnesaemia may be associated with hyporeflexia and respiratory depression (Lipsitz 1971) but in general what evidence there is (Green et al 1983, Pruett et al 1988) suggests that Apgar scores are unaffected; but the fetal state before delivery may be modified towards less reactive fetal heart rates and less fetal breathing movements (Peaceman et al 1989). It should be noted that the latter were uncontrolled observations of the use of magnesium sulphate as a tocolytic agent to treat preterm labour.

The problem for those who wish to use the best available treatment is to form an assessment of how magnesium sulphate compares to other therapies of which none is ideal. There is a notable lack of good controlled trials. In the United Kingdom eclampsia is now so rare that nobody can do a single-centre study; but multi-centre trials would be extremely difficult to organize.

Diazepam is a good preparation to terminate a fit. However it is short acting and it is not suitable for longer term prophylaxis (that is over a time period of several hours or days). It is likely that many of its problems in obstetric use relate to ill-advised attempts to prolong its action by continuous or repeated intravenous administrations. Thus a small trial suggested that magnesium sulphate could be better than diazepam (Crowther 1990), causing less neonatal depression and associated with fewer recurrent fits after the first hour, but the numbers of cases were too small for the conclusions to be certain and the only maternal death occurred in a woman allocated to magnesium sulphate. A randomized comparison of phenytoin with magnesium sulphate infusions to treat pre-eclampsia and eclampsia suggested that phenytoin had certain advantages including easier attainment of therapeutic blood concentrations, and more rapid labour with a smaller blood loss after vaginal delivery (Friedman et al 1990). The latter effects could be related to the tocolytic action of magnesium sulphate. In comparison, in a smaller trial magnesium sulphate seemed more effective in preventing fits than phenytoin (Dommisse 1990).

Clearly more work needs to be done to define the relative merits of these different treatments. The major disadvantages of magnesium sulphate are the risk of toxicity and the lack of an understanding of its mode of action.

Phenytoin

There is little experience of the use of phenytoin in obstetrics (Slater et al 1987), whereas it is routinely prescribed in medical practice to treat and prevent convulsions. It has a long half-life so that after an adequate loading dose it needs to be given only once a day. It is absorbed slowly, variably and sometimes incompletely from the gut. To prevent recurrent fits acutely it has been recommended that 18 mg/kg is given intravenously at the rate of not more than 50 mg/min, with an onset of action after 20 minutes, but in pre-eclamptic or eclamptic patients this is associated with an unacceptably high incidence of side effects including choreoathetosis and hypotension (Ryan et al 1989). This was ascribed to hypoalbuminaemia which would be expected to increase the availability of free phenytoin comprising only 10% of the blood concentration. 10 mg/kg administered at once and 5 mg/kg 2 hours later was associated with acceptable blood levels and few side effects. The intravenous preparation is very alkaline and therefore causes burning at the site of infusion and sometimes later phlebitis. The major advantages are that conscious levels are unimpaired and the effect is prolonged. However, it is not an easy drug to administer. The dose must be adjusted to body weight, it is desirable to monitor the electrocardiogram during administration because dysrhythmias are a side effect and blood concentrations need to be checked to ensure that the therapeutic range has been achieved. Even if blood levels are adequate recurrent convulsions can occur (Tuffnell et al 1989). As already mentioned, magnesium sulphate was found to be more effective in a small trial (Dommisse et al 1990), but marginally inferior in another (Friedman et al 1990). A large randomized controlled trial to compare intravenous magnesium sulphate with phenytoin is needed. If undertaken in the United Kingdom it would need to involve most of the large maternity units in the country. A major problem is that obstetricians in this country have little experience of using either preparation and skillful administration is clearly an important part of the drugs' effectiveness. However, phenytoin should not become an accepted part of the prophylaxis or treatment of eclampsia before such systematic evaluations are completed.

REFERENCES

Allen J, Maigaard S, Forman A et al 1987 Acute effects of nitrendipine in pregnancy-induced hypertension. Br J Obstet Gynaecol 94: 222–226
Altura B M, Altura B T 1981 Magnesium ions and contraction of vascular smooth muscles: relationship to some vascular diseases. Federation Proc 40: 2672–2679
Altura B M, Altura B T, Carella A 1983 Magnesium deficiency-induced spasms of umbilical vessels: relation to preeclampsia, hypertension, growth retardation. Science 221: 376–378

Beaufils M, Uzan S, Donsimoni R, Colau J C 1985 Prevention of pre-eclampsia by early antiplatelet therapy. Lancet i: 840–842

Belfort M, Uys P, Dommisse J, Davey D A 1989 Haemodynamic changes in gestational proteinuric hypertension: the effects of rapid volume expansion and vasodilator therapy. Br J Obstet Gynaecol 96: 634–641

Benigni A, Gregorini G, Frusca T et al 1989 Effect of low-dose aspirin on fetal and maternal generation of thromboxane by platelets in women at risk for pregnancy-induced hypertension. N Engl J Med 321: 357–362

Bertel O, Conen D, Radu E W, Muller J, Lang C, Durbach U C 1983 Nifedipine in hypertensive emergencies. Br Med J 286: 19–21

Bourgeois F J, Thiagarajah S, Harbert G M, DiFazio C 1986 Profound hypotension complicating magnesium therapy. Am J Obstet Gynecol 154: 19–20

Braunwald E 1982 Mechanism of action of calcium-channel-blocking agents. N Engl J Med 307: 1618–1627

Breckenridge A, Dollery C T, Parry E H O 1970 Prognosis of treated hypertension. Q J Med 39: 411–429

Broughton Pipkin F, Turner S R, Symonds E M 1980 Possible risk with captopril in pregnancy: some animal data. Lancet i: 1256

Broughton Pipkin F, Symonds E M, Turner S R 1982 The effect of captopril (SQ14,225) upon mother and fetus in the chronically cannulated ewe and in the pregnant rabbit. J Physiol 323: 415–422

Byrom F B 1954 Pathogenesis of hypertensive encephalopathy and its relation to the malignant phase of hypertension: experimental evidence from the hypertensive rat. Lancet ii: 201–211

Cockburn J, Moar V A, Ounsted M, Redman C W G 1986 Final report of study on hypertension during pregnancy: the effects of specific treatment on the growth and development of the children. Lancet i: 647–649

Collins E, Turner G 1975 Maternal effects of regular salicylate ingestion in pregnancy. Lancet ii: 335–337

Constantine G, Beevers D G, Reynolds A L, Luesley D M 1987 Nifedipine as a second line antihypertensive drug in pregnancy. Br J Obstet Gynaecol 94: 1136–1142

Cork R C, James M F M 1985 Magnesium pre-treatment at C-section for pregnancy-induced hypertension. Anesth Analg 64: 202

Cotton D B, Gonik B, Dorman K F 1984 Cardiovascular alterations in severe pregnancy-induced hypertension: acute effects of intravenous magnesium sulfate. Am J Obstet Gynecol 148: 162–165

Cranford R E, Leppik I E, Patrick B, Anderson C B, Kostick B 1978 Intravenous phenytoin: clinical and pharmacokinetic aspects. Neurology 28: 874–880

Crowther C 1990 Magnesium sulphate versus diazepam in the management of eclampsia: a randomized controlled trial. Br J Obstet Gynaecol 97: 110–117

Cruikshank D P, Pitkin R M, Donnelly E, Reynolds W A 1981 Urinary magnesium, calcium, and phosphate excretion during magnesium infusion. Obstet Gynecol 58: 430–434

Cunningham F G, Grant N F 1989 Prevention of preeclampsia—a reality. New Engl J 321: 606–607

Dale J, Landmark K H, Myhre E 1983 The effects of nifedipine, a calcium antagonist, on platelet function. Am Heart J 105: 103–105

Department of Health and Social Security 1989 Report on Confidential Enquiries into Maternal Deaths in England and Wales 1982–84. Her Majesty's Stationery Office, London, pp 10–19

Department of Health and Social Security 1986 Report on confidential enquiries into maternal deaths in England and Wales 1979–81. Her Majesty's Stationery Office, London, pp 13–21

Dinsdale H B 1988 Does magnesium sulfate treat eclamptic seizures? Yes. Arch Neurol 45: 1360–1361

Dommisse J 1990 Phenytoin sodium and magnesium sulphate in the management of eclampsia. Br J Obstet Gynaecol 97: 104–109

Donaldson J O 1986 Does magnesium sulfate treat eclamptic convulsions? Clin Neuropharmacol 9: 37–45

Editorial 1986 Aspirin: what dose? Lancet i: 592–593

Edvinsson L, Brandt L, Andersson K-E, Bengtsson B 1979 Effect of calcium antagonist on experimental constriction of human brain vessels. Surg Neurol 11: 327–330

Eisenbud E, Lobue C C 1976 Hypocalcemia after therapeutic use of magnesium sulfate. Arch Intern Med 136: 688–691

Fidler J, Smith V, de Swiet M 1983 Randomised controlled comparative study of methyl dopa and oxprenolol for the treatment of hypertension in pregnancy. Br Med J 286: 1927–1930

Fitzgerald G A, Oates J A, Hawiger J et al 1983 Endogenous biosynthesis of prostacyclin and thromboxane and platelet function during chronic administration in man. J Clin Invest 71: 676–688

Fitzgerald D J, Entman S S, Mulloy K, Fitzgerald D A 1987 Decreased prostacyclin biosynthesis preceding clinical manifestations of pregnancy-induced hypertension. Circulation 75: 956–963

Friedman S A, Lim K-H, Baker C A, Repke J T 1990 A comparison of phenytoin infusion versus magnesium sulfate infusion in preeclampsia. Soc Perinatal Obstet, Abstr 12: 16

Gallery E D M, Ross M E, Gyory A Z 1985 Antihypertensive treatment in pregnancy: analysis of different responses to oxprenolol and methyldopa. Br Med J 291: 563–566

Gant N F, Daley G L, Chand S, Whalley P J, MacDonald P C 1973 A study of angiotensin II pressure response throughout primigravid pregnancy. J Clin Invest 52: 2682–2689

Ghoneim M M, Long J P 1970 The interaction between magnesium and other neuromuscular blocking agents. Anesthesiology 32: 23–27

Goodlin R C, Haesslin H O, Fleming J 1978 Aspirin for the treatment of recurrent toxaemia. Lancet ii: 51

Green K W, Key T C, Coen R, Resnik R 1983 The effects of maternally administered magnesium sulfate on the neonate. Am J Obstet Gynecol 146: 29–33

Guignard J P, Burgerner F, Calame A 1981 Persistent anuria in a neonate: a side effect of captopril? Int J Pediatr Nephrol 2: 133

Hann P, Boatwright C, Ardlie N G 1983 Effect of calcium entry blocking agent nifedipine on activation of human platelets and comparison with verapamil. Thromb Haemostas 50: 513–517

Hanretty K P, Whittle M J, Howie C A, Rubin P C 1989 Effect of nifedipine on Doppler flow velocity waveforms in severe preeclampsia. Br Med J 299: 1205–1206

Harake B, Gilbert R D, Ashwal S, Power G G 1987 Nifedipine: effects on fetal and maternal hemodynamics in pregnant sheep. Am J Obstet Gynecol 157: 1003–1008

Hibbard L T 1973 Maternal mortality due to acute toxemia. Obstet Gynecol 42: 263–270

Hilmy M I, Somjen G G 1986 Distribution and tissue uptake of magnesium related to its pharmacological effects. Am J Physiol 214: 406–413

Iseri L T, French J H 1984 Magnesium: nature's physiologic calcium blocker. Am Heart J 108: 188–194

Jouppila P, Kirkinen P, Koivula A, Ylikorkala O 1986 Labetolol does not alter the placental and fetal blood flow or maternal prostanoids in pre-eclampsia. Br J Obstet Gynaecol 93: 543–547

Kaplan P W, Lesser R P, Fisher R S, Repke J T, Hanley D F 1988 No, magnesium sulfate should not be used in treating eclamptic seizures. Arch Neurol 45: 1361–1364

Klebanoff M A, Berendes H W 1988 Aspirin exposure during the first 20 weeks of gestation and IQ at 4 years of age. Teratology 37: 249–255

Koontz W L, Reid K H 1985 Effect of parenteral magnesium sulfate on penicillin-induced seizure foci in anesthetized cats. Am J Obstet Gynecol 153: 96–99

Kreft-Jais C, Plouin P F, Tchobroutsky C, Boutry M J 1988 Angiotensin converting enzyme inhibitors during pregnancy: a survey of 22 patients given captropril and nine given enalapril. Br J Obstet Gynaecol 95: 420–422

Larkin J G, Butler E, Brodie M J 1988 Nifedipine for epilepsy? A pilot study. Br Med J 296: 530–531

Lenz T, Haller H, Ludersdorf M et al 1987 Effects of cute hypermagnesaemia on intracellular calcium concentration and adrenergic activity. Clin Sci 72: 131–134

Lindow S W et al 1988 The effect of sublingual Nifedipine on uteroplacental blood flow in hypertensive pregnancy. Br J Obstet Gynaecol 95: 1276–1281

Lipman J, James M F M, Erskine J, Plit M L, Eidelman J, Esser J D 1987 Autonomic dysfunction in severe tetanus: magnesium sulfate as an adjunct to deep sedation. Crit Care Med 15: 987–988

Lipsitz P J 1971 The clinical and biochemical effects of excess magnesium in the newborn. Pediatrics 47: 501–509

Lopez-Jaramillo P, Narvaez M, Weigel R M, Yepez R 1989 Calcium supplementation reduces the risk of pregnancy-induced hypertension in an Andes population. Br J Obstet Gynaecol 96: 648–655

McCubbin J H, Sibai B M, Abdella T N, Anderson G D 1981 Cardiopulmonary arrest due to acute maternal hypermagnesaemia. Lancet i: 1058

McParland P J, Pearce J M F, Chamberlain G V P 1990 Doppler ultrasound and aspirin in recognition and prevention of pregnancy-induced hypertension. Lancet 335: 1552–1555

MacPherson M, Broughton Pipkin F, Rutter N 1986 The effect of maternal labetolol on the newborn infant. Br J Obstet Gynaecol 93: 539–542

Mordes J P, Wacker W E 1978 Excess magnesium. Pharmacol Rev 29: 253–300

Mordes J P, Swartz R, Arky R A 1975 Extreme hypermagnesemia as a cause of refractory hypotension. Ann Int Med 83: 657–658

Mroczek W J, Lee W R, Davidov M E 1977 Effect of magnesium sulfate on cardiovascular hemodynamics. Angiology 19: 720–724

Nyrop M, Zweifler A J 1988 Platelet aggregation in hypertension and the effects of antihypertensive treatment. J Hypert 6: 262–269

Parisi V M, Salinas J, Stockmar E J 1989 Fetal vascular responses to maternal nicardipine administration in the hypertensive ewe. Am J Obstet Gynecol 161: 1035–1039

Peaceman A M, Meyer B A, Thorp J A, Parisi V M, Creasy R K 1989 The effect of magnesium sulfate tocolysis on the fetal biophysical profile. Am J Obstet Gynecol 161: 771–774

Pickles C J, Symonds E M, Broughton Pipkin F 1989 The fetal outcome in a randomized double-blind controlled trial of labetalol versus placebo in pregnancy-induced hypertension. Br J Obstet Gynaecol 96: 38–43

Plouin P-F, Breart G, Llado J et al 1990 A randomized comparison of early with conservative use of antihypertensive drugs in the management of pregnancy-induced hypertension. Br J Obstet Gynaecol 97: 134–141

Pritchard J A 1955 The use of the magnesium ion in the management of eclamptogenic toxemias. Surg Gynecol Obstet 100: 131–140

Pritchard J A, Stone S R 1967 Clinical and laboratory observations on eclampsia. Am J Obstet Gynecol 99: 754–765

Pritchard J A, Cunningham F G, Pritchard S A 1984 The Parkland Memorial Hospital protocol for treatment of eclampsia: evaluation of 245 cases. Am J Obstet Gynecol 148: 951–960

Pruett K M, Kirshon B, Cotton D B, Adam K, Doody K J 1988 The effects of magnesium sulfate therapy on Apgar scores. Am J Obstet Gynecol 159: 1047–1048

Ramanathan J, Sibai B M, Pillai R, Angel J J 1988 Neuromuscular transmission studies in preeclamptic women receiving magnesium sulfate. Am J Obstet Gynecol 158: 40–46

Redman C W G 1984 The management of hypertension in pregnancy. Sem Nephrol 4: 270–282

Redman C W G 1988 Eclampsia still kills. Br Med J 296: 1209–1210

Redman C W G 1989 Hypertension in pregnancy. In: de Swiet M (ed) Medical disorders of pregnancy. Blackwell Scientific, London, pp 249–305

Redman C W G, Beilin L J, Bonnar J, Ounsted M K 1976 Fetal outcome in trial of antihypertensive treatment in pregnancy. Lancet ii: 753–756

Redman C W G, Beilin L J, Bonnar J 1977 Treatment of hypertension in pregnancy with methyldopa: blood pressure control and side effects. Br J Obstet Gynaecol 84: 419–426

Redman C W G, Bonnar J, Beilin L J 1978 Early platelet consumption in pre-eclampsia. Br Med J 1: 467–469

Redman C W G, Kelly J G, Cooper W D 1990 The excretion of enalapril and enalaprilat in human breast milk. Eur J Clin Pharmacol 38: 99

Reynolds B, Butters L, Evans L, Adams T, Rubin P C 1984 First year of life after the use of atenolol in pregnancy associated hypertension. Arch Dis Child 59: 1061–1063

Roberts J M, Taylor R N, Musci T J, Rodgers D M, Hubel C A, McLaughlin M K 1989 Preeclampsia: an endothelial cell disorder. Am J Obstet Gynecol 161: 1200–1204

Robson R H, Vishwanath M C 1982 Nifedipine and beta-blockade as a cause of cardiac failure. Br Med J 284: 104

Rosa F W, Bosco L A, Graham C F, Milstien J B, Dreis M, Creamer J 1989 Neonatal anuria with maternal angiotensin-converting enzyme inhibition. Obstet Gynecol 74: 371–374

Rubin P C, Butters L, Clark D M et al 1983 Placebo-controlled trial of atenolol treatment of pregnancy-associated hypertension. Lancet i: 431–434

Rubin P C, Butters L, Clark D et al 1984 Obstetric aspects of the use in pregnancy-associated hypertension of the beta-adrenoceptor antagonist atenolol. Am J Obstet Gynecol 150: 389–392

Rubin P C, Butters L, McCabe R 1988 Nifedipine and platelets in preeclampsia. Am J Hypert 1: 175–177

Rubin P C, Butters L, Kennedy S 1990 Atenolol in the management of essential hypertension during pregnancy. Br Med J 301: 587–589

Rumack C M, Guggenheim M A, Rumack B H, Peterson R G, Johnson M L, Braithwaite W R 1981 Neonatal intracranial hemorrhage and maternal use of aspirin. Obstet Gynecol 58 (suppl): 52S–55S

Ryan G, Lange I R, Naugler M A 1989 Clinical experience with phenytoin prophylaxis in severe preeclampsia. Am J Obstet Gynecol 161: 1297–1304

Sanchez-Ramos L, O'Sullivan M J, Garrido-Calderon J 1987 Effect of low-dose aspirin on angiotensin II pressor response in human pregnancy. Am J Obstet Gynecol 156: 193–194

Schiff E, Peleg E, Goldenberg M et al 1989 The use of aspirin to prevent pregnancy-induced hypertension and lower the ratio of thromboxane A2 to prostacyclin in relatively high risk pregnancies. N Engl J Med 321: 351–356

Sibai B M, McCubbin J H, Anderson G D, Lipshitz J, Dilts P V 1981 Eclampsia. I. Observations from 67 recent cases. Obstet Gynecol 58: 609–613

Sibai B M, Spinnato J A, Watson D L, Lewis J A, Anderson G D 1984 Effect of magnesium sulfate on electroencephalographic findings in preeclampsia-eclampsia. Obstet Gynecol 64: 261–266

Sibai B M, Mirro R, Chesney C M, Leffler C 1989 Low-dose aspirin in pregnancy. Obstet Gynecol 74: 551–557

Sinatra R S, Philip B K, Naulty J S, Ostheimer G W 1985 Prolonged neuromuscular blockade with vecuronium in a patient treated with magnesium sulfate. Anesth Analg 64: 1220–1222

Slater R M, Wilcox F L, Smith W D et al 1987 Phenytoin infusion in severe pre-eclampsia. Lancet i: 1417–1420

Spitz B, Magness R R, Cox S, Brown C E L, Rosenfeld C R, Gant N F 1988 Low-dose aspirin. I. Effect on angiotensin II pressor responses and blood prostaglandin concentrations in pregnant women sensitive to angiotensin II. Am J Obstet Gynecol 159: 1035–1043

Streissguth A P, Treder R P, Barr H M et al 1987 Aspirin and acetaminophen use by pregnant women and subsequent child IQ and attention decrements. Teratology 35: 211–219

Stuart M J, Gross S J, Elrad H, Graeber J E 1982 Effects of acetylsalicylic-acid ingestion on maternal and neonatal hemostasis. N Engl J Med 307: 909–912

Swales J D, Ramsay L E, Coope J R et al 1989 Treating mild hypertension. Agreement from the large trials. Br Med J 298: 694–696

Thorp J M, Katz V L, Campbell D, Cefalo R C 1989 Hypersensitivity to magnesium sulfate. Am J Obstet Gynecol 161: 889–890

Thurnau G R, Kemp D B, Jarvis A 1987 Cerebrospinal fluid levels of magnesium in patients with preeclampsia after treatment with intravenous magnesium sulfate: a preliminary report. Am J Obstet Gynecol 157: 1435–1438

Tuffnell D, O'Donovan P, Lilford R J, Prys-Davies A, Thornton J G 1989 Phenytoin in pre-eclampsia. Lancet ii: 273–274

Ulmsten U 1984 Treatment of normotensive and hypertensive patients with preterm labor using oral nifedipine, a calcium antagonist. Arch Gynecol 236: 69–72

von Euler U S, Lishajko F 1973 Effects of Mg^{2+} and Ca^{2+} on noradrenaline release and uptake in adrenergic nerve granules in different media. Acta Physiol Scand 89: 415–422

Waisman G D, Mayorga L M, Camera M I, Vignola C A, Martinotti A 1988 Magnesium plus nifedipine: potentiation of hypotensive effect in preeclampsia. Am J Obstet Gynecol 159: 308–309

Wallenburg H C S, Dekker G A, Makovitz J W, Rotmans P 1986 Low-dose aspirin prevents pregnancy-induced hypertension and pre-eclampsia in angiotensin-sensitive primigravidae. Lancet i: 1–3

Walsh S W 1985 Preeclampsia: an imbalance in placental prostacyclin and thromboxane production. Am J Obstet Gynecol 152: 335–340

Walters B N J, Redman C W G 1984 Treatment of severe pregnancy-associated hypertension with the calcium antagonist nifedipine. Br J Obstet Gynaecol 91: 330–336

Watson K V, Moldow C F, Ogburn P L, Jacob H S 1986 Magnesium sulfate: rationale for its use in preeclampsia. Proc Soc Nat Acad Sci USA 83: 1075–1078

Werler M M, Mitchell A A, Shapiro S 1989 The relation of aspirin use during the first trimester of pregnancy to congenital cardiac defects. N Engl J Med 321: 1639–1642

Yaari Y, Selzer M E, Pincus J H 1986 Phenytoin: mechanisms of its anticonvulsant action. Ann Neurol 20: 171–184

Yamaguchi M, Mori N 1985 6-keto prostaglandin F1alpha, thromboxane B2, and 13,14-dihydro-15-keto prostaglandin F concentrations of normotensive and preeclamptic patients during pregnancy, delivery, and the postpartum period. Am J Obstet Gynecol 151: 121–127

Ylikorkala O, Makila U-M, Kaapa P, Viinikka L 1986 Maternal ingestion of acetylsalicylic acid inhibits fetal and neonatal prostacyclin and thromboxane in humans. Am J Obstet Gynecol 155: 345–349

Zierler S, Rothman K J 1985 Congenital heart disease in relation to maternal use of Bendectin and other drugs in early pregnancy. N Engl J Med 313: 347–352

6. Prelabour spontaneous rupture of the membranes

C. O'Herlihy   M. Turner

Spontaneous rupture of the membranes (SROM) commonly coincides with the onset of labour. It precedes labour by a latent interval of at least several hours in about 10% of term pregnancies and in a much greater proportion of cases when delivery occurs preterm (Mead 1980). SROM before labour has sometimes been called 'premature', regardless of the length of gestation. The clinical approach to management, however, is very different when the fetus is immature. Therefore, we would recommend instead the more specific title 'prelabour' SROM and would suggest that the ambiguous term 'premature' be dropped.

A perceptible shift has taken place in the management of SROM in recent years, away from a general policy of early induction of labour towards an increasingly conservative approach in clearly defined clinical circumstances. Despite a large number of recent reports dealing with the topic, a clear consensus on the clinical approach to rupture of the membranes before labour has not been established. Nevertheless, sufficient re-evaluation of practice has taken place to justify a review which reassesses some aspects of this frequent clinical syndrome, while highlighting areas where uncertainty persists, especially in respect of aetiology, diagnosis and methods of induction of labour. Most investigators have devoted attention to prelabour SROM before term, which, although less common, is associated with considerable perinatal mortality and morbidity. SROM at term is less hazardous but can lead to increased obstetric intervention and will be discussed separately.

AETIOLOGY

The collagen content of the amnion decreases progressively in later pregnancy (Skinner et al 1981) so that spontaneous rupture in labour can be considered a physiological event. It has not been established whether SROM before term is the result of a collagen deficiency (Al-Zaid 1980), although it is true that physical overdistension of the uterus, due to polyhydramnios or multiple pregnancy, increases the risk of early rupture (Gibbs 1987).

The relationship of several other extraneous factors to inappropriate early SROM is also problematic. Coital activity and repeated vaginal digital examinations have been reported to increase the risk (Lenihan 1984). Alternatively, evidence for a bacteriological cause (rather than infection as a consequence of membrane rupture) appears to have been established in at least some cases, with E. *coli*, bacteroides and Group B haemolytic streptococci most frequently implicated (Naeye 1982, Lamont et al 1986). Bacterial overgrowth is associated with an increase in vaginal pH (Gleeson et al 1989), which may weaken the protective cervical mucus operculum and permit dissolution of the membranes; in addition, bacterially-stimulated phospholipase A_2 may mediate premature cervical effacement via prostaglandin intermediates. Although immunological evidence that infection can precede rather than follow preterm SROM has been provided (Cederqvist et al 1979), when the majority of patients are managed conservatively for days or even weeks after SROM, ascending chorioamnionitis does not develop. This would discount an infective aetiology in all cases.

DIAGNOSIS AND MONITORING

The recognition of SROM is based on the logical triad of history, physical examination and investigation. In most cases, the patient's description of a gush of fluid followed by an intermittent uncontrollable trickle leaves little doubt. Since leakage is generally greater at first, confirmation of rupture is expedited if the woman attempts initially to collect some of the fluid; this advice has been incorporated into our antenatal education programme and we would recommend it as a useful exercise, especially since the volume of fluid draining usually decreases with time. In any event, the diagnosis is facilitated by obtaining a specimen of amniotic fluid where the presence of free floating vernix (after 32–34 weeks' gestation), or even meconium, will differentiate it from urine or vaginal discharge.

If doubt persists, simple dipstick assessment of pH (7·1 or higher with liquor amnii) and protein (rarely present in urine), together with visualization of the fern-like pattern of dried amniotic fluid on a glass slide, is usually diagnostic (Friedman & McElin 1969). Nitrazine yellow paper turns dark blue in the higher pH range but can also give false positive results in the presence of blood, semen and vaginitis. Invasive methods such as dye injection should be avoided because of their documented fetal hazards (Cowett et al 1976). Laboratory analysis of the fluid discharge may be warranted in a few cases, including determination of creatinine, urea, uric acid and the concentration of nile-blue staining cells; to some extent gestational age may influence these results, whereas the presence of alpha-fetoprotein in the fluid draining is specific for SROM (Rochelson et al 1987).

A controversial area of current practice centres on the clinical method chosen to identify amniotic fluid leakage. Many obstetricians still favour an invasive approach, using either vaginal digital or speculum examination, despite the increased risk of precipitating ascending chorioamnionitis through disturbance of the lower genital flora (Schutte et al 1983). Our practice over many years which has tended to avoid vaginal examination following prelabour SROM (except in the unusual circumstances of abnormal fetal lie or heart rate pattern) has shown that an adequate specimen for analysis can be collected at the vulva within 24 hours of admission in almost every case (Egan & O'Herlihy 1988). A digital or speculum examination is unlikely to contribute to diagnosis or management in patients in whom the presenting part is in the pelvis and the fetal heart is normal. In addition, there is evidence that invasive examination is not only uncomfortable but also limits the option of expectant management, with quoted infection rates of 50% within 72 hours (Lebherz et al 1963, Fayez et al 1978): this is a particular disadvantage when the fetus is immature, when prolonged expectancy is desirable.

It has been suggested that ultrasound might be an ideal non-invasive technique for confirming membrane rupture (Larsen 1979) but its systematic evaluation in term pregnancies has recently proved disappointing (Robson et al 1990). This study found that the patient's history of SROM was erroneous in one third of cases, based on a 2-day period of hospital observation and subsequent obstetric outcome. Before term, urinary incontinence is less likely to confuse the diagnosis. Following SROM at term, amniotic fluid measurements using ultrasound overlap with those found in pregnancies with intact membranes (Table 6.1): in addition, the quantity of residual liquor is of no value in predicting the duration of the prelabour latent interval. In preterm pregnancies on the other hand, ultrasound may have a significant role, particularly in serial biophysical monitoring during a prolonged latent interval, in the exclusion of lethal malformations, in the assessment of fetal lung function and in the prediction of pulmonary hypoplasia (Blott et al 1987).

Table 6.1 The analysis of depth of amniotic fluid pool (AFP) measured by ultrasound in patients with confirmed and non-confirmed spontaneous rupture of membranes (SROM) at term. Reproduced with permission from Robson et al 1990

Confirmed SROM			Non-confirmed SROM		
Weeks' gestation n = patients	Mean ± s.d. AFP (mm)	Range	Weeks' gestation n = patients	Mean ± s.d. AFP (mm)	Range
37–38 (n = 24)	48 ± 19	15–87	37–38 (n = 17)	64 ± 16	42–84
39–40 (n = 52)	48 ± 16	20–100	39–40 (n = 21)	55 ± 17	25–88
41–42 (n = 24)	50 ± 16	31–89	41–42 (n = 13)	62 ± 18	28–89

Infection is the principal hazard for both mother and fetus during the latent interval between SROM and delivery. Patients with ruptured membranes, therefore, are best observed in hospital. We have found that clinical surveillance—namely, 4-hourly recordings of maternal and fetal heart rates and maternal temperature—provides satisfactory early evidence of ascending infection and facilitates expeditious and safe delivery. The onset of meconium-staining of the fluid draining is almost diagnostic of sepsis in preterm pregnancies (Davies et al 1972). Uterine tenderness and offensive smelling vaginal discharge tend to occur as late signs of infection (Gibbs et al 1980). Laboratory estimations of white cell counts, sedimentation rate and C-reactive protein can be performed serially or on clinical suspicion but are non-specific and generally provide information too late for prompt clinical action. Once infection is apparent, delivery must be effected quickly, usually by Caesarean section unless spontaneous labour has been stimulated by the infection and high dosage intravenous antibiotic therapy should be simultaneously commenced. We would not advise induction of labour in clinically infected patients.

The level of the amniotic rupture may have a significant bearing on both the risk of ascending chorioamnionitis and the duration of the prelabour interval. A high hind water leak occurs in a small proportion of cases and can lead to dystocia when induction is attempted at term, if formal amniotomy is not first performed. Hind water rupture should be suspected when a diagnostic fluid sample has been obtained but drainage subsequently ceases. At preterm gestations, apparent 'resealing' of the membranes may rarely occur with hind water ruptures. This is followed by reaccumulation of amniotic fluid and may even permit the patient's discharge from hospital to await spontaneous labour, although we would advise caution in such cases. Techniques for artificially resealing with fibrin (Baumgarten & Moser 1986), while theoretically attractive, are as yet clinically unproven.

PRELABOUR SROM BEFORE TERM

SROM precedes delivery in 40–60% of singleton spontaneous preterm births (Keirse et al 1989). Once the diagnosis is likely, early maternal transfer to a unit with neonatal intensive-care facilities is essential, so as to obviate the hurried disturbance later of a mother already in labour or a neonate already unwell. The balance of risks between immaturity and infection depends upon gestational age at the time of membrane rupture but, in general, the risk of prematurity predominates. Before 26 weeks' gestation the chance of survival is negligible, while after 35 weeks perinatal outcome differs little from that at term. Although the latent period before labour is said to vary inversely with the length of gestation (Mead 1980), most infants will deliver within 7–10 days of amniorrhexis. Nevertheless, survival of a number of infants has been documented when SROM has occurred as early as 20–22 weeks, followed by latent intervals of up to 18 weeks before delivery (Blott et al 1987, McIntosh 1988).

It is likely that strict avoidance of invasive vaginal examination will enhance maturity by minimizing the risk of ascending chorioamnionitis. Should infection occur, a broad spectrum antibiotic regimen in high dosage (for example, an intravenous combination of cephradine and metronidazole) should be combined with expedited delivery. Prophylactic antibiotics do not appear to alter the incidence of intra-uterine infection (Keirse et al 1989) although maternal febrile morbidity is reduced; antibiotics carry the potential disadvantage of genital colonization with resistant strains. Whether they prolong the prelabour interval by deferring bacterial ascent awaits further evaluation. In the presence of infection, antibiotics provide better neonatal and maternal results when started intrapartum than after delivery (Gilstrap et al 1988). This is particularly true when the mother is a carrier of Group B haemolytic streptococci. Where the prevalence of this organism is high, screening of the antenatal population is advisable, although the infant is normally safe provided antimicrobial therapy is begun before delivery.

Amniocentesis has been recommended during the prelabour interval following SROM to identify bacteria and to measure surfactant activity in the residual amniotic pool (Cotton et al 1984). It has, however, a high failure rate when the membranes are ruptured and the amniotic fluid sampled can be bacteria-free even in the presence of ascending infection. The value of amniocentesis is more obvious in the assessment of functional lung maturity but an adequate specimen can generally be obtained non-invasively at the vulva when phosphatidylglycerol measurement is the analysis of choice (Stedman et al 1981). Knowledge that the fetal lungs are mature is not necessarily of great assistance in management, since prolongation of the expectant interval until the onset of spontaneous labour is associated with fewer maternal complications during labour without concomitant fetal morbidity than when early stimulation of labour is practised (Garite et al 1981).

The use of corticosteroids to stimulate surfactant production following SROM, and before suspected or documented fetal pulmonary maturity, has generated considerable debate. Caution has been urged by those who fear the masking of intra-uterine infections but a recent metanalysis of several trials by Crowley et al (1990) suggests that the maturational benefits of a 48-hour course of dexamethasone in pregnancies between 28 and 34 weeks considerably outweigh the disadvantage of any increase in sepsis. The use of tocolytic agents, either oral or intravenous, beta-mimetic or anti-prostaglandin, cannot be supported following preterm SROM (Keirse et al 1989). There is no data to suggest an improvement in perinatal outcome following their use (Garite et al 1987) and in the doubtful event that tocolysis did postpone labour, this could theoretically trap the fetus in an infected environment. A possible but unproven advantage of tocolysis may

Table 6.2   Suggested protocol of management of patients with prelabour spontaneous rupture of membranes before 37 weeks gestation

Avoid vaginal examination—unless unstable lie/abnormal fetal heart rate
Confirm diagnosis by collection of fluid specimen at vulva
Early maternal transfer to unit with neonatal intensive care facilities

Monitor with maternal pulse, temperature and fetal heart rate 4-hourly
Avoid tocolytics
Avoid prophylactic antibiotics
Corticosteroid therapy for 48 hours, if 28–34 weeks
Regular ultrasound assessment—presentation, growth, fetal breathing, amniotic fluid volume

Immediate delivery (+antibiotics) if clinical signs of infection
Vaginal examination at onset of labour
Caesarean delivery in breech presentation <36 weeks

lie in the postponement of labour in order to facilitate in utero transfer following early SROM.

Pulmonary hypoplasia is the other potentially disastrous fetal respiratory complication following preterm SROM. The continued circulation of amniotic fluid promoted by fetal breathing movements (FBM) is essential for the completion of alveolar growth, at least until the end of the second trimester. Oligohydramnios following SROM before that time is likely to lead to hypoplastic lung development and early neonatal death. The detection, however, of FBM with ultrasound is reassuring that normal development is continuing and that infection is absent (Blott et al 1987). Our experience of scanning 15 cases in the mid-trimester following membrane rupture revealed FBM in only 1 of 6 fetuses with gross oligohydramnios (4 of whom had hypoplastic lungs), compared with 7 of 9 fetuses with adequate residual liquor, none of whom had hypoplasia. An improvement on the previously dismal results of resuscitating infants with these dry lungs has recently been reported, using very high early ventilation pressures (McIntosh 1988). This development suggests that antepartum ultrasound identification of these pregnancies, together with skilled neonatal attendants at delivery, may improve the hitherto poor prognosis.

At the onset of labour a careful reassessment of every patient with preterm SROM is advisable, even in the absence of signs of infection. Cord accidents tend to cluster either after the initial membrane rupture or when uterine activity begins, particularly when the breech presents (Fayez et al 1978). Fetal distress is also more common because of cord compression, secondary to oligohydramnios. Amnioinfusion has been suggested as a means of countering this effect (Nageotte et al 1985) but the usual rapidity of preterm labour is unlikely to permit this intervention frequently. Although placental abruption may be associated with preterm SROM, it is more likely to occur after the sudden release of polyhydramnios, rather than at the onset of labour (Vintzileos et al 1987). Consideration should be given to delivery by Caesarean section when the fetal presentation is other than cephalic at gestations between 26 and 36 weeks; mechanical difficulties with breech delivery are especially likely in association with antecedent oligo-hydramnios.

Table 6.2 outlines a suggested protocol for management following prelabour SROM before term. Our practice is to attempt induction of labour with intravenous oxytocin after 36–37 weeks' gestation in that minority of preterm SROM pregnancies in whom prior delivery has not yet occurred. Induction then is generally successful but can, in any case, be deferred and attempted later provided vaginal examination is avoided until after regular uterine activity has been established. Earlier intervention is likely to lead to more prolonged neonatal hospitalization because of immaturity and more prolonged maternal discomfort during induction.

PRELABOUR SROM AT TERM

The management of prelabour SROM at term is less complicated than preterm because considerations of fetal immaturity become irrelevant, obviating the principal indication for prolonged expectancy. Most patients will labour spontaneously, so that in the absence of intervention only about 2–5% remain undelivered after 48 hours (Egan & O'Herlihy 1988, Grant & Keirse 1989). This uncomplicated natural outcome has not, however, discouraged a predominantly interventional obstetric approach once the diagnosis of SROM is made. Early induction leads to greater analgesic requirements and longer labours, culminating in higher incidences of operative vaginal and Caesarean delivery and associated infectious morbidity (Conway et al 1984, Gibbs 1987).

Immediate induction of labour following prelabour SROM would therefore seem a bad idea. At term, however, the risk of maternal infection correlates directly with the duration of the latent interval and prophylactic antibiotic therapy is of no proven benefit (Mead 1980). Nevertheless, provided digital and speculum examinations are avoided, the risk of intra-

Table 6.3   The clinical outcome in patients ($n = 88$) with prolonged prelabour spontaneous rupture of membranes (> 24 h) after 37 weeks' gestation. Reproduced with permission from Egan & O'Herlihy 1988

	Nulliparae	Multiparae
Total—prolonged membrane rupture	37	51
Oxytocin induction (at 24–48 h)	21	20
duration (h, mean ± s.d.)	5.5 ± 2.9	3.6 ± 2.1
failed induction	2	0
Caesarean section	3 (8%)	1 (2%)
Positive vaginal bacterial culture	28	34
Positive neonatal blood culture	9	7
Neonatal antibiotic therapy	4	1

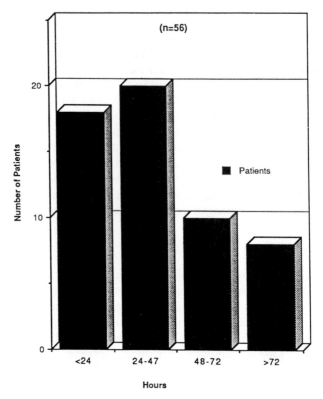

Fig. 6.1   Duration of membrane rupture to delivery in 56 patients with SROM and one previous Caesarean section managed expectantly. Reproduced with permission from Carroll et al 1990.

uterine infection is very low for at least 3 days following membrane rupture. By that time all but a small number of patients have delivered and the results of induction in the remainder are good (Table 6.3). The rationale for prelabour vaginal assessment is difficult to understand, since at term the fetal lie is almost invariably longitudinal and stable and immediate Caesarean delivery rather than induction of labour is more appropriate in the small number of cases with an abnormal lie or fetal heart pattern following SROM.

Monitoring of the prelabour interval can be performed adequately using the clinical parameters of maternal temperature and fetal and maternal heart rates already discussed, following an initial non-stress cardiotocograph. In the absence of infection, fetal distress and abnormal lie, our policy at term is to offer oxytocin induction once 24 hours have elapsed from SROM. In some circumstances, such as previous Caesarean delivery, breech presentation, high parity or a maternal request to avoid induction, a longer latent period is allowed in anticipation of spontaneous labour (Egan & O'Herlihy 1988).

In this era of escalating abdominal delivery rates, the approach to SROM following one previous Caesarean section merits particular consideration. Early induction not only increases the likelihood of dystocia and repeated Caesarean section but uterine stimulation with oxytocics may possibly precipitate scar dehiscence. Alternatively, if induction is avoided altogether most patients deliver within 72 hours (Fig. 6.1) and a vaginal delivery rate of over 90% can be achieved, with Caesarean section confined to patients who had not previously delivered vaginally (Carroll et al 1990).

Oxytocin has long been established as the first choice induction agent following SROM at term; its intravenous administration permits safe titration of dosage against uterine response. Several studies, summarized by Grant & Keirse (1989) have compared its efficacy with prostaglandin (PGE$_2$) given in various dosages and routes, most commonly intravaginally. PGE$_2$ induction is followed less frequently by Caesarean section, possibly because it mimics more closely the onset of spontaneous labour. Many women find PGE$_2$ induction more acceptable but there is a need for careful randomized comparison with oxytocin following SROM before its widespread use can be advocated. Intravenous oxytocin retains an advantage over locally administered PGE$_2$ when induction fails; a later attempt to stimulate contractions is still possible whereas vaginal therapy once started cannot be abandoned because of its almost inevitable precipitation of ascending genital infection.

CONCLUSIONS: QUESTIONS ANSWERED AND UNANSWERED

The re-evaluation during the past decade of the important clinical syndrome of prelabour SROM reflects its significance as a precursor of a large minority of labours, both at term and especially preterm. Some redefinition of management can currently be suggested but many interventions require further evaluation. Long-standing fears concerning ascending infection have lessened. In particular, maternal death from sepsis is extremely rare (Daikoku et al 1981). Diagnosis can generally be confirmed by simple inspection of the amniotic fluid specimen and vaginal digital examination provides no advantage over sterile speculum inspection (Munson et al 1985). An expectant approach can be adopted almost indefinitely, provided any vaginal examination is avoided and careful clinical monitoring is conducted in hospital: laboratory investigations provide little additional help in early warning of infection. Routine prophylactic antibiotics are not as effective in controlling maternal and neonatal infectious morbidity as prompt intrapartum parenteral therapy in cases of suspected infection.

When the membranes rupture in the mid or early third trimester, maternal transfer should be immediately effected to an obstetric unit where third level neonatal resuscitation and intensive care are available. Tocolytics appear to do no good in such cases but the fetus may benefit from corticosteroid therapy if surfactant production is suspected to be immature. Amniocentesis is not recommended and the value of amnioinfusion remains uncertain. Ultrasound is of value in assessing fetal presentation, growth and well-being and lung development, especially preterm, but at term it is of little help in confirming the diagnosis of SROM.

Obstetric measures to effect delivery may do more harm than good. Preterm expectancy is almost always rewarded by spontaneous labour and delivery before 37 weeks' gestation. Early induction following prelabour SROM at term represents a significant contribution to the increasing incidence of Caesarean delivery for dystocia and certainly increases maternal intrapartum morbidity. Induction of the 5–10% of mothers undelivered more than 24 hours after SROM represents a reasonable compromise and is followed in a high proportion by vaginal delivery. Whether oxytocin or PGE_2 is most effective for such inductions still needs to be clarified.

Further studies are needed to document the natural history of very preterm SROM and to collect data on the most appropriate methods of prolonging the latent interval, while avoiding pulmonary hypoplasia; quantitation of the residual amniotic fluid volume may help in this respect. At term, investigations which better predict patients susceptible to dystocic complications in labour may allow modifications of management, as exemplified by expectancy following previous Caesarean delivery.

REFERENCES

Al-Zaid N S 1980 Bursting pressure and collagen content of fetal membranes and their relation to premature rupture of the membranes. Br J Obstet Gynaecol 87: 227–229

Baumgarten K, Moser S 1986 Technique of fibrin adhesion for premature rupture of membranes during pregnancy. J Perinat Med 14: 43–49

Blott M, Greenough A, Nicolaides K H, Moscoso G, Gibb D, Campbell S 1987 Fetal breathing movements as predictor of favourable pregnancy outcome after oligohydramnios due to membrane rupture in second trimester. Lancet 2: 129–131

Carroll S G, Turner M J, Stronge J M, O'Herlihy C 1990 Management of antepartum spontaneous membrane rupture after one previous caesarean section. Eur J Obstet Gynaecol Reprod Biol 35: 173–178

Cederqvist L L, Zervoudakis I A, Ewool L C, Litwin S D 1979 The relationship between prematurely ruptured membranes and fetal immunoglobulin production. Am J Obstet Gynecol 134: 784–788

Conway D I, Prendiville W J, Morris A, Speller D C, Stirrat G M 1984 Management of spontaneous rupture of the membranes in the absence of labour in primigravid women at term. Am J Obstet Gynecol 150: 947–951

Cotton D B, Gonik B, Bottoms S F 1984 Conservative versus aggressive management of preterm rupture of membranes. A randomised trial of amniocentesis. Am J Obstet Gynecol 63: 38–43

Cowett R M, Hakanson D O, Kocon R W, Oh W 1976 Untoward neonatal effect of intra amniotic administration of methylene blue. Obstet Gynecol 48: 745–755

Crowley P, Chalmers I, Keirse M J 1990 The effect of corticosteroid administration before preterm delivery: an overview of the evidence from controlled trials. Br J Obstet Gynaecol 97: 11–25

Daikoku N H, Kaltreider F, Johnson T R, Johnson J W, Simmons M A 1981 Premature rupture of membranes and preterm labour; neonatal infection and perinatal mortality risks. Obstet Gynecol 58: 417–425

Davies P A, Robinson R J, Scopes J W, Tizard J P, Wigglesworth J S 1972 Medical care of newborn babies, SIMP, London, p 29

Egan D, O'Herlihy C 1988 Expectant management of spontaneous rupture of membranes at term. J Obstet Gynaecol 8: 243–247

Fayez J A, Hassan A A, Jonas H S, Miller G L 1978 Management of premature rupture of the membranes. Obstet Gynecol 52: 17–21

Friedman M L, McElin T W 1969 Diagnosis of ruptured fetal membranes. Am J Obstet Gynecol 104: 545–550

Garite T J, Freeman R K, Linzey E M, Braly P S, Dorchester W L 1981 Prospective randomised study of corticosteroids in the management of premature rupture of the membranes and the premature gestation. Am J Obstet Gynecol 141: 508–515

Garite T J, Keegan K A, Freeman R K, Nageotte M P 1987 A randomised trial of ritodrine tocolysis versus expectant management in patients with premature rupture of membranes at 25 to 30 weeks of gestation. Am J Obstet Gynecol 157: 388–393

Gibbs R S 1987 Premature rupture of the membranes. In: Pauerstein C J (ed) Clinical obstetrics. Wiley, New York, pp 367–381

Gibbs R S, Castillo M S, Rodgers P J 1980 Management of acute chorioamnionitis. Am J Obstet Gynecol 136: 709–713

Gilstrap L C, Leveno K J, Cox S M, Burris J S, Mashburn M, Rosenfeld C R 1988 Intrapartum treatment of acute chorioamnionitis: impact on neonatal sepsis. Am J Obstet Gynecol 159: 579–583

Gleeson R P, Elder A M, Turner M J, Rutherford A J, Elder M G 1989 Vaginal pH in pregnancy in women delivered at and before term. Br J Obstet Gynaecol 96: 183–187

Grant J, Keirse M J 1989 Prelabour rupture of the membranes at term. In: Chalmers I, Enkin M, Keirse M J N C (eds) Effective care in pregnancy and childbirth. Oxford University Press, Oxford, pp 1112–1117

Keirse M J, Ohlsson A, Treffers P, Kanhai H H 1989 Prelabour rupture of the membranes preterm. In: Chalmers I, Enkin M, Keirse M J N C (eds) Effective care in pregnancy and childbirth. Oxford University Press, Oxford, pp 666–693

Lamont R F, Taylor-Robinson D, Newman M, Wigglesworth J S, Elder M G 1986 Spontaneous early preterm labour associated with abnormal genital bacterial colonization. Br J Obstet Gynaecol 93: 804–810

Larsen J W 1979 Premature amniorrhexis. Obstet Gynecol Ann 8: 203–221

Lebherz T B, Hellman L P, Madding R, Anctil A, Arje A R 1963 Double blind study of premature rupture of the membranes. Am J Obstet Gynecol 106: 469–483

Lenihan J P 1984 Relationship of antepartum pelvic examinations to premature rupture of the membranes. Obstet Gynecol 63: 33–37

McIntosh N 1988 Dry lung syndrome after oligohydramnios. Arch Dis Child 63: 190–193

Mead P B 1980 Management of the patient with premature rupture of the membranes. Clinics in Perinatol 7: 243–255

Munson L A, Graham A, Koos B J, Valenzuela G J 1985 Is there a need for digital examination in patients with spontaneous rupture of the membranes? Am J Obstet Gynecol 153: 562–563

Naeye R L 1982 Factors that predispose to premature rupture of the fetal membranes. Obstet Gynecol 60: 83–98

Nageotte M P, Freeman R K, Garite T J, Dorchester W 1985 Prophylactic intrapartum amnioinfusion in patients with preterm premature rupture of the membranes. Am J Obstet Gynecol 153: 557–562

Robson M S, Turner M J, Stronge J M, O'Herlihy C 1990 Is amniotic fluid quantification of value in the diagnosis and conservative management of premature membrane rupture at term? Br J Obstet Gynaecol 97: 324–328

Rochelson B L, Rodke G, White R, Bracero L, Baker D A 1987 A rapid colorimetric AFP monoclonal antibody test for the diagnosis of preterm rupture of the membranes. Obstet Gynecol 69: 163–166

Schutte M R, Treffers P E, Kloosterman G, Soepatmi S 1983 Management of premature rupture of membranes: the risk of vaginal examination to the infant. Am J Obstet Gynecol 146: 395–400

Skinner S J, Campos G A, Liggins G C 1981 Collagen content of human amniotic membranes: effect of gestation length and premature rupture. Obstet Gynaecol 146: 395–400

Stedman C M, Crawford S, Staten E, Chirny W B 1981 Management of preterm premature rupture of the membranes; assessing amniotic fluid in the vagina for phosphatidylglycerol. Am J Obstet Gynecol 140: 34–38

Turner M J, Macauley J, Gordon H 1986 Induction of labour in primigravidae with ruptured membranes and an unfavourable cervix at term using vaginal prostaglandin E_2 pessaries. J Obstet Gynaecol 7: 151–152

Vintizileos A M, Campbell W A, Nochimson D J, Weinbaum P J 1987 The use and misuse of the nonphysical profile. Am J Obstet Gynecol 156: 527–533

7. Massive obstetric haemorrhage

G. Burke   N. M. Duignan

Massive obstetric haemorrhage continues to be an important cause of maternal mortality, even though the maternal mortality rate due to haemorrhage has declined. The Report on Confidential Enquiries into Maternal Death in England and Wales, 1979–1981 (DHSS 1986), recorded only 14 deaths as being directly attributed to haemorrhage (7·3 per million maternities); however, in addition, there were 20 deaths due to ectopic pregnancy, 4 due to uterine rupture and 2 deaths from abortion associated with haemorrhage. An important finding of the report was that care was considered substandard in 12 of the 14 deaths directly attributed to haemorrhage. The most recent report, for the years 1982–1984 (DoH 1989), showed a further fall in the number of maternal deaths directly due to haemorrhage, with 9 in the 3-year period. This represented a marked improvement, particularly as the obstetric management was criticized in only 3 of the 9 cases. However, haemorrhage complicated a further 15 deaths from other causes and it also contributed to several of the 10 deaths from ectopic pregnancy.

In the United States, between 1974 and 1978, 331 maternal deaths (13·4%) were associated with obstetric haemorrhage: of these, 114 were due to postpartum haemorrhage; 71 to uterine rupture; 55 to abruption; 39 to non-uterine haemorrhage; 33 were associated with retained placenta (including placenta percreta and increta) and 19 with placenta praevia. It was noted that the rate of fatal obstetric haemorrhage appeared to be particularly high in women delivering in hospitals with less than 300 deliveries per annum (Kaunitz et al 1985). More recently, Sachs et al (1987) reported that maternal mortality due to obstetric haemorrhage in Massachusetts had declined by over 90% between the periods 1954–1957 and 1982–1985, and that trauma (suicide, accidents and homicide) had become the main cause of maternal death. In Sweden, between 1971 and 1980, there were 68 maternal deaths (a maternal mortality rate of 6·6 per 100 000 live births); only 9 were due to haemorrhage, with uterine rupture (4) being the commonest cause (Hogberg 1986). Duthie et al (1989) showed that maternal mortality in Hong Kong had fallen from 45 to 5 per 100 000 between 1961 and 1985. Haemorrhage and ectopic pregnancy accounted for nearly 50% of cases in this period, during which the death rate due to haemorrhage fell by 86%.

Table 7.1 Maternal mortality rate (MMR) in a selection of countries and regions. (Reproduced with permission from Royston and Armstrong 1989b)

Country or region	MMR
Cuba	32
Czechoslovakia	8
France	13
Germany (Federal Republic)	11
Greece	12
Japan	15
Portugal	15
Romania	149
USA	9
USSR	48
Africa	640
Asia	420
Latin America	270

In spite of these improvements in the West, and in parts of the East, the situation in some developing countries may only be described as grim. The maternal mortality rates for a selection of Western countries and developing regions are listed in Table 7.1. In some areas, the maternal mortality rate (per 100 000 live births) is over 1000, and haemorrhage probably accounts for between one-third and two-thirds of these. For example, Greenwood et al (1987a), reporting on pregnancy outcome in a rural area of the Gambia, found a maternal mortality rate of 2200 per 100 000. There were 15 deaths in the small area surveyed (with a population of about 12 000) in 1 year, more than twice the expected number of maternal deaths in all of Sweden in 1 year. Postpartum haemorrhage was responsible for one third of these deaths, and none had the benefit of even the most basic medical assistance. El Kady et al (1989) reported the maternal mortality rate in Menoufia Governorate, Egypt, between 1981 and 1983 to be 190 per 100 000, with haemorrhage being the commonest cause. Boes (1987a) who studied only patients delivered in hospital, in southern Africa between 1980 and 1982, still found a maternal mortality rate of 83 per 100 000. Haemorrhage accounted for 20% of the 737 deaths reviewed (Boes 1987b), with postpartum haemorrhage and abruption being the commonest occurrences. Not surprisingly, Adetoro (1987) identified cumbersome and ineffective blood transfusion services as one of the main preventable factors in maternal mortality in a Nigerian hospital, which had a maternal mortality rate of 450 per 100 000. The overwhelming inadequacy of maternity services in many parts of the world is reflected in the estimated 500 000 deaths that occur annually from causes related to pregnancy and childbirth: all but 6000 occur in the developing world (Royston & Lopez 1987).

Massive obstetric haemorrhage has been defined as the loss of a patient's blood volume in a few hours (Findley 1987). However, complications are likely to develop long before such a loss, particularly if the loss is rapid: indeed, patients may not survive the acute loss of more than 50% of the blood volume (Seeley 1987). It therefore seems appropriate to describe haemorrhage of more than 1500 ml (25–30% of the blood volume in pregnancy) as massive.

The replacement of very large volumes of blood poses particular technical problems which require special consideration. In this chapter, we will describe the causes of massive obstetric haemorrhage and discuss practical methods of treatment which can be implemented in the ordinary obstetric unit; more sophisticated techniques, available only in larger centres, will also be discussed, but operative techniques will not be described in any detail, as these are very well dealt with in the more appropriate setting of an atlas of operative surgery (e.g. Lees & Singer 1982).

CAUSES OF OBSTETRIC HAEMORRHAGE

While the source of bleeding in massive obstetric haemorrhage is usually readily apparent, the diagnosis may not be so obvious when the bleeding is occult; indeed, the severity of the haemorrhage may be seriously under-estimated. This is more likely in cases of abruptio placentae, uterine rupture, broad ligament haematomas or rarer causes of intra-abdominal haemorrhage.

Haemorrhage in early pregnancy

In the first 20 weeks, severe haemorrhage may be associated with abortion, ectopic pregnancy, or molar pregnancy, particularly when such pregnancy is relatively advanced. Early diagnosis is essential for preventing serious haemorrhage. At the Coombe Lying-In Hospital, we have noted a decrease in the incidence of severe haemorrhage associated with spontaneous abortion as a result of improved management of bleeding in the first trimester based on ultrasound (Drumm & Clinch 1975). All such cases have an ultrasonic examination within 24 hours, which provides an accurate diagnosis and enables early treatment to be carried out. Similarly, the early diagnosis of ectopic pregnancy should reduce the incidence of severe haemorrhage in this condition: this is shown to be the case in the most recent triennial report (DoH 1989), in which the maternal mortality rate from ectopic pregnancy fell despite an increase in the number of cases.

Haemorrhage is the commonest complication of therapeutic abortion, although, according to official statistics, it occurred in only 0·23% of legal abortions in England and Wales in 1986 (Abortion Statistics 1986). It was found most frequently when the procedure was performed between 13 and

19 weeks gestation. In the United States, there was an eight-fold decrease in mortality from abortion between 1972 and 1981, and haemorrhage has overtaken infection as the main cause of death (0·21 per 100 000 abortions, Binkin 1986). Abortions performed by curettage had the lowest mortality, while hysterotomy/hysterectomy had the highest. Serious haemorrhage may also occur in cases of missed abortion, when coagulopathy can complicate the situation.

Trauma must also be recognized as a cause of severe haemorrhage. Such trauma may be due, on the one hand, to a cervical laceration extending upwards into the broad ligament as a result of over-vigorous dilatation; on the other hand, perforation of the uterus may result in intraperitoneal bleeding or in an expanding broad ligament haematoma, particularly if the perforation is lateral, where the uterine vessels may be injured. Vaginal prostaglandin, administered some hours before the procedure, may facilitate operative dilatation and reduce trauma (Darney 1986, Nyholm et al 1988). When oxytocic drugs are used in the second trimester, either for therapeutic or missed abortion, it is important to realize that the pregnant uterus may rupture, particularly if previously scarred, and a diagnosis of uterine rupture should always be considered when unexpected bleeding or collapse occurs in these patients.

Abruptio placentae

In cases of severe abruption, the diagnosis is seldom in doubt: the patient is shocked, the uterus is tense and the fetus is dead, even though there may be little or no revealed bleeding. Abruption is frequently associated with hypertension, and disordered coagulation (disseminated intravascular coagulation) is a common complication (Gilabert et al 1985). When the fetus is dead, the management is directed at replacing blood loss and achieving a vaginal delivery. If the fetus is still alive, Caesarean section will be required to deliver it safely but surgery should not be attempted until the mother has been adequately resuscitated, coagulation defects have been excluded or reversed, and adequate blood is available. Accurate haemodynamic monitoring is required as many patients have co-existent pre-eclampsia, but the insertion of a central venous line should be deferred until the results of the coagulation tests are known: if these are not readily available, subclavian insertion of the line should be avoided. Frequent re-evaluation of the patient's haemodynamic and haematological status is mandatory in severe abruption. Massive post-partum haemorrhage is not uncommon even after vaginal delivery, while intra-operative bleeding may complicate Caesarean section, particularly when there is extensive extravasation of blood into the myometrium (the Couvelaire uterus).

Occasionally, rare causes of intra-abdominal bleeding may mimic abruption. Spontaneous rupture of uterine or ovarian veins classically present with sudden onset of abdominal pain accompanied by signs of hypovolaemic shock (Ginsburg et al 1987). In addition, the signs of haemo-peritoneum (including shoulder tip pain) will usually be present. Similar clinical presentations are found in spontaneous rupture of other vessels (e.g. splenic or adrenal). Conditions where bleeding is not a feature, but where some signs and symptoms, suggestive of abruption, may be present, include acute hydramnios and red degeneration of a fibroid.

Placenta praevia and accreta

Placenta praevia continues to be one of the commonest causes of massive obstetric haemorrhage and the expectant management of this condition is well established. Diagnosis is rarely a problem provided ultrasound is available. Delivery will usually be by elective Caesarean section at about 38 weeks for all but minor grades where, ultrasonically, there is only a small portion of the placenta on the lower segment of the uterus. If the clinical behaviour of the condition suggests increased risk (i.e. repeated significant antepartum haemorrhages) it may be necessary to deliver the baby at an earlier gestation. Even in experienced hands, there is great potential for serious peroperative bleeding and this operation should not be left to an inexperienced trainee. A major degree of placenta praevia on the anterior wall of the uterus poses particular difficulty. Four units of blood should be available before commencing the operation electively and a vertical incision used to enter the abdomen. The surgeon may be alarmed to find very large veins running along the lower segment: these may be ligated before incising the lower segment. Only very rarely is it necessary to make other than a transverse incision in the lower segment and it is often possible to open the amniotic cavity above the placenta. Sometimes it may be necessary to cut through the placenta, but even then, provided the fetus is delivered promptly, blood loss may be relatively small. However, on occasions, bleeding from the placental site in the lower segment may be excessive because this thin muscle layer is not as haemostatically effective as that of the upper segment and hysterectomy may be required because of uncontrollable haemorrhage. Placenta accreta is now being encountered more frequently following previous Caesarean section (Clark et al 1985a, DHSS 1986, DoH 1989, McShane et al 1985, Weckstein et al 1987). Clark et al (1985a) cited an incidence as high as 24% among patients with placenta praevia who had had only one previous Caesarean operation. Two of the three maternal deaths reported as being due to placenta praevia in the triennial report for 1979–1981 (DHSS 1986) were associated with placenta accreta and, on each occasion, the operation was undertaken by a junior doctor. Compression of both uterine arteries between thumb and forefinger while the uterus is elevated through the abdominal wound is helpful in controlling initial haemorrhage, while aortic compression is a further invaluable temporary technique until definitive treatment has been effected (DHSS 1986).

Uterine rupture

Uterine rupture is uncommon. It occurs in parous women, is more common among those who have had a previous Caesarean section or hysterotomy, and may be precipitated by the injudicious use of oxytocin.

Molloy et al (1987) found the incidence of uterine rupture among patients with a previous lower segment Caesarean section to be significantly increased when such patients were given oxytocic drugs and epidural analgesia.

The main danger in cases of uterine rupture is that the diagnosis may be delayed, particularly when the bleeding is occult. This is especially likely when intra-abdominal bleeding occurs after vaginal delivery, as in one of the three cases of maternal death from uterine rupture recorded in the most recent triennial report (DoH 1989). The uterus may rupture before the onset of labour in patients who have had a Classical section and it should be borne in mind that antepartum haemorrhage in these patients may be due to scar rupture. A diagnosis of uterine rupture must always be considered in cases of intrapartum or postpartum collapse and the management consists of prompt volume replacement, together with laparotomy and uterine repair or hysterectomy.

Postpartum haemorrhage

Postpartum haemorrhage (PPH) is still a cause of massive obstetric haemorrhage. In the 7 years 1978–1984, a total of 1050 patients among 49 300 deliveries at the Coombe Lying-In Hospital were noted to have had a postpartum haemorrhage, an incidence of 2·1% (Clinical Report 1984). Sixteen (1·5%) of these 1050 patients required hysterectomy to control severe haemorrhage. The most recent British report on maternal mortality (DoH 1989) includes 5 deaths due to postpartum haemorrhage or 'other obstetrical trauma'. Gilbert et al (1987), who reported an incidence of postpartum haemorrhage of 11% in a British department, suggested that the high rate was due to changes in labour ward practice; they found primiparity, induction of labour, prolonged labour, forceps delivery and the prophylactic use of oxytocin rather than Syntometrine to be contributory factors. The lower incidence recorded in our own practice may be associated with a more active management of labour or a different method of assessing blood loss after delivery; it is of interest that the recorded rate of PPH was similar among primiparae and multiparae.

The most recent British report on maternal mortality (DoH 1989) included 5 deaths due to PPH or other obstetrical trauma. Serious PPH may be caused by uterine atony, by a morbidly adherent placenta or by trauma, which includes uterine rupture and lacerations to the vagina and cervix. The diagnosis of uterine atony is straightforward, and this usually responds to treatment with intravenous ergometrine and/or oxytocin infusion. If significant bleeding persists despite such therapy, the diagnosis of atony must be reviewed and other causes considered: these include retained placental cotyledon, trauma, uterine rupture and coagulation defects. These patients need examination under general anaesthesia and uterine exploration to exclude retained placental tissue, uterine rupture or trauma to the uterus, cervix or vagina. If uterine rupture is found or if bleeding persists, a laparotomy will be necessary, with hysterectomy likely.

ASSESSMENT

It is imperative that each patient be assessed carefully. Failure to evaluate (and re-evaluate) the collapsed or bleeding patient properly may result in a serious under-estimate of the blood loss. Shweni et al (1987) reported that 6 of 13 patients with severe secondary postpartum haemorrhage after Caesarean section were not actively bleeding at presentation, because of hypovolaemic shock. It is vital, therefore, that the bleeding patient is assessed at an early stage by an experienced team, which should involve a senior anaesthetist and a senior obstetrician. This assessment should provide a good estimate of the amount and rate of blood loss, the degree of shock and a likely diagnosis of the cause of the bleeding, and it should be carried out in a suitably equipped area with sufficient lighting and space to allow the resuscitation to proceed smoothly. Emergency rooms, labour wards and operating theatres usually (but not always) fulfill these basic criteria: it is the responsibility of the medical staff to ensure that these facilities are available at all times and that essential equipment is properly maintained and in adequate supply. The medical staff must also ensure that appropriate back-up laboratory and blood transfusion services are available and that these services are structured to cope with emergencies requiring multiple transfusions and frequent haematological tests.

Shock is defined as a circulation inadequate to satisfy overall cellular metabolic requirements (Seeley 1987) and while this definition does not include any reference to blood pressure or pulse rate, maintenance of a circulation that will perfuse the tissues adequately is dependent upon both pressure and volume: the mean systemic arterial pressure is the product of the cardiac output multiplied by the systemic vascular resistance. Pressure is maintained in the earliest phase of hypovolaemic shock through increased sympathetic tone which results in a reflex tachycardia, maintaining cardiac output when stroke volume falls, and an increase in systemic vascular resistance. The so-called 'classic' signs (e.g. tachycardia) may be absent, however, and the diagnosis may be missed: it is a common misconception that a bradycardia or a normal heart rate excludes a diagnosis of hypo-volaemic shock. Sander-Jensen et al (1986) found that a vagally mediated decrease in heart rate is, in fact, a regular finding during hypotensive, severe haemorrhage and they considered that this might be a protective mechanism, allowing for improved diastolic filling when venous return to the heart is critically reduced. In their series of 273 patients with acute haemorrhagic shock, Barriot & Riou (1987) found that 7% had paradoxical bradycardia with undetectable systolic blood pressure and they noted that this was more likely to occur in more severe and rapid haemorrhages. Furthermore, drugs, epidural anaesthesia and pain may affect the signs of shock.

It is simply not possible to reliably measure the amount of blood loss when haemorrhage is severe: minor inaccuracies are compounded as the patient continues to bleed and it can be readily appreciated that management based on 'eye-balling' the loss is potentially lethal. Replacement must be guided by other means. O'Driscoll & McCarthy (1966) were the first to recommend monitoring of central venous pressure (c.v.p.) in cases of placental abruption, and demonstrated that renal failure could be prevented by rapid transfusion guided in this way. Subsequently, similar reports came from the US (Wilson et al 1968). The jugular venous pulse (j.v.p.) may be quite useful in the initial assessment of the patient, but central venous pressure monitoring is essential when conducting volume replacement in serious haemorrhage. The technique for insertion of the c.v.p. catheter is described by Lees & Singer (1982). Therapy should be directed at achieving and maintaining a central venous pressure of 8–10 cm of water. It has been suggested that the c.v.p. will aid in measuring colloid overload, but not crystalloid overload, and that measurement of the pulmonary capillary wedge pressure (p.c.w.p.) with a Swan-Ganz catheter is more reliable (Barry et al 1980). This catheter is most useful in special circumstances, such as co-existing cardiac disease (class 3 and 4; pulmonary hypertension), sepsis, severe pre-eclampsia, adult respiratory distress syndrome, or shock unresponsive to initial fluid therapy (Berkowitz 1983), and its use is probably best reserved for these situations. Arterial lines are desirable when frequent blood gas analyses and blood pressure measurement are required. However, invasive monitoring techniques can be hazardous and should only be used when necessary. The authors are aware of a maternal death where haematoma formation at the site of a jugular vein cannula resulted in complete air-way obstruction, complicating the resuscitation (Clinical Report 1979). Other early complications of c.v.p. lines include pneumothorax, haemothorax, subcutaneous emphysema, arterial damage, pleural effusion and hydromediastinum, brachial plexus injury, air embolism and cardiac perforation, while infection and thrombosis are later hazards (Kaye & Smith 1988).

Adult respiratory distress syndrome (ARDS) may develop in the shocked patient. In this condition, breathing is laboured and the respiratory rate is more than 20 per minute; initially a chest X-ray may show a diffuse interstitial pulmonary infiltrate and blood gases show a low oxygen tension (less than 50 mm Hg) which is unresponsive to oxygen therapy. When refractory hypoxaemia is present, mechanical ventilation is necessary. Ventilation is also required when there is carbon dioxide retention, impaired consciousness or an inability to clear secretions (Rafferty & Niederman 1983).

It is difficult to establish the prognosis in shock, particularly in the early stages. It appears that outcome is related to duration rather than severity and that the onset of cardiac, respiratory or renal failure, persistent jaundice and clouding of consciousness augur badly, particularly in older patients, whereas the ability to increase standardized stroke work in response to intravenous fluids seems to herald a good outcome (Ledingham et al 1982).

RESUSCITATION

We all know that transfusion has saved the lives of many patients, and I believe that it would have saved the lives of many more had not men, in view of its risks and the circumstances attending it, deferred its performance till they were sure that their patients were going to die. Then the operation 'did no good'.

Bull's citation in the *Medical Record* of January, 1884, on early experience with blood substitutes in haemorrhage (Oberman 1986) remains valid.

The immediate danger to the haemorrhaging patient is inadequate circulation, not inadequate oxygen-carrying capacity, and the first task is to restore circulating volume. To do this, a number of solutions may be employed. Fresh whole blood is the ideal solution, since it will carry out nearly all of the functions of the blood that has been lost—it will restore the circulation, it will provide appropriate osmotic and oncotic pressure, it will carry oxygen and carbon dioxide and, in addition, it will restore the essential elements of coagulation which have been depleted. Fresh whole blood is, for practical purposes, unavailable, however, but its individual components are readily available in areas with a good transfusion service. However, neither blood nor its components are required for the immediate restoration of the circulating volume: this can be accomplished with crystalloid (such as normal saline or Hartmann's solution—non-salt crystalloids such as 5% dextrose are ineffective) or colloid solutions (solutions that contain substances with molecular weights of more than 40 000, which have significant oncotic properties). An intravenous cannula of adequate bore should be inserted into a good vein. A 14-gauge cannula is the smallest that should be employed and ideally a second line should be established. If there is difficulty in finding a suitable vein, a sphygmomanometer cuff should be inflated over the arm and saline may be injected into a hand vein using a syringe and a small needle: this will result in the distension of a vein suitable for cannulation. Blood warming devices and pressure infusion bags are essential equipment.

There is controversy regarding the use of crystalloids or colloids for initial resuscitation. Paull (1987) found an incidence of severe reactions in 1 of 821 patients treated prophylactically with dextran 70, including a cardiac arrest in one woman about to undergo Caesarean section. There is general agreement that the dextrans should be avoided altogether because of their interference with platelet function and blood cross-matching: they should be regarded as contraindicated in obstetric haemorrhage. Colloids remain in the circulation longer, a potential advantage if blood is not available quickly, but this advantage is of less relevance in the patient who is continuing to bleed rapidly. This longer half-life becomes a disadvantage if fluid overload and pulmonary oedema develop. While colloids may exert a favourable oncotic pressure in the presence of an intact pulmonary circulation, if there is any damage to the pulmonary capillary endothelium, as may be the case in severe shock, colloids may cross the capillary wall and draw more fluid out of the vessels. Pearl et al (1988), however, using an experimental animal model to compare saline, 5% albumin and 6% hydroxyethyl starch, concluded that crystalloid and colloid have similar pulmonary effects when used for resuscitation from haemorrhagic shock in the presence of pulmonary capillary injury. Crystalloids have been said to have advantages over colloids in preserving and restoring renal function (Rafferty et al 1983) by promoting a diuresis, but it may be argued that renal function is best protected by simply ensuring an adequate circulation. Crystalloid (Hartmann's solution) and the polygeline colloid, Haemaccel, are both used at the Coombe Lying-In Hospital for immediate restoration of volume. Haemaccel appears to have a relatively short duration of action and it contains significant amounts of calcium which, in the healthy patient, may have a beneficial, positive ionotrophic effect (this would be a hazard in a patient with significant coronary artery disease). The availability of rapid cross-matching at the hospital normally provides packed cells within 20 minutes for further volume replacement. In the haemorrhaging patient there is little use in transfusing crystalloids or colloids once a good circulation has been restored. Thereafter, blood component therapy—packed cells and fresh frozen plasma—should be employed to maintain the circulation, to provide oxygen-carrying capacity and to restore coagulation factors.

There is a good case to be made for using fresh frozen plasma in the initial stage of resuscitation in patients with severe haemorrhage since it is an excellent volume-expander and it also promptly restores deficient clotting factors. This is particularly useful in the management of major placental abruption, and it is current practice at the Coombe Lying-In Hospital in treating this condition.

Hypertonic saline has been little used in resuscitation of patients with hypovolaemic shock. De Felippe et al (1980) used 100–400 ml of a 7·5% sodium chloride solution to treat 12 patients with terminal hypovolaemic shock who had not responded to vigorous volume replacement and corticosteroid and dopamine infusions, with prompt reversal of shock in 11. Layon et al (1987) found that 3% saline effected resuscitation without compromising cardiopulmonary function in another animal model of haemorrhagic shock. These reports are interesting but data are insufficient at present to assess properly the merit of this type of treatment.

The patient needs the capacity to transport oxygen and carbon dioxide, as well as an adequate circulation and, while the use of crystalloid or colloid is appropriate initial therapy, blood is required. While blood is being prepared, oxygen should be administered. If a large volume of colloid has been given before the blood is available, there may be a reluctance to give blood quickly because of the risk of overload: this is almost never a problem in the healthy obstetric patient and the importance of obtaining an adequate circulating volume cannot be over-emphasized, the major risk being under-transfusion. Cross-matched blood should be available by the time 1500–2000 ml (25–35% of the blood volume) of crystalloid have been infused. If it is not, and bleeding is continuing, consideration should be given to the use of group O rhesus-negative (except in patients known to have anti-c antibodies) or, preferably, typed, uncross-matched blood of the patient's own group: usually the blood group of obstetric patients is known. Modern blood transfusion services provide blood as its individual components, and used correctly, these are adequate for most circumstances. The essential elements required are packed red cells, fresh frozen plasma and, sometimes, platelet concentrate. Packed cells may be transfused rapidly if they are first diluted with normal saline. Blood filters are irrelevant in the patient who is bleeding profusely, but should be used in less serious haemorrhages. Therapy should be directed at achieving a haematocrit of 30%.

Blood substitutes, such as Fluosol-DA 20%, have the ability to carry oxygen and carbon dioxide as well to provide osmotic and oncotic pressure. Their development was reviewed in a recent editorial (Editorial 1986), where their considerable potential for adverse effects was noted. Karn et al (1985) used Fluosol-DA 20% successfully in two Jehovah's Witnesses with haemoglobins of 3·0 g/dl or less following massive postpartum haemorrhage and they suggested that these agents may prove to have a role in the management of patients with haemorrhage where blood transfusion is not available or not acceptable, when tissue hypoxia is developing. However, Gould et al (1986) found that, after haemorrhage, Fluosol-DA was unnecessary in moderate anaemia and ineffective in severe anaemia (75% of these patients died), with only a very small increment in arterial oxygen content being achieved.

Massive blood transfusion carries increased risks: these include the risk of transmission of both viral and bacterial infection and of transfusion reactions, both immediate and delayed. The risk of transfusion-transmitted infection is unlikely to ever be completely eliminated (Bove 1987) but steps to exclude high-risk donors and to test for HIV antibody, antibody to hepatitis B core antigen and alanine aminotransferase are likely to minimize the risks. If a severe haemolytic reaction occurs, respiratory distress and collapse occur promptly. The transfusion should be stopped and the patient given crystalloid or plasma instead. After initial fluid loading, fresh blood may be transfused after repeated, accurate cross-matching (Findley 1987).

In addition to these potential hazards, transfused blood is deficient in coagulation factors and in 2,3 diphosphoglycerate, which will cause a shift to the left in the oxygen saturation curve, so that oxygen is yielded less easily to the tissues. Microaggregates in stored blood have been implicated in the pathogenesis of adult respiratory distress syndrome, but micro-filtration is not recommended in very severe haemorrhage because it slows the rate of infusion. Hypocalcaemia and hyperkalaemia can also complicate massive transfusion but they rarely reach clinical significance. The need to monitor electrolytes during resuscitation is obvious.

Haemostasis

The association between obstetric haemorrhage, particularly placental abruption, and coagulation defects, including disseminated intravascular coagulation (DIC), is well established.

Abnormalities of coagulation were detected or suspected in six of the nine maternal deaths due to haemorrhage reported in the most recent Maternal Mortality Report (DoH 1989). Massive transfusion itself will cause changes in the same coagulation tests, notably prolongation of the prothrombin and partial thromboplastin times, and reduction in the platelet count. However, disseminated intravascular coagulation can be recognized by a prolonged thrombin time or a reduction in the fibrinogen level, with prolongation of the thrombin time being the most important and rapid test for DIC (Letsky 1987).

Continued haemorrhage, especially that associated with abruption, depletes stores of clotting factors, particularly fibrinogen. Fresh blood and fresh frozen plasma should be given to correct these coagulation defects, including DIC, since they contain both fibrinogen and clotting factors. Transfusion of one unit of fresh frozen plasma for every four to five units of packed cells is recommended.

Platelet transfusion may be required when massive blood loss occurs but, as was pointed out by the NIH Consensus Conference on platelet transfusion therapy (NIH 1987), there is a shortage of scientific information on which to base precise guidelines. Following replacement of one blood volume, 35–40% of the platelets usually remain and the con-ference suggested that, in the absence of documented thrombocytopenia and clinically abnormal bleeding time, platelets should not be admin-istered. Platelet transfusion carries a risk of infection because the platelets are generally prepared by pooling concentrates from multiple donors. Thompson (1985) noted that large platelets, which are haemostatically more effective, are selectively consumed in massive haemorrhage and for this reason, the platelet count may not be an accurate reflection of the true severity of thrombocytopenia. According to Miller & Brzica (1986), patients who have undergone trauma or require surgery probably need a platelet count of 100 000 to maintain adequate haemostasis. One unit will generally elevate the count by 7000–10 000. Microaggregate blood filters should not be used for platelet administration. In view of the above, and in the absence of sufficient precise information on which to base management, it would seem reasonable to transfuse platelets when the count falls below 50 000 and as a routine in very large haemorrhages.

Rarely, chronic defects of haemostasis are encountered in pregnancy. These include von Willebrand's disease, Christmas disease (Factor IX deficiency), the carrier state for haemophilia (Factor VIII deficiency) and immune thrombocytopenic purpura (ITP). Cryoprecipitate is required in the management of the first three of these conditions. Immune thrombocytopenic purpura is the most commonly encountered of these conditions in pregnancy, since it usually affects young women. High-dose intravenous gamma-globulin (IVIgG) is becoming established as the best form of management in pregnancies complicated by ITP, as it appears to be the only treatment offering protection to both the mother and the fetus. It is generally administered to provide protection at time of delivery, but in severe ITP (for example, where splenectomy has been required), there may be considerable risk to both mother and fetus before delivery, and repeated courses may be required (Burke et al 1989). The effect of a 5-day course usually lasts for 2 to 3 weeks, but the optimal dosage schedule remains to be defined. Platelets should be available for transfusion at time of delivery.

METHODS OF ARRESTING HAEMORRHAGE

It may not be possible to stabilize the patient who is bleeding profusely until the haemorrhage has been arrested. In this situation, the attending staff must be alert to the seriousness of the patient's condition and, having instituted the initial resuscitative procedures, act swiftly and skilfully, if tragedy is to be averted. In the majority of cases encountered, however, the patient's general condition will have been stabilized by the initial measures, and procedures to stop the bleeding can be selected and implemented without the same degree of urgency.

Medical treatment

Atonic postpartum haemorrhage may be treated medically with intravenous ergometrine or synthetic oxytocin and these agents are effective in most cases. If atony fails to respond to such treatment, another cause for the bleeding must be excluded and an examination under anaesthesia should be performed. There is no evidence that uterine packing is of any value.

Analogues of prostaglandin F2, given intramuscularly (Toppozada et al 1981, Hayashi et al 1981), have been used successfully to control intractable postpartum haemorrhage due to uterine atony and the direct intramyometrial method has also been effective (Bruce et al 1982). The intravenous administration of prostaglandin E2 has been reported in the management of persistent primary PPH (Henson et al 1983), but, since these drugs decrease peripheral resistance, the authors warned that hypovolaemia must be corrected before the drug is given. Recently, Hankins et al (1988) have noted a marked arterial oxygen desaturation in some patients treated for postpartum haemorrhage with analogues of prostaglandin F2α but it was not clear whether this temporary phenomenon was due to the drug or other factors; other authors have reported minimal side effects (Hayashi et al 1981, Toppozada et al 1981).

Obstetric hysterectomy

If medical treatment fails to control postpartum haemorrhage, hysterectomy may be necessary. This procedure is the most effective method for dealing with haemorrhage due to persistent uterine atony, a morbidly adherent placenta or uterine rupture; these were the commonest indications for such therapy cited by Giwa-Osagie et al (1983), Clark et al (1984), Thonet (1986) and Sturdee & Rushton (1986). As it is an irrevocable step, it is reserved for the management of conditions where conservative measures have failed, but its performance should not be delayed until the patient is *in extremis*. Neither should its performance be delayed while less difinitive procedures with which the surgeon has little experience are attempted. Subtotal hysterectomy was performed in 54% of the patients in the series reported by Clark et al, and this is the simpler and speedier operation to perform. Usually, it will be effective in dealing with haemorrhage due to uterine atony and to a morbidly adherent placenta, when the placental site does not involve the lower uterine segment. Rupture of a lower segment uterine incision can often be dealt with by simply repairing the rupture, but traumatic rupture (i.e. rupture not involving a previous Caesarean section scar) or rupture of a classical section scar will frequently require hysterectomy. Whether a total hysterectomy is required will depend on extension of the rupture into the lower uterine segment. As was pointed out by Clark et al (1984), it is the clinical situation in which hysterectomy is performed, and not the type of hysterectomy, that determines the amount of blood loss and operating time. For instance, Giwa-Osagie et al (1983) reported a higher maternal mortality in those patients who had had a total hysterectomy but they attributed this to the fact that such surgery was needed in the more serious conditions. Total hysterectomy is more frequently performed in cases of placenta accreta, a condition which is becoming increasingly important (Clark et al 1985a, Weckstein et al 1987). The need for the involvement of senior personnel is emphasized by the report of Smith (1982) where 3 out of 14 patients having obstetric hysterectomy in a district general hospital died: in all 3 cases anaesthesia was administered by a registrar and in 2, the operation was performed by a registrar. Ureteric injury occurred in 4 of the 14 patients.

We recommend subtotal hysterectomy as the operation of choice in most instances of obstetric haemorrhage requiring hysterectomy and we concur with the view of Lees & Singer (1982) that 'the surgeon should not attempt total hysterectomy in most circumstances'. The risk of neoplasia developing in the cervical stump several years later is not relevant in the context of life-threatening haemorrhage.

Internal iliac artery ligation

Internal iliac (or hypogastric) artery ligation has received considerable attention lately. The technique (Lees & Singer 1982, Tosson & Richardson 1986) involves a transperitoneal approach to the vessels. A longitudinal 4–5 cm incision is made in the pelvic peritoneum at the level of the bifurcation of the common iliac artery inferior and lateral to the ureter. The peritoneum, with the ureter attached, is then gently reflected medially. The internal iliac is now exposed by careful blunt dissection and two ligatures of non-absorbable material are placed around the anterior division with an aneurysm needle, 0·5 cm apart. The vessel is not divided and the femoral pulse should be identified after ligation. Techniques involving the use of absorbable suture material have also been described, and these can allow re-canalization of vessels (Dubay et al 1980). Because of the extensive anastomoses of the pelvic vessels, most authors recommend bilateral ligation. The operation results in a reduction in pulse pressure distal to the ligatures rather than in a complete interruption of the blood supply because of collateral circulation, and pelvic ischaemia is said to be uncommon. However, in their series of 18 patients who had the procedure carried out, Evans & McShane (1985) reported one patient with postischaemic motor neuron damage and ischaemia of the central pelvic area with breakdown of the perianal region and the episiotomy site. Another patient had a right common iliac obstruction postoperatively and needed a bypass graft. These authors concluded that internal iliac ligation appears to be effective for uterine atony and midline perforation, but is less so for placenta accreta and is totally ineffective for uterine lacerations. Clark et al (1985b) found the procedure to be effective in controlling bleeding in less than half of their 19 patients, including patients with uterine atony. They felt, however, that complications associated with the procedure were due to a delay in carrying out the definitive treatment (hysterectomy) rather than to the procedure itself.

Angiographic embolization

Angiographic embolization of bleeding vessels with gelatin sponge shavings (Gelfoam—Upjohn) has been used to treat postpartum and post-abortal haemorrhage (Greenwood et al 1987b, Ito et al 1986, Shweni et al 1987, Brown et al 1979). It is usually performed via the femoral artery. The dye is first injected into the aorta below the renal arteries and filming over the pelvis allows identification of the bleeding vessels which are then catheterized and embolized. If the bleeding artery cannot be catheterized, the Gelfoam is injected at the distal end of the anterior division of the internal iliac artery, relying on the flow to direct the emboli towards the bleeding vessels. The aortography is repeated to confirm that the bleeding has been arrested. The iliac arteries can also be catheterized directly. However, the rate of bleeding must be at least 2 ml per minute for angiographic detection and this may not be the case in profoundly shocked patients. The number of patients reported in the literature to have been managed with angiographic embolization is relatively small, however, and this method will be available only in centres with appropriately trained personnel. Greenwood et al (1987b), however, consider that it should be used when conservative and minor surgical procedures have failed to arrest postpartum haemorrhage, as major surgery may be avoided and reproductive capacity maintained. The available literature suggests that this technique represents a real advance in the management of obstetric haemorrhage.

The intra-arterial injection of vasoconstrictive agents has also been described in the management of haemorrhage: Mud et al (1987) successfully used intra-arterial infusions of dopamine HCl in the initial management of haemorrhaging patients and vasopressin has also been used in this way (Magrina et al 1981).

The MAST suit

In some circumstances, a patient with massive obstetric haemorrhage will have been treated initially in a non-specialist unit and will require transport, after stabilization, to an appropriate centre. The Vietnam war produced advances in the early management of trauma, including the development of a pneumatic suit to stabilize patients during transport. This suit was subsequently improved and is now known as the military anti-shock trouser or MAST suit. It consists of double-layered polyvinyl and has three separate chambers (one abdominal and two leg compartments) which are inflated by a foot pump. Pearse et al (1984) reviewed the use of this device in obstetrics and gynaecology. Use of the suit results in an 'autotransfusion' of only 150–300 ml but probably the major mechanism of action is the increase in peripheral resistance which application of the suit causes. This results in a rapid increase in blood pressure (in one series of 70 patients cited by Pearse et al a mean rise in blood pressure of 65 mm Hg was achieved with the suit alone) and a slowing of active bleeding, with improved perfusion of vital organs. A decrease in the incidence of adult respiratory distress and acute tubular necrosis would therefore be expected. The MAST suit has been used effectively in patients with pelvic fracture and it has also been used to good effect in the management of postoperative patients where surgical intervention has failed to control the bleeding. Uses in obstetrics include peroperative use in ectopic pregnancy, preoperatively in postpartum haemorrhage, and in rarer situations such as rupture of the liver and abdominal pregnancy. The suit is not without potential hazards, however, which include hypoventilation, lactic acidosis, hyperkalaemia, diminished urinary output and skin breakdown. The risk of these potential hazards is probably reduced by using the lowest suit pressures that will result in acceptable blood pressure. Suit pressures below 40 mm Hg are well tolerated. It is recommended that the suit should remain inflated for 12–24 hours after bleeding has ceased and the suit must then be deflated gradually. Obviously, rapid deflation may cause severe hypotension. The main advantage of the suit would appear to be in the transport of haemorrhaging patients before definitive treatment, but it may also be useful when treatment has not controlled the bleeding completely.

CONCLUSIONS

Mothers still die from haemorrhage, and while the number of maternal deaths from haemorrhage has fallen to very low rates in the West, the situation in parts of the developing world is appalling. Harrison (1989), in a recent editorial, believed that training and proper utilization of midwives, rather than the retraining of traditional birth attendants, was essential in order to reduce maternal mortality in the developing world, but he also emphasized the importance of the eradication of mass illiteracy in this regard. The decline in the direct maternal death rate due to haemorrhage in Cuba from 32 to 2 per 100 000 between 1960 and 1984 (Farnot Cardoso 1986) demonstrates what can be achieved in developing countries by making maternal and child health a priority. It should be appreciated that the problem in the developing world is related to the availability of services and is not simply the result of poor pre-pregnancy health: Kaunitz et al (1984) reported a maternal mortality rate of 870 per 100 000 live births among a religious group in the United States who refused obstetric care.

Effective management of obstetric haemorrhage depends upon prompt restoration of circulating volume, accurate diagnosis of the cause of bleeding and early and appropriate therapy to arrest the bleeding. Under-estimation of the amount of blood loss, delay in instituting definitive therapy and the performance of difficult operations by inexperienced staff (such as Caesarean section for anterior placenta praevia in patients with previous sections) appear to be frequent contributory factors to poor outcome. The resources of even well equipped and staffed units may be stretched by massive obstetric haemorrhage and staff should be familiar with an agreed protocol that can be implemented quickly and smoothly.

REFERENCES

Abortion Statistics 1986 Her Majesty's Stationery Office, London

Adetoro O O 1987 Maternal mortality: a 12-year survey at the University of Ilorin Teaching Hospital, Ilorin, Nigeria. Int J Gynaecol Obstet 25: 93–98

Barriot P, Riou B 1987 Haemorrhagic shock with paradoxical bradycardia. Intensive Care Med 13: 203–207

Barry A P, Bonnar J, Browne A D H et al 1980 IMA Maternal Mortality Report 1979. Ir Med J 73: 448–452

Berkowitz R L 1983 The Swan-Gantz catheter and colloid-osmotic pressure determinations. In: Berkowitz R L (ed) Critical care of the obstetric patient. Churchill Livingstone, New York, Ch 1

Binkin N J 1986 Trends in induced legal abortion morbidity and mortality. Clin Obstet Gynecol 13: 83–93

Boes E G M 1987a Maternal mortality in southern Africa, 1980–1982. Part 1. Pregnancy can be lethal. S Afr Med J 71: 158–160

Boes E G M 1987b Maternal mortality in southern Africa, 1980–1982. Part 2. Causes of maternal deaths. S Afr Med J 71: 160–161

Bove J R 1987 Transfusion associated hepatitis and AIDS: what is the risk? N Engl J Med 317: 242–245

Brown B J, Heaston D K, Poulson A M, Gabert H A, Mineau D E, Miller F J 1979 Uncontrollable postpartum bleeding: a new approach to haemostasis through angiographic arterial embolization. Obstet Gynecol 54: 361–365

Bruce S L, Paul R H, Van Dorsten J P 1982 Control of post-partum uterine atony by intramyometrial prostaglandin. Obstet Gynecol 59 (suppl): 47–50

Burke G, Casey C, Chamberlain P F, Egan E, Meehan F P 1989 Refractory immune thrombocytopenic purpura in pregnancy, managed with multiple courses of high-dose gammaglobulin. Ir J Med Sci 158: 69–70

Clark S L, Koonings P P, Phelan J P 1985a Placenta praevia/accreta and prior Caesarean section. Obstet Gynecol 66: 89–92

Clark S L, Phelan J P, Sze-Ya Y, Bruce S R, Paul R H 1985b Hypogastric artery ligation for obstetric haemorrhage. Obstet Gynecol 66: 353–356

Clark S L, Sze-Ya Y, Phelan J P, Bruce S R, Paul R H 1984 Emergency hysterectomy for obstetric haemorrhage. Obstet Gynecol 64: 376–380

Clinical Report 1979 The National Maternity Hospital, Holles St, Dublin 2

Clinical Report 1984 The Coombe Lying-In Hospital, Dolphin's Barn, Dublin 8

Darney P D 1986 Preparation of the cervix: hydrophilic and prostaglandin dilators. Clin Obstet Gynecol 13: 43–51

De Felippe J, Timoner J, Velasco I T, Lopes O U, Rocha e Silva M 1980 Treatment of refractory hypovolaemic shock by 7·5% sodium chloride injections. Lancet ii: 1002–1004

DHSS 1986 Report on Confidential Enquiries into Maternal Deaths in England and Wales, 1979–1981. Her Majesty's Stationery Office, London

DoH 1989 Report on Confidential Enquiries into Maternal Deaths in England and Wales, 1982–1984. Her Majesty's Stationery Office, London

Drumm J E, Clinch J 1975 Ultrasound in management of clinically diagnosed threatened abortion. Br Med J 2: 424

Dubay M L, Holshauser C A, Burchell R C 1980 Internal iliac artery ligation for postpartum haemorrhage: recanalization of vessels. Am J Obstet Gynecol 136: 689–691

Duthie S J, Ghosh A, Ma H K 1989 Maternal mortality in Hong Kong 1961–1985. Br J Obstet Gynaecol 96: 4–8

Editorial 1986 Blood substitutes: has the right solution been found? Lancet ii: 717–718

El Kady A A, Saleh S, Gadalla S, Fortney J, Bayoumi H 1989 Obstetric deaths in Menoufia Governorate, Egypt. Br J Obstet Gynaecol 96: 9–14

Evans S, McShane P 1985 The efficacy of internal iliac artery ligation in obstetric haemorrhage. Surg Gynecol Obstet 160: 250–253

Farnot Cardoso U 1986 Giving birth is safer now. World Health Forum 7: 348–354

Findley I R 1987 Problems of treating massive blood loss. In: Morgan B (ed) Problems in obstetric anaesthesia (perinatal practice vol 3) Wiley, London, Ch 5

Gilabert J, Estelles A, Aznar J, Galbis M 1985 Abruptio placentae and disseminated intra-vascular coagulation. Acta Obstet Gynecol Scand 64: 35–39

Gilbert L, Porter W, Brown V A 1987 Postpartum haemorrhage—a continuing problem. Br J Obstet Gynaecol 94: 67–71

Ginsburg K A, Valdes C, Schnider G 1987 Spontaneous utero-ovarian rupture during pregnancy: 3 case reports and a review of the literature. Obstet Gynecol 69: 474–476

Giwa-Osagie O F, Uguru V, Akinla O 1983 Mortality and morbidity of emergency obstetric hysterectomy. J Obstet Gynaecol 4: 94–96

Gould S A, Rosen A L, Laksham R S et al 1986 Fluosol-DA as a red-cell substitute in acute anaemia. N Engl J Med 314: 1653–1656

Greenwood A M, Greenwood B M, Bradley A K et al 1987a A prospective survey of the outcome of pregnancy in a rural area of the Gambia. Bull WHO 65: 635–643

Greenwood L H, Glickman M G, Schwartz P E, Morse S S, Denny D F 1987b Obstetric and non-malignant gynaecologic bleeding: treatment with angiographic embolization. Radiology 164: 155–159

Hankins G D V, Berryman G K, Scott R T, Hood D 1988 Maternal arterial desaturation with 15-methyl prostaglandin F2α for uterine atony. Obstet Gynecol 72: 367–370

Harrison K A 1989 Maternal mortality in developing countries. Br J Obstet Gynaecol 96: 1–3

Hayashi R H, Castillo M S, Noah M L 1981 Management of severe postpartum haemorrhage due to uterine atony using an analogue of prostaglandin F2α. Obstet Gynecol 58: 426–429

Henson G, Gough J D, Gillmer M D G 1983 Control of persistent primary postpartum haemorrhage due to uterine atony with intravenous prostaglandin E2. Case report. Br J Obstet Gynaecol 90: 280–282

Hogberg U 1986 Maternal deaths in Sweden, 1971–1980. Acta Obstet Gynecol Scand 65: 161–167

Ito M, Matsui K, Mabe K, Katabuchi H, Fujisaki S 1986 Transcatheter embolization of pelvic arteries as the safest method for postpartum haemorrhage. Int J Gynaecol Obstet 24: 373–378

Karn K E, Ogburn P L, Julian T, Cerra F B, Hammerschmidt D E, Vercellotti G 1985 Use of a whole blood substitute, Fluosol-DA 20%, after massive postpartum haemorrhage. Obstet Gynecol 65: 127–130

Kaunitz A M, Spence C, Danielson T S, Rochat R W, Grimes D A 1984 Perinatal and maternal mortality in a religious group avoiding obstetric care. Am J Obstet Gynecol 150: 826–831

Kaunitz A M, Hughes J M, Grimes D A, Smith J C, Rochat R W, Kafrissen M E 1985 Causes of maternal mortality in the United States. Obstet Gynecol 65: 605–612

Kaye C G, Smith D R 1988 Complications of central venous cannulation. Br Med J 297: 572–573

Layon J, Duncan D, Gallagher T J, Banner M J 1987 Hypertonic saline as a resuscitation solution in haemorrhagic shock: effects on extravascular lung water and cardiopulmonary function. Anesth Analg 66: 154–158

Ledingham I McA, Cowan B N, Burns H J G 1982 Prognosis in severe shock. Br Med J 284: 433

Lees D H, Singer A 1982 A colour atlas of gynaecological surgery. Vol 6: surgery of conditions complicating pregnancy. Wolfe Medical, London

Letsky E 1987 Haemostasis in pregnancy. In: Morgan B M (ed) Foundations of obstetric anaesthesia. Farrand Press, London, Ch 12

Magrina J F, Moffat R E, Masterson B J, Krantz K E 1981 Selective arterial infusion of Pitressin for the control of puerperal haemorrhage after hypogastric artery ligation. Obstet Gynecol 58: 646–648

McShane P, Heyl P S, Epstein M F 1985 Maternal and perinatal morbidity resulting from placenta praevia. Obstet Gynecol 65: 176–182

Miller R D, Brzica S M Jr 1986 Blood, blood components, colloids and autotransfusion therapy. In: Miller R D (ed) Anesthesia, vol 2. 2nd edn. Churchill Livingstone, New York, Ch 39

Molloy B, Sheil O, Duignan N M 1987 Delivery after caesarean section: review of 2176 consecutive cases. Br Med J 294: 1645–1647

Mud H J, Schattenkerk M E, de Vries J E, Bruining H A 1987 Non-surgical treatment of pelvic haemorrhage in obstetric and gynaecologic patients. Crit Care Med 15: 534–535

NIH 1987 Platelet transfusion therapy. JAMA 257: 1777–1780

Nyholm H C J, Mikkelsen A L, Secher N J 1988 Pretreatment of the cervix with 9-deoxy-16, 16-dimethyl-9-methylene-prostaglandin E2 (Metenprost) vaginal pessaries before first trimester legal abortion in nulliparae. J Obstet Gynaecol 8: 210–213

Oberman H A 1986 Transfusion classic. Transfusion 26, 5: 404

O'Driscoll K, McCarthy J R 1966 Abruptio placentae and central venous pressures. J Obstet Gynaecol Br Commonwealth 73: 923–929

Paull J 1987 A prospective study of dextran-induced anaphylactoid reactions in 5754 patients. Ann Intensive Care 15: 163–167

Pearl R G, Halperin B D, Mihm F G, Rosenthal M H 1988 Pulmonary effects of crystalloid and colloid resuscitation from haemorrhagic shock in the presence of oleic acid-induced pulmonary capillary injury in the dog. Anesthesiology 68: 12–20

Pearse C S, Magrina J F, Finley B 1984 Use of MAST suit in obstetrics and gynaecology. Obstet Gynecol Surv 39: 416–422

Rafferty T D, Niederman M S 1983 Ventilator therapy and care of the patient with ARDS. In: Berkowitz R L (ed) Critical care of the obstetric patient. Churchill Livingstone, New York, Ch 2

Rafferty T D, Keefer J R, Barash P G 1983 Fluid management in the massively bleeding obstetric patient. In: Berkowitz R L (ed) Critical care of the obstetric patient. Churchill Livingstone, New York, Ch 3

Royston E, Armstrong S 1989 Preventing maternal deaths. World Health Organization, Geneva

Royston E, Lopez A D 1987 On the assessment of maternal mortality. World Health Stat Q 40: 214–224

Sachs B P, Brown D A J, Driscoll S G et al 1987 Maternal mortality in Massachusetts: trends and prevention. N Engl J Med 316: 667–672

Sander-Jensen K, Secher N H, Bie P, Warberg J, Scwartz T W 1986 Vagal slowing of the heart during haemorrhage: observations from 20 consecutive hypotensive patients. Br Med J 292: 364–366

Seeley H F 1987 Pathophysiology of haemorrhagic shock. Br J Hosp Med 37: 14–20

Shweni P M, Bishop B B, Hansen J N, Subrayen K T 1987 Severe postpartum haemorrhage after Caesarean section. S Afr Med J 72: 617–619

Smith A M 1982 Emergency obstetric hysterectomy. J Obstet Gynaecol 2: 245–248

Sturdee D W, Rushton D I 1986 Caesarean and postpartum hysterectomy 1968–1983. Br J Obstet Gynaecol 93: 270–274

Thompson C B 1985 Selective consumption of large platelets during massive bleeding. Br Med J 291: 95–96

Thonet R G N 1986 Obstetric hysterectomy—an 11-year experience. Br J Obstet Gynaecol 93: 794–798

Toppozada M, El-Bossaty M, El-Rahman H A, Shams El-Din A H 1981 Control of intractable atonic postpartum haemorrhage by 15-methyl prostaglandin F2 alpha. Obstet Gynecol 58: 327–330

Tosson S R, Richardson J A 1986 Internal iliac artery ligation in obstetric and gynaecologic practice. J Obstet Gynaecol 6: 268–270

Weckstein L N, Masserman J S H, Garite T J 1987 Placenta accreta: a problem of increasing clinical significance. Obstet Gynecol 69: 480–482

Wilson F, Nelson J H, Moltz A 1968 Methods and indications for central venous pressure monitoring. Am J Obstet Gynecol 101: 137–151

8. Pain relief in labour

F. Reynolds

It is surprising that analgesia in labour should be in any way a controversial subject, considering what a painful experience labour can be—yet epidural blockade, the most reliable means of providing pain relief, is often associated in the consumer's mind with other forms of obstetric intervention which all tend to be regarded as interference in what would otherwise be a satisfying natural event.

That there may be sound medical reasons for obstetric intervention tends to be overlooked by the critical consumer. Likewise the extreme pain that leads the labouring woman to request analgesia tends to be forgotten after the event. In fact Morgan et al (1982) showed that, of those mothers experiencing what was judged at the time to be severe pain, more than 90% viewed the experience with satisfaction in retrospect. So effective pain relief in labour is not provided in order to incur lasting gratitude, but rather to treat distress with compassion *at the time*, and to minimize the resulting stress for both mother and baby. That labour pain may later be forgotten does not lessen present suffering. Moreover effective pain relief can have sound medical advantages, particularly to the baby.

FRINGE METHODS OF ANALGESIA

I hope that devotees of the methods I mention here will not take exception to this title. I merely wish to group together methods outside the mainstream of inhalational, narcotic and regional analgesia. Research into fringe methods has not been recorded extensively in the traditional medical literature in recent years, and their detailed description is beyond the scope of this review.

Suffice it to say that a friendly atmosphere, homely surroundings (Chapman et al 1986) and a good midwife (Waldeström 1988) are all believed to reduce the need for analgesia in labour. Self hypnosis has anecdotally been found successful in individual cases, but a randomized controlled trial in primipara (Freeman et al 1986) found that although producing maternal satisfaction after the event (a poor index of successful analgesia, vide supra), the technique had no effect on the need for traditional analgesia, or on delivery type, and was associated with a significant prolongation of labour.

Acupuncture has been investigated sporadically in labour using abdominal (Abouleish & Depp 1975) or sacral (Umeh 1986) acupuncture points but both these studies lacked placebo controls. It is probably the most time consuming method of analgesia and the results are inconsistent and unpredictable. In about 2/3 of women it may produce partial analgesia for about 2 hours (Abouleish & Depp 1975), and electro-acupuncture introduces extra wires and machinery and may interfere with fetal monitoring while also further limiting the patient's movement.

Transcutaneous electrical nerve stimulation (TENS)

As the poor man's acupuncture, or a labour saving method of back rubbing for the bureaucratic age, TENS has been widely used. Being non-invasive and relatively harmless it has become popular in minimalist circles.

The electrodes are placed over the posterior primary rami of T10–L1 and S2–4 and the strength of the current can be adjusted gradually to the maximum amplitude producing a pleasant sensation. The level can be increased during contractions (Robson 1979). In theory this should be an effective means of relieving pain, by stimulating large sensory fibres whose collaterals appear to activate interneurons in the substantia gelatinosa (lamina II in the posterior horn) which in turn inhibit transmitter release in the pain pathways (Fig. 8.1, Reynolds 1984). Early uncontrolled trials suggested that about 3/4 of women in labour found TENS helpful (Robson 1979, Stewart 1979), but more recently controlled trials using dummy TENS have been less positive. Harrison et al (1986) found that TENS did not reduce the need for other forms of analgesia or improve the normal delivery rate, though both midwives and mothers in the treatment group made more favourable comments about it. Thomas et al (1988) detected no difference in pain score between treatment and control groups and whether the TENS apparatus was switched on or off. Again there was no reduction in the need for supplementary analgesia, but again an increased element of consumer satisfaction in that more women in the active TENS group said that they would like the treatment next time. There was a suggestion that TENS was effective for back pain, but many patients had no back pain.

INHALATIONAL ANALGESIA

Inhalational agents have been in use in obstetrics since the mid nineteenth century. When Queen Victoria received chloroform from John Snow during the birth of her eighth child, this was not anaesthesia but analgesia. Volatile agents (chloroform, ether and more recently trichloroethylene) and nitrous oxide have been used. For many years nitrous oxide had the serious disadvantage that for midwife administration it was mixed with air and the

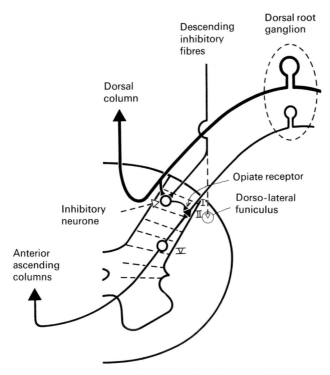

Fig. 8.1   A much simplified representation of the pain pathways and the factors that modulate pain transmission. Pain is conducted by the smaller sensory fibres (Aδ and C) whose cell bodies are in the dorsal route ganglion and whose central projections synapse principally in lamina II, the substantia gelatinosa. Transmission in this synapse may be inhibited by neurones activated both by collaterals from the large sensory fibres which ascend in the dorsal column and also by fibres in the dorso-lateral funiculus which descend from the brain stem from areas where opiate receptors are dense. Opiate receptors are also found in the substantia gelatinosa and play a part principally in the pre-synaptic inhibition of pain transmission.

words 'fit for gas and air' were rubber-stamped onto the notes of patients who were free from cardiorespiratory disease—as if *any* mother were 'fit' to breathe a mixture containing, when the apparatus was functioning correctly, only 10% oxygen. Until the 1960s we were all under the misapprehension that nitrous oxide, normally stored as a liquid, and oxygen, which is gaseous in cylinders, could not be mixed in a single cylinder. Thus if a non-hypoxic mixture were to be given, separate cylinders were necessary. It was Tunstall (1961) who showed us that at 2000 p.s.i. oxygen would dissolve nitrous oxide in the gas phase, and that therefore a safe mixture of the two could be used for analgesia by a process which depended neither on a fallible mixing device, nor on using two cylinders with different rates of emptying. This represented significant progress in obstetric analgesia and has greatly broadened the scope and availability of nitrous oxide, which is now the single most widely used agent in the UK.

Trichloroethylene, a volatile agent which enjoyed a vogue during the 'gas and air' era, is no longer used despite the fact that it is an effective analgesic in subanaesthetic concentrations, while the more recently introduced volatile anaesthetics probably act at least in part by an enhanced sedative effect. The halogenated ethers methoxyflurane then more recently enflurane (Abboud et al 1981) and isoflurane (McLeod et al 1985) have all been investigated, though showing little advantage over nitrous oxide. Indeed the pungent odour of the ethers, and their expense, both mitigate against their wide acceptance.

However nitrous oxide itself, even in the 50:50 mixture with oxygen as Entonox, has its shortcomings, not least of which is poor analgesia (Levack & Tunstall 1984). The effort to obtain pain relief provokes even more hyperventilation than that induced by pain, and the resulting hypocapnia may be associated with dizziness and even tetany. Theoretically fetal hypoxia could also result, from negation of the double Bohr effect by maternal hyperventilation and from uterine vasoconstriction, but these are offset by the 50% oxygen in Entonox. Efforts have been made to enhance the analgesia by continuous nasal administration of Entonox (Arthurs & Rosen 1979) and by adding trichloroethylene to it (Levack & Tunstall 1984). The latter combination can even be too powerful and hence unsuitable for unsupervised administration by midwives, and moreover the manufacture of trichloroethylene for medical use has since been discontinued. Lightheadedness and nausea make nitrous oxide unacceptable to a proportion of mothers, while inhibition of methionine synthetase activity by prolonged use of the agent is generally regarded as clinically unimportant in this context.

SYSTEMIC OPIOID ANALGESICS

Pethidine

It is an accident of history that pethidine came to be the standard drug in this category. In 1950 the decision was taken that midwives should be allowed to administer a narcotic analgesic without a doctor's prescription, and pethidine was at the time the latest wonder drug believed to be as effective as morphine but without the side effects. In fact, of course, this has not turned out to be the case, but its one important advantage over morphine is a more rapid onset of action due to greater lipid solubility.

In the mother pethidine is a powerful sedative, and it increases the incidence of nausea and vomiting, but its analgesic efficacy is not great, there being only about a 20% reduction in pain score (Vella et al 1985). The emetic effect is readily counteracted by metoclopramide, which also helps prevent oesophageal reflux (Hey et al 1981) while promethazine is inappropriate since it prolongs the sedative effect but antagonizes what little analgesia might result (Vella et al 1985).

Though pethidine has a sedative effect it is inappropriate in fulminating pre-eclampsia, since the major metabolite norpethidine has convulsant properties (Kaiko et al 1983), and the phenothiazine derivatives chlorpro-mazine and promethazine are similarly unhelpful. It may therefore be more appropriate to provide pain relief in these circumstances with an epidural block (see later).

The most serious maternal side effect of pethidine, however, which is probably shared by other opiate agonists, is to delay gastric emptying (Nimmo et al 1975). Whenever pethidine is used in labour it should probably therefore be accompanied by ranitidine given prophylactically to inhibit gastric acid production, in case general anaesthesia should become necessary.

Though hypoxic episodes have been reported more commonly with pethidine than with epidural analgesia in the first stage of labour (Reed et al 1989), respiratory depression following pethidine is not a major problem in the labouring mother in whom the persisting pain normally continues to stimulate respiration. Not so the baby. In early years pethidine was withheld in late labour for fear of neonatal respiratory depression. This tradition of withholding analgesia when labour pain is at its height has of course tended to be perpetuated into the realm of epidural analgesia. In neither case is it appropriate on any grounds. Pethidine does indeed depress respiration, suckling and other neurobehavioural responses in the newborn (Wiener et al 1977), but its effects are greatest when maternal administration precedes delivery by several hours (Morrison et al 1973) and negligible if only given within an hour of birth. This is not because it traverses the placenta slowly but rather because the drug itself and its active metabolites accumulate slowly in fetal tissues (Kuhnert et al 1979). The detrimental effects of pethidine are readily counteracted by naloxone, though Narcan neonatal should not be used as the dose is inadequate and lasts only about half an hour. A dose of 0·2 mg i.m. has a lasting effect (Wiener et al 1977) and should probably be given to every newborn whose mother has received pethidine in labour, irrespective of timing. On no account should it be given to the mother before delivery when its antianalgesic effect would be quite inappropriate.

Patient controlled analgesia (PCA) has been employed in an attempt to improve analgesia from pethidine. Robinson et al (1980a) demonstrated reduced dose requirement and improved maternal satisfaction when mothers were allowed to self-administer intravenous boluses of pethidine 0·25 mg/kg at 10 minute intervals compared to 150 mg given intra-muscularly as required by the midwife. By contrast Rayburn et al (1989) using smaller PCA doses at longer intervals, compared with nurse admin-istration of 25–50 mg 3 hourly on request, found PCA doses were higher (perhaps not surprisingly) but pain relief equivalent. Neonatal naloxone was needed more often with PCA, and the authors felt the technique had little to recommend it.

Partial opioid agonists

Over the years substitutes for pethidine have been sought that would be less likely to depress neonatal respiration. To this end a series of partial agonists have been produced, that is agents whose maximum effects are limited. Unfortunately it is generally the case that the low ceiling applies not only to side effects but also to analgesia. This particularly applied to *pentazocine* (Fortral) which has the added drawback that it may produce dysphoria. Ventilatory depression in the newborn was however more short lived than following pethidine (Refstad & Lindbaek 1980).

Later *meptazinol*, an agent said to be particularly free from respiratory depressant effects, entered the field. Its potency, efficacy and duration of action are similar to those of pethidine in labour (Nicholas & Robson 1982, Sheikh & Tunstall 1986). Nausea is a fairly prominent feature but the

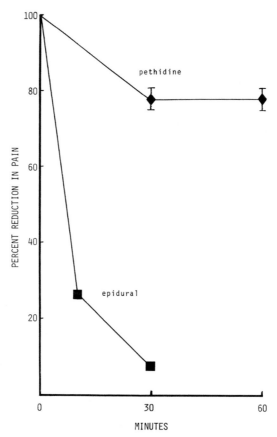

Fig. 8.2 The percentage reduction in pain measured using a visual analogue score in 161 patients given 100 mg of pethidine (diamonds) and 52 patients given epidural bupivacaine (squares). Vertical bars represent standard errors. In the epidural population these are too small to be shown.

newborn appear to fare somewhat better after meptazinol (Nicholas & Robson 1982, Jackson & Robson 1983).

Recently some interest has centred on *nalbuphine*. A dose of 20 mg is equianalgesic with 100 mg of pethidine, while nalbuphine is associated with less nausea and vomiting but more maternal sedation and neonatal depression (Wilson et al 1986). The use of a PCA system with a 2–4 mg loading dose and the mother able to self-administer 1 mg intravenously every 6–10 minutes has been found to be associated with lower dose requirement, fewer side effects and more maternal satisfaction than 10–20 mg i.v. boluses (Podlas & Breland 1987).

There would appear to be no immediate prospect of major progress in the field of systemic analgesia in labour, with PCA giving equivocal results and no real competitor for pethidine after half a century of use. Two randomized controlled trials of epidural blockade versus intramuscular pethidine demonstrate the improved analgesia with epidural, particularly in the first stage of labour (Robinson et al 1980b, Philipsen & Jensen 1989). Indeed using contemporary visual analogue scores there is little comparison (Fig. 8.2) and even when viewed after the event the difference persists (Robinson et al 1980b). The average consumer recognizes this difference (Morgan et al 1984), but pethidine continues to have a role because it is more readily available than epidural analgesia and with the advent of the effective antagonist naloxone for the baby, carries little danger except that of delayed gastric emptying in the parturient. Moreover, when viewed in retrospect over half the mothers who receive it regard the pain relief it provides as satisfactory (Vella et al 1985, Robinson et al 1980b). Also, a misplaced fear of epidural analgesia makes many women hesitate to choose it until they experience the severity of the pain.

EPIDURAL ANALGESIA

An enormous amount of research interest has focused on epidural analgesia in labour and has in recent years centred on certain areas, namely: special indications, safety and safeguards (test doses etc.), improving the analgesia (infusions, epidural opioids), management of the second stage and welfare of the neonate.

The contraindications are well established as coagulopathy and sepsis, since epidural haematoma and abscess can both endanger the spinal cord. Nowadays previous Caesarean section is regarded as an indication (vide infra) and even placental praevia is managed under epidural blockade in some centres. The advantages and disadvantages of epidural analgesia in obstetrics have been summarized in a recent review (Reynolds 1989).

Indications

Anaesthetic literature abounds with reports of rare diseases in which epidural analgesia has been used successfully in obstetrics. Indeed in units where a successful epidural service is established almost any medical or obstetric complication may be regarded as an indication for regional analgesia. This is largely because it may be desirable to avoid both the stress of painful labour, and the risk of general anaesthesia should operative delivery be necessary. In recent years epidural blockade has been used increasingly for emergency Caesarean section since by giving a single large bolus of up to 20 ml of bupivacaine 0·5% a pre-existing analgesic block may very quickly be extended to provide regional anaesthesia suitable for surgery. Moreover, should an epidural catheter not be in place, spinal is used in preference to general anaesthesia in many centres, though skill and experience are required to avoid dramatic hypotension, and a very fine needle must be used to minimize the incidence of headache postpartum.

Hypertension

Pregnancy induced hypertension is the commonest obstetric indication for epidural analgesia. Epidural blockade is of little value in the absence of pain, but in labour it has generally been found to control hypertension successfully and better than hydralazine and magnesium sulphate (Neri et al 1986) though one report, in which the nature of the epidural block was not described, the technique was said not to affect maximum blood pressure (Greenwood & Lilford 1986). There can be little doubt however of its value in pre-eclampsia, provided the catheter is inserted *before the onset of any coagulopathy*. Epidural analgesia prevents the sympathoadrenal over-activity that is characteristic of pre-eclampsia (Abboud et al 1982), produces favourable haemodynamic changes (Newsome et al 1986) and a consistent improvement in intervillous blood flow (Jouppila et al 1982). Early work also showed how the complete analgesia it could provide could minimize the chance of seizures (Moir et al 1972). Moreover general anaesthesia, which is particularly risky in the presence of laryngeal oedema, can be avoided.

Thus when delivery is indicated for pre-eclampsia, the course of action in many large centres on both sides of the Atlantic is to check the platelet count, and if it is greater than 80–100 000 to site an epidural catheter which can then be used for labour or Caesarean section. If the platelet count later falls, it should have returned to normal before the catheter is removed.

Trial of scar

Reviews of labour in several hundred women with previous Caesarean sections suggest that epidural anaesthesia in no way masks the danger (Carlsson et al 1980, Uppington 1983). In fact because pain from a scar and pain from uterine contractions are felt at the same site and the scar is most likely to be stressed *during* a contraction, and because epidural local anaesthetic more readily blocks the pain of uterine contraction (which is conducted by Aδ fibres) than pathological pain (predominantly C fibre stimulation), it may aid in the diagnosis of scar dehiscence. The same phenomenon has been observed with placental abruption, in which epidural blockade does not abolish the pain (Paterson 1979). Pathological pain in the presence of a working epidural can be distinguished from a failed epidural because in the former case the feet are warm and dry.

Preterm labour

It has been suggested that the use of epidural analgesia in preterm labour can improve the outlook for the baby (Osbourne et al 1984). Labour is less stressful and delivery less traumatic; indeed many years ago it was shown that epidural analgesia was associated with a reduced neonatal mortality rate among low birthweight babies (David & Rosen 1976). Likewise the outlook in twin pregnancy, particularly for the second twin, is improved (Crawford 1987).

Safety and safeguards

Misplacement of the epidural needle or catheter has a number of unfortunate sequelae which concentrate the efforts of anaesthetists. Apart from missing the epidural space altogether, which is the result of totally inadequate training, the catheter may be misplaced in a vein, the subarachnoid or, as is less frequently recognized, the subdural space. Avoiding these complications is largely a matter of skill and appropriate technique. While aspiration down the catheter and the test dose are designed to detect the first two misplacements they cannot recognize the third.

Gentle aspiration down a catheter or lowering the open end may reveal it to be intravascular or subarachnoid, and is more likely to be reliable with a multi-holed than with a single-holed catheter, since the latter is more readily occluded (Morrison & Buchan 1990). Aspiration is probably the most appropriate safeguard before topping up an epidural (Prince & McGregor 1986). The dead space of a catheter is much less than 1 ml thus, provided the filter is in view, blood can readily be seen entering it. Cerebrospinal fluid is less easily recognized but can be distinguished from free fluid in the epidural space because it keeps coming unabated.

Test doses have been the subject of some controversy in recent years. A test dose of 2 ml of local anaesthetic (for example bupivacaine 0·5%) will not produce unequivocal symptoms if injected intravenously, and for this reason the inclusion of adrenaline in the test dose has been advocated. Moore & Batra (1981) showed that in non-obstetric patients 15 micrograms of adrenaline given intravenously produced a tachycardia which could be detected by continuous ECG monitoring. However during labour in as many as 25% of women the heart rate may increase after a correctly placed test dose (Cartwright et al 1986) while even i.v. adrenaline may not produce a tachycardia (Leighton et al 1987), and moreover is not totally harmless. *There can therefore be no justification for including adrenaline in the test dose in obstetrics.*

A test dose of local anaesthetic is primarily designed to detect intrathecal (subarachnoid) catheter placement. It has been argued that 2 ml of 0·5% bupivacaine may either be too slow, or produce a dangerously high block, and heavy (hyperbaric) lignocaine has been advocated. In fact heavy lignocaine is not available in the UK and evidence from subarachnoid block shows that 1·5–2 ml of bupivacaine 0·5% reliably produces both pain relief in labour and tingly feet extremely rapidly. A test dose might not be so reliable prior to topping-up however, when the pre-existing epidural might well mask or mimic subarachnoid block. Aspiration is more easily interpreted in these circumstances (Prince & McGregor 1986).

Continuous infusion (vide infra) is a third form of safeguard.

If *intravascular* placement of the catheter is not recognized and more than the test dose of local anaesthetic is administered, the patient may feel light-headed and experience tingling in lips and fingers, then if the injection continues, convulsions may follow and in extreme cases dysrhythmias have been reported, particularly with bupivacaine (Albright 1979). The mother should be given oxygen plus artificial respiration and cardiac massage if necessary and the anaesthetist called immediately. This mishap has caused maternal death in the USA but not in England and Wales (Reynolds 1989). Recovery may be dependent on (1) *slow* injection, so that the mistake is detected before a large dose is given, (2) appropriate resuscitative measures while ensuring the mother is *not placed supine.*

If *subarachnoid* catheterization is unrecognized and a full epidural dose of local anaesthetic is administered, this is 3 to 6 times the dose that is necessary to produce subarachnoid anaesthesia, and a 'total spinal' ensues. In this case the woman may report rapidly rising numbness and dyspnoea then become unconscious, pulseless and apnoeic. With prompt resuscitation this should not result in death or permanent damage, but four such deaths were reported over 15 years in England and Wales (Reports on Confidential Enquiries). Regrettably epidurals have sometimes been used where skilled resuscitation was not readily available.

In practice occasionally both aspiration and the test dose give negative results, yet a subarachnoid block results. Moreover the phenomenon has also been reported after a top-up; a 'delayed total spinal' (Phillips & Brown 1976). Such phenomena are commonly attributed to catheter migration, yet a catheter cannot by itself penetrate intact dura mater, and it has been suggested that partial or complete *subdural* catheter insertion is a more likely explanation (Reynolds & Speedy 1990). Local anaesthetic injected into the subdural space may remain there, and slowly spread giving rise to a block which is characteristically slow in onset and extensive. The injection of fluid may on the other hand tear the much less substantial arachnoid mater, and this is more likely the larger the volume and the quicker the injection. Thus occasionally a test dose may be positive after negative aspiration, or the main dose may produce a total spinal after a negative test dose, or a subsequent dose, particularly a large one, may produce a total spinal after a normal response from earlier doses.

It must be emphasized that a total spinal should be extremely rare, particularly after a top-up, but because it is so dangerous, it is essential to be alert to the possibility.

Continuous infusion

The increasing availability of simple and reliable infusion pumps has popularized continuous infusions in recent years. Epidural analgesia by continuous infusion has been advocated for a number of reasons. Pain relief is smoother and, though it is seldom possible to avoid the need for top-ups completely, the number that are required is greatly reduced, and midwives' and doctors' time is saved (Gaylard et al 1987). Though hypotension occurs most frequently with the first epidural dose, reducing the number of top-ups reduces the risk of late hypotension. It is also apparent that should the catheter enter a vein or the subarachnoid space, the onset of trouble should be gradual and so with vigilance serious problems can be avoided.

Numerous versions of the technique are reported, but all involve giving an initial loading dose and proceeding after a short interval to an infusion of bupivacaine in any concentration from 0·0625 to 0·25% in volumes from 5 to 25 ml/hour. In general for a given total dose larger volumes work better than smaller ones (Li et al 1985, Ewan et al 1986, Flynn et al 1988) and all give better analgesia than intermittent administration (Hicks et al 1988). There is a tendency however for effective fixed dose infusion regimens to rely on a larger dose of bupivacaine than that found necessary by intermittent administration, and this may increase the forceps delivery rate (Smedstad & Morison 1988). A method of overcoming this blunderbuss approach is to vary the infusion rate according to symptoms and height of block (Gaylard et al 1987). Another approach is to use patient controlled epidural analgesia, with a background low dose infusion (Gambling et al 1988, Lysak et al 1990). These workers successfully used a background infusion of 4 to 6 ml/hour of 0·125% bupivacaine with 4 ml on demand boluses, though Lysak et al found that bupivacaine dose requirement was reduced when fentanyl 1 μg/ml was added to the solution.

Recently continuous subarachnoid infusion, using an extremely fine catheter, has become popular in the US. Here dose requirement is extremely small, thus obviating the risk from i.v. injection or total spinal anaesthesia.

Spinal opioids

Another method of improving the reliability of epidural analgesia is to add an opioid to the local anaesthetic. Stimulation of opiate receptors in the substantia gelatinosa of the posterior horn (see Fig. 8.1) appears principally to act presynaptically to inhibit transmitter release in the pain pathways. Opioids placed intrathecally, or even epidurally, are better situated to achieve high concentrations at these receptors, than they are if given systemically. Thus intense analgesia can be achieved with relatively low doses. During the early days it was hoped that spinal opioids would provide complete and long lasting analgesia that was free from side effects. Regrettably this has not turned out to be the case, though they may have a place in controlling perineal pain (Reynolds & O'Sullivan 1989) and in enhancing analgesia from an epidural infusion.

Epidural morphine, the longest acting agent, is successful in the control of chronic pain but very slow in onset owing to its poor lipid solubility, and remarkably ineffective on its own in labour (Booker et al 1980), while it may actually counteract the analgesia from bupivacaine (Lirzin et al 1989). Intrathecal morphine is effective however, but side effects, particularly pruritus and emesis, are prohibitive (Baraka et al 1981) and only partially counteracted by systemic naloxone (Dailey et al 1985). It has been suggested, moreover, that spinal morphine may reactivate herpes simplex virus.

Pethidine is unsuitable for epidural use. It is effective only in large doses (25–100 mg) which produce some local anaesthesia. Its duration of action is brief, particularly if repeated, but cannot be prolonged by the addition of adrenaline (Perriss & Malins 1981, Skjoldebrand et al 1982).

Epidural diamorphine though suitable for postoperative analgesia is ineffective on its own in labour, but a bolus of 5 mg with a loading dose of bupivacaine can reduce the subsequent bupivacaine dose requirement (McGrady et al 1989).

In labour the most successful agents to date are fentanyl and sufentanil, which, when added to a small dose of bupivacaine produce analgesia that is quicker in onset, more intense and longer lasting than bupivacaine alone (Milon et al 1986, Van Steenberge et al 1987) though if used on their own they have little to offer (Reynolds & O'Sullivan 1989).

It has frequently been demonstrated that a combination of opioid and bupivacaine produces better analgesia than the same dose of local anaesthetic on its own (Desprats et al 1983, Milon et al 1986, Phillips 1988, Cohen et al 1987, Van Steenberge et al 1987). This is hardly surprising. Moreover if an opioid is added to a dose of bupivacaine that would normally be effective on its own, then the subjective benefits are less and the local anaesthetic side effects of hypotension, leg weakness and poor expulsive effort are not avoided, while pruritus is added. However, good results are obtained by adding fentanyl (Justins et al 1982) or sufentanil (Naulty et al 1989) to extremely low doses of bupivacaine while very low dose epidural infusions are rendered effective by the addition of either of these agents (Chestnut et al 1988).

Evidence to date suggests however that hypotension, mild leg weakness and instrumental delivery are not avoided even with *low* dose bupivacaine (Van Steenberge et al 1987, Reynolds & O'Sullivan 1989) though improved management of perineal pain, and shivering (Holcombe et al 1988) are distinct advantages of epidural fentanyl and sufentanil.

Fentanyl has a long terminal half-life however, and if given continuously will accumulate in mother and baby (Leveque et al 1987). Neonatal effects should be considered therefore, or naloxone given empirically to the baby at birth. In this respect sufentanil, which is not yet available in the UK, may have an advantage over fentanyl, but direct evidence is as yet not available.

Management of the second stage of labour

The effect of epidural analgesia on the instrumental delivery rate is a controversy that refuses to die down. Much depends on management.

Epidural analgesia does not prolong the first stage of labour (Fairley et al 1988), but it reduces uterine activity in the second (Bates et al 1985) when an oxytocin infusion may be required to make good a relative deficiency (Goodfellow et al 1983), though this has not always been found beneficial (Saunders et al 1989). Patience during the second stage may help reduce the forceps delivery rate (Studd et al 1980) though waiting beyond 3 or 4 hours is unlikely to be helpful (Kadar et al 1986).

Voluntary expulsive efforts before the presenting part has descended have long been regarded as inappropriate and have been associated with an increase in the need for rotational forceps in the presence of epidural analgesia (Maresh et al 1983). It is clear, moreover, that if the second stage is to be allowed to be prolonged the mother's energy should be conserved for the latter part when pushing is more likely to be beneficial.

The belief dies hard that if epidural analgesia 'causes' forceps, then withholding it as the second stage approaches should favour a spontaneous delivery. There is little evidence to bear out this hypothesis. Indeed in a randomized trial in which one group of women received a top-up at the start of the second stage while in the other it was withheld, the normal delivery rate was higher in the former group (Phillips & Thomas 1983). Many women find that if analgesia is withheld at this time of greatest pain, they are unable to co-operate. Moreover should delivery need to be expedited because of fetal distress, the mother is ill-prepared for forceps in the absence of analgesia.

Minimal doses of local anaesthetic do however favour normal delivery, though at the cost in some cases of perfect analgesia (Thorburn & Moir 1981), while an infusion should perhaps be discontinued during the second stage (Chestnut et al 1987). Preliminary verbal reports from the US, however, claim that sufentanil infusion with minute bupivacaine doses allows not only spontaneous delivery but even ambulation in labour

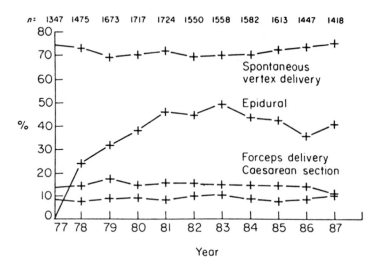

Fig. 8.3   Graph showing annual trends in the types of delivery and the effect of the introduction of an epidural service in one unit in Doncaster Royal Infirmary. (Reproduced with permission from Bailey 1989.)

(Naulty, personal communication, 1989). We await the evidence with interest.

It is clear therefore that to minimize the possibility that epidural analgesia *causes* instrumental delivery, time and patience, possibly oxytocin, modest doses of local anaesthetic with early topping up and late pushing are necessary. Because women at high risk of abnormal delivery tend to be over represented in the epidural population, it is difficult to determine by comparison with a non-epidural group of mothers, if the forceps delivery rate is actually increased by epidural analgesia. It is only possible to know this by comparing the total population of parturients with one for whom epidural analgesia is not available. Such a comparison was possible in Doncaster, where with a change of consultant obstetrician an epidural service was introduced de novo over a short space of time (Bailey & Howard 1983). Apart from a brief hiccup while experience was gained, the forceps delivery rate in the trial population was unchanged (Fig. 8.3). This was dependent on the ideal management outlined above.

THE BABY

Finally, much has been written about the effects of analgesia in labour on the baby. In essence, provided severe persistent hypotension and the supine position are avoided, epidural analgesia is if anything of benefit to the baby in several ways (Reynolds 1989). It is a pity that more of the mothers who are consumed with doubts and worries are not told this.

REFERENCES

Abboud T K, Shnider S M, Wright R G et al 1981 Enflurane analgesia in obstetrics. Anesth Analg 60: 133–137

Abboud T K, Artal R, Sarkis F et al 1982 Sympathoadrenal activity, maternal, fetal and neonatal responses after epidural anesthesia in the preeclamptic patient. Am J Obstet Gynecol 144: 915–918

Abouleish E, Depp R 1975 Acupuncture in obstetrics. Anesth Analg 54: 83–88

Albright G A 1979 Cardiac arrest following regional anesthesia with etidocaine or bupivacaine. Editorial. Anesthesiology 51: 285–287

Arthurs G J, Rosen M 1979 Self administered intermittent nitrous oxide analgesia for labour. Enhancement of effect with continuous nasal inhalation of 50% nitrous oxide (Entonox). Anaesthesia 34: 301–309

Bailey P W 1989 Epidural anaesthesia and instrumental delivery (letter). Anaesthesia 44: 171–172

Bailey P W, Howard F A 1983 Epidural analgesia and forceps delivery: laying a bogey. Anaesthesia 38: 282–285

Baraka A, Noueihid R, Hajj S 1981 Intrathecal injection of morphine for obstetric analgesia. Anesthesiology 54: 136–140

Bates R G, Helm C W, Duncan A, Edmonds D K 1985 Uterine activity in the second stage of labour and the effect of epidural analgesia. Br J Obstet Gynaecol 92: 1246–1250

Booker P D, Wilkes R G, Bryson T H L, Beddard J 1980 Obstetric pain relief using epidural morphine. Anaesthesia 35: 377–379

Carlsson C, Nybell-Lindahl G, Ingemarsson I 1980 Extradural block in patients who have previously undergone caesarean section. Br J Anaesth 52: 827–830

Cartwright P D, McCarrol S M, Antzaka C 1986 Maternal heart rate changes with a plain epidural test dose. Anesthesiology 65: 226–228

Chapman M G, Jones M, Spring J E et al 1986 The use of a birthroom: a randomized controlled trial comparing delivery with that in the labour ward. Br J Obstet Gynaecol 93: 182–187

Chestnut D H, Vandewalker G E, Owen C L et al 1987 The influence of continuous epidural bupivacaine analgesia on the second stage of labor and method of delivery in nulliparous women. Anesthesiology 66: 774–780

Chestnut D H, Owen C L, Bates J N et al 1988 Continuous infusion epidural analgesia during labor: a randomized, double-blind comparison of 0·0625% bupivacaine/0·0002% fentanyl versus 0·125% bupivacaine. Anesthesiology 68: 754–759

Cohen S E, Tan S, Albright G A, Halpern J 1987 Epidural fentanyl/bupivacaine for obstetric analgesia. Anesthesiology 67: 403–407

Crawford J S 1987 A prospective study of 200 consecutive twin deliveries. Anaesthesia 42: 33–43

Dailey P A, Brookshire G L, Shnider S M et al 1985 The effects of naloxone associated with the intrathecal use of morphine in labor. Anesth Analg 64: 658–666

David H, Rosen M 1976 Perinatal mortality after epidural analgesia. Anaesthesia 33: 1054–1059

Desprats R, Mandry J, Grandjean H et al 1983 Analgésie péridurale au cours du travail: étude comparative de l'association fentanyl-marcaine et du marcaine seule. J Gynecol Obstet Biol Reprod 12: 901–905

Ewan A, McLeod D D, MacLeod D M et al 1986 Continuous infusion epidural analgesia in obstetrics: a comparison of 0·08% and 0·25% bupivacaine. Anaesthesia 41: 143–147

Fairley F M, Phillips G F, Andrews B J et al 1988 An analysis of uterine activity in spontaneous labour using a microcomputer. Br J Obstet Gynaecol 95: 57–64

Flynn R J, McMurray T J, Dwyer R, Moore J 1988 Comparison of plasma bupivacaine concentrations during continuous extradural infusion for labour. Br J Anaesth 61: 382–384

Freeman R M, Macaulay A J, Eve L et al 1986 Randomised trial of self hypnosis for analgesia in labour. Br Med J 292: 657–658

Gambling D R, Yu P, McMorland G H, Palmer L 1988 A comparative study of patient controlled epidural analgesia (PCEA) and continuous infusion epidural analgesia (CIEA) during labour. Canad J Anaesth 35: 249–254

Gaylard D G, Wilson I H, Balmer H G R 1987 An epidural infusion technique for labour. Anaesthesia 42: 1098–1101

Goodfellow C F, Hull M G R, Swaab D F et al 1983 Oxytocin deficiency at delivery with epidural analgesia. Br J Obstet Gynaecol 90: 214–219

Greenwood P A, Lilford R J 1986 Effect of epidural analgesia on maximum and minimum blood pressures during the first stage of labour in primigravidae with mild/moderate gestational hypertension. Br J Obstet Gynaecol 93: 260–263

Harrison R F, Woods T, Shore M et al 1986 Pain relief in labour using transcutaneous electrical nerve stimulation (TENS). A TENS/TENS placebo controlled study in two parity groups. Br J Obstet Gynaecol 93: 739–746

Hey V M F, Ostick D G, Mazumder J K, Lord W D 1981 Pethidine, metoclopramide and the gastro-oesophageal sphincter. A study in healthy volunteers. Anaesthesia 36: 173–176

Hicks J A, Jenkins J G, Newton M C, Findley I L 1988 Continuous epidural infusion of 0·075% bupivacaine for pain relief in labour. Anaesthesia 43: 289–292

Holcombe J, Johnson M D, Sevarino F B et al 1988 Effect of epidural sufentanil on temperature regulation in the parturient. Regional Anesthesia 13 supple: 55

Jackson M B A, Robson P J 1983 Preliminary clinical and pharmacokinetic experiences in the newborn when meptazinol is compared with pethidine as an obstetric analgesic. Postgrad Med J 59 suppl 1: 47–51

Jouppila P, Jouppila R, Hollmen A, Koivula A 1982 Lumbar epidural analgesia to improve intervillous blood flow during labor in severe preeclampsia. Obstet Gynecol 59: 158–161

Justins D, Francis D M, Houlton P G, Reynolds F 1982 A controlled trial of extradural fentanyl in labour. Br J Anaesth 54: 409–414

Kadar N, Cruddas M, Campbell S 1986 Estimating the probability of spontaneous delivery conditional on time spent in the second stage. Br J Obstet Gynaecol 93: 568–576

Kaiko R F, Foley K M, Grabinski P Y et al 1983 Central nervous system excitatory effects of meperidine in cancer patients. Ann Neurol 13: 180–185

Kuhnert B R, Kuhnert P M, Tu A-S L et al 1979 Meperidine and normeperidine levels following meperidine administration during labor. II Fetus and neonate. Am J Obstet Gynecol 133: 909–914

Leighton B L, Norris M C, Sosis M et al 1987 Limitations of epinephrine as a marker of intravascular injection in laboring women. Anesthesiology 66: 688–691

Levack I D, Tunstall M E 1984 Systems modification in obstetric analgesia. Anaesthesia 34: 183–185

Leveque C, Garen C, Pathier D et al 1987 Le fentanyl dans l'analgésie obstetricale par voir péridural. J Gynecol Obstet Biol Reprod 16: 113–121

Li D F, Rees G A D, Rosen M 1985 Continuous extradural infusion of 0·0625% or 0·125% bupivacaine for pain relief in primigravid labour. Br J Anaesth 57: 264–270

Lirzin J D, Jacquinot P, Dailland P et al 1989 Controlled trial of extradural bupivacaine with fentanyl, morphine or placebo for pain relief in labour. Br J Anaesth 62: 641–644

Lysak S, Eisenach J C, Dobson C E 1990 Patient controlled epidural analgesia during labor: a comparison of three solutions with a continuous infusion control. Anesthesiology 72: 44–49

McGrady E M, Brownhill D K, Davis A G 1989 Epidural diamorphine and bupivacaine in labour. Anaesthesia 44: 400–403

McLeod D D, Ramayya G P, Tunstall M E 1985 Self-administered isoflurane in labour. A comparative study with Entonox. Anaesthesia 40: 424–426

Maresh M, Choong K H, Beard R W 1983 Delayed pushing with lumbar epidural analgesia in labour. Br J Obstet Gynaecol 90: 623–627

Milon D, Levenac G, Noury D et al 1986 Analgésie péridurale au cours du travail: comparaison de trois associations fentanyl-bupivacaine et de la bupivacaine seule. Ann Fr Anesth Réanim 5: 18–23

Moir D D, Victor-Rodrigues L, Willocks J 1972 Epidural analgesia during labour in patients with preeclampsia. J Obstet Gynaecol Br Commonwth 79: 465–469

Moore D C, Batra M S 1981 The components of an effective test dose prior to epidural block. Anesthesiology 55: 693–696

Morgan B M, Bulpitt C J, Clifton P, Lewis P J 1982 Analgesia and satisfaction in childbirth (The Queen Charlotte's 1000 mother survey). Lancet ii: 808–810

Morgan B M, Bulpitt C J, Clifton P, Lewis P J 1984 The consumers' attitude to obstetric care. Br J Obstet Gynaecol 91: 624–628

Morrison L M M, Buchan A S 1990 Comparison of complications associated with single-holed and multi-holed extradural catheters. Br J Anaesth 64: 183–185

Morrison J C, Wiser W L, Rosser S I et al 1973 Metabolites of meperidine related to fetal depression. Am J Obstet Gynecol 15: 1132–1137

Naulty J S, Ross R, Bergen W 1989 Epidural sufentanil-bupivacaine for analgesia during labor and delivery. Anesthesiology 71: A842

Neri A, Nitke S, Lauchman E, Ovadia J 1986 Lumbar epidural analgesia in hypertensive patients during labour. Eur J Obstet Gynecol Reprod Biol 22: 1–6

Newsome L R, Bramwell R S, Curling P E 1986 Severe preeclampsia: hemodynamic effects of lumbar epidural anesthesia. Anesth Analg 65: 31–36

Nicholas A D G, Robson P J 1982 Double-blind comparison of meptazinol and pethidine in labour. Br J Obstet Gynaecol 89: 318–322

Nimmo W S, Wilson J, Prescott L F 1975 Narcotic analgesia and delayed gastric emptying during labour. Lancet i: 890–893

Osbourne G K, Patel N B, Howat R C L 1984 A comparison of the outcome of low birth weight pregnancy in Glasgow and Dundee. Health Bull (Edin) 42: 68–77

Paterson M E L 1979 The aetiology and outcome of abruptio placentae. Acta Obstet Gynecol Scand 58: 31–35

Perriss B W, Malins A F 1981 Pain relief in labour using epidural pethidine with adrenaline. Anesthesia 36: 631–633

Philips J H, Brown W U 1976 Total spinal anesthesia late in the course of obstetric bupivacaine epidural block. Anesthesiology 44: 340–341

Philipsen T, Jensen N H 1989 Epidural block or parenteral pethidine as analgesic in labour: a randomized study concerning progress in labour and instrumental deliveries. Eur J Obstet Gynaecol Reprod Biol 30: 27–33

Phillips G 1988 Continuous infusion epidural analgesia in labor: the effect of adding sufentanil to 0·125% bupivacaine. Anesth Analg 67: 462–465

Phillips K C, Thomas T A 1983 Second stage of labour with or without extradural analgesia. Anaesthesia 38: 972–976

Podlas J, Breland B D 1987 Patient controlled analgesia with nalbuphine during labor. Obstet Gynecol 70: 202–204

Prince G, McGregor D 1986 Obstetric epidural test doses. A reappraisal. Anaesthesia 41: 1240–1250

Rayburn W, Leuschen M P, Earl R et al 1989 Intravenous meperidine during labor: a randomized comparison between nursing- and patient-controlled administration. Obstet Gynecol 74: 702–706

Reed P N, Colquhoun A D, Hanning C D 1989 Maternal oxygenation during normal labour. Br J Anaesth 62: 316–318

Refstad S D, Lindbaek E 1980 Ventilatory depression of the newborn of women receiving pethidine or pentazocine. A double-blind comparative trial. Br J Anaesth 52: 265–271

Reports on Confidential Enquiries into Maternal Deaths in England and Wales. London, Her Majesty's Stationery Office 1970–1972, 1973–1975, 1976–1978, 1979–1981, 1982–1984

Reynolds F 1984 Pain and the analgesic drugs: spinal opiates. In: Churchill Davidson H C (ed) A practice of anaesthesia 5th edn, Lloyd Luke, London, pp 821–829

Reynolds F 1989 Epidural analgesia in obstetrics. Pros and cons for mother and baby. Br Med J 299 (editorial): 751–752

Reynolds F, O'Sullivan G 1989 Epidural fentanyl and perineal pain in labour. Anaesthesia 44: 341–344

Reynolds F, Speedy H 1990 The subdural space: the third place to go astray. Anaesthesia 45: 120–123

Robinson J O, Rosen M, Evans J M et al 1980a Self-administered intravenous and intramuscular pethidine. A controlled trial in labour. Anaesthesia 35: 763–770

Robinson J O, Rosen M, Evans J M et al 1980b Maternal opinion about analgesia for labour. A controlled trial between epidural block and intramuscular pethidine combined with inhalation. Anaesthesia 35: 1173–1181

Robson J E 1979 Transcutaneous nerve stimulation for pain relief in labour. Anaesthesia 34: 357–360

Saunders N J St G, Spiby H, Gilbert L et al 1989 Oxytocin infusion during second stage of labour in primiparous women using epidural analgesia: a randomised double-blind placebo controlled trial. Br Med J 299: 1423–1426

Sheikh A, Tunstall M E 1986 Comparative study of meptazinol and pethidine for the relief of pain in labour. Br J Obstet Gynaecol 93: 264–269

Skjoldebrand A, Garle M, Gustafsson L L et al 1982 Extradural pethidine with and without adrenaline during labour: wide variation in effect. Br J Anaesth 54: 415–420

Smedstad K G, Morison D H 1988 A comparative study of continuous and intermittent epidural analgesia for labour and delivery. Can J Anaesth 35: 234–241

Stewart P 1979 Transcutaneous nerve stimulation as a method of analgesia in labour. Anaesthesia 34: 361–364

Studd J W W, Crawford J S, Duignan N M et al 1980 The effect of lumbar epidural analgesia on the rate of cervical dilatation and the outcome of labour of spontaneous onset. Br J Obstet Gynaecol 87: 1015–1021

Thomas I L, Tyle V, Webster J, Neilson A 1988 An evaluation of transcutaneous electrical nerve stimulation for pain relief in labour. Aust NZ J Obstet Gynaecol 28: 182–189

Thorburn J, Moir D D 1981 Extradural analgesia: the influence of volume and concentration of bupivacaine on the mode of delivery, analgesic efficacy and motor block. Br J Anaesth 53: 933–939

Tunstall M E 1961 Obstetric analgesia. The use of a fixed nitrous oxide and oxygen mixture from one cylinder, Lancet ii: 964

Umeh B U O 1986 Sacral acupuncture for pain relief in labour: initial clinical experience in Nigerian women. Acupuncture and electro-therapeutics. Res Int J 11: 147–151

Uppington J 1983 Epidural analgesia and previous caesarean section. Anaesthesia 38: 336–341

Van Steenberge A, Debroux H C, Noorduin H 1987 Extradural bupivacaine with sufentanil for vaginal delivery. A double-blind trial. Br J Anaesth 59: 1518–1522

Vella L, Francis D, Houlton P, Reynolds F 1985 Comparison of the antiemetics metoclopramide and promethazine in labour. Br Med J 290: 1173–1175

Waldenström U 1988 Midwives' attitudes to pain relief during labour and delivery. Midwifery 4: 48–57

Wiener P C, Hogg M I J, Rosen M 1977 Effects of naloxone on pethidine-induced neonatal depression. Br Med J 2: 228–231

Wilson C M, McClean E, Moore J, Dundee J W 1986 A double-blind comparison of intramuscular pethidine and nalbuphine in labour. Anaesthesia 41: 1207–1213

9. Symphyseotomy—a re-appraisal for the developing world

J. van Roosmalen

The need to have an alternative to caesarean section for delivering the dead fetus was one of the subjects in *Progress in Obstetrics and Gynaecology*, volume 6 (Giwa-Osagie & Azzan 1987).

Arguments in favour of destructive operations were:

1. The great dangers of caesarean section after prolonged and neglected labour in women who invariably already have genital infection;
2. The socio-cultural needs of women to have a vaginal delivery (often making the woman or her relatives refuse consent for caesarean delivery);
3. The risks of scar rupture in an unattended subsequent pregnancy at home.

These arguments can also be brought up when there is mechanical difficulty during labour and the fetus is still alive. Maternal mortality after caesarean section in developing countries, especially in rural hospitals where most caesareans are performed by generalist doctors or even by medical auxiliaries, is high, with a range from 0.6 to 5.0% in a recent review (Van Roosmalen 1988). The same holds true for the incidence of uterine scar rupture in subsequent pregnancies: 0.3–6.8% (Van Roosmalen 1988).

In this chapter, the value of symphyseotomy for the management of cephalopelvic disproportion (CPD) is examined as compared with use of caesarean section. It is based on a search of the literature and on personal experience of the author with symphyseotomy in two rural hospitals in the south-western highlands of Tanzania.

Symphyseotomy is the artifical separation of the symphysis pubis with a scalpel in order to enlarge the pelvic diameters to facilitate the process of birth. This relatively simple procedure has been very popular in predominantly Roman Catholic countries, where sterilization after repeated caesarean birth—a practice which limits the number of offspring—was condemned. Thirty years ago, E. Zarate (1955), the most ardent enthusiast of symphyseotomy in Latin America, even thought that use of the procedure would result in the abolition of caesarean section.

In most western countries, however, symphyseotomy never became popular. Shorter (1982), for example, in his extensive history of western childbirth, devotes only one sentence to the subject, as do many contemporary textbooks of obstetrics, Munro Kerr's *Operative Obstetrics* (1982) being the only exception.

HISTORY OF SYMPHYSEOTOMY

Ever since Hippocrates, childbirth was thought to be accompanied by spontaneous pelvic enlargement by separation of the symphysis pubis (Eastham 1948). This view was held by Ambroise Pare in the sixteenth century and by William Harvey in the seventeenth century (Gebbie 1982, Thiery 1985).

Andreas Vesalius was the first to question the notion of spontaneous pelvic enlargement in his *De Humani Corporis Fabrica* in 1543 (Fasbender 1906). It is logical that, only after Vesalius' correct view was accepted that the symphysis pubis is an unseparable unit during the process of birth, could the idea of artificial separation of the symphysis take shape.

In 1655, the first symphyseotomy was performed as an alternative to post-mortem caesarean section. At that time Percival Willughby reported: 'The wild Irish women do break the pubic bones of the female infant, so soon as it is born. And I have heard some wandering Irish women affirm the same to be true, and that they have ways to keep these bones from uniting. It is for certain, that they be easily, and soon, delivered. And I have observed that many wanderers of that nation have had a waddling and lamish gesture in their going' (Shorter 1982). From this statement, one may guess that the general public in Ireland was aware of the existence of symphyseotomy in a negative connotation long before the first symphyseotomy on a living woman was reported in the literature.

In 1777, Jean Rene Sigault, in Paris, performed the first symphyseotomy on a living woman, who was very stunted in growth and had a history of four stillborn babies after difficult labours. The woman survived and had her first liveborn baby. She suffered, however, from a vesicovaginal fistula for the rest of her life (de Feyfer 1934, Gebbie 1982).

Though welcomed as a great innovation, the early results were not very promising. Fourteen mothers and 18 newborns of the first 36 symphyseotomies died (Wright 1963). These bad results may be partly explained by the extremely prolonged labour, for which symphyseotomy was performed, but this was still preferable to caesarean section which, at that time, had an almost 100% maternal mortality rate.

The first symphyseotomy in the Netherlands was performed by Groshans (1934) in 1778, and between 1778 and 1831 at least 20 symphyseotomies were reported with three maternal deaths (de Feyfer 1934).

After initial enthusiasm the operation fell into discredit. In the late nineteenth century a revival took place in Italy. Morisani, among others, reported many cases with a maternal mortality under 5% and a perinatal mortality just under 12% (Gebbie 1982).

Van der Linden (1961) reviewed 2801 symphyseotomies, performed between 1900 and 1960. Maternal mortality in his series was as low as 14 per 1000; maternal morbidity (such as vesicovaginal fistulae, vaginal lacerations and orthopaedic complications), occurred in 7%. The perinatal mortality rate was 86 per 1000 births. Van der Linden concluded in 1961 that he felt 'justified in stating that, although symphyseotomy is not an ideal operation it certainly does not deserve the unfavourable reputation which it has in the Netherlands. In some areas it even constitutes an indispensable intervention which affords good possibilities'.

These symphyseotomies were almost exclusively performed in the predominantly Roman Catholic countries of Italy, Spain, France, Ireland and in some Latin American countries. An explanation of this may lie in the condemnation of sterilization by the Roman Catholic church. This religion also put the interest of the newborn above that of the mother (Young 1944). Caesarean section prevented the potential for large families, where tubal ligation was performed after repeated caesarean deliveries.

Even in non-Catholic countries like Great Britain, symphyseotomy was performed in the first half of the twentieth century (Munro Kerr 1948).

Bowesman (Gebbie 1982) and Pereira (1964) mentioned that symphyseotomy was practised by traditional healers in several parts of Africa. Approximately 10% of the symphyseotomies reported by Van der Linden (1961) were performed in Africa.

REVIEW OF THE RECENT LITERATURE

Since 1960, most communications on symphyseotomy (Seedat & Crichton 1962, Lasbrey 1963, Gebbie 1966, Bird & Bal 1967, Gordon 1969, Mottiar & Saria 1970, Hartfield 1973a, Kairuki 1975, Onsrud 1976, Armon & Philip 1978, Norman 1978, Van Roosmalen 1987) have stemmed from Africa, although one has recently been published from Papua New Guinea (Mola et al 1981).

MATERNAL MORTALITY

Maternal mortality after symphyseotomy has decreased dramatically since 1960 and is almost negligible (Table 9.1). In the different series of symphyseotomies mentioned in Table 9.1, there were three maternal deaths from a total of 1752 symphyseotomies: a rate of 1.7 per 1000 births. None of these was related to the procedure of symphyseotomy: two were caused by eclampsia and one occurred after caesarean section in a woman with a failed symphyseotomy.

Table 9.1   Maternal and perinatal mortality in symphyseotomy in different communities

Country/year	Author	Symphyseotomies (no.)	Maternal mortality	Perinatal mortality	
				No.	Rate
South Africa (1962)	Seedat & Crichton	505	0	42/505	83
South Africa (1963)	Lasbrey	151	0	3/151	19
Uganda (1963)	Gebbie	108	0	16/108	148
Kenya (1967)	Bird & Bal	104	0	22/104	212
South Africa (1969)	Gordon	201	0	20/201	100
Zambia (1970)	Mottiar & Saria	75	1	18/75	240
Nigeria (1973a)	Hartfield	138	1	23/138	167
Uganda (1975)	Kairuki	30	0	3/30	100
Zaïre (1976)	Onsrud	34	0	7/34	296
Tanzania (1978)	Armon & Philip	105	1	9/105	86
Zimbabwe (1978)	Norman	161	0	16/161	99
Papua New Guinea (1981)	Mola et al	86	0	7/86	81
Tanzania (1987)	Van Roosmalen	54	0	11/54	204
All studies (1962–1987)		1752	3	197/1752	112

MATERNAL MORBIDITY

Serious maternal morbidity after symphyseotomy, described in Table 9.2, did not differ much from the rate reported between 1900 and 1960: 7% in 1900–1960 and 8% from 1960 onwards (Van der Linden 1961).

Fifteen of the 30 vesico-vaginal fistulae appeared to be the result of pressure-necrosis of the bladder neck due to obstructed labour rather than to symphyseotomy. The latter present immediately after birth, while those due to obstructed labour develop only some days after delivery when necrotic tissue is shed. Some of the immediate fistulae were the result of the application of forceps after symphyseotomy in order to assist birth. After the introduction of vacuum extraction, this practice was abandoned and the

Table 9.2 Serious maternal morbidity following symphyseotomy in different communities (total no. of symphyseotomies = 1752)

Vesico-vaginal fistula	30 (1.7%)
Vestibular and/or urethral lesions	33 (1.9%)
Osteitis pubis/retropubic abscess	10 (0.6%)
Long-term walking disability and/or pain	32 (1.8%)
Stress incontinence	36 (2.1%)
All complications*	141 (8.1%)

* Note that more than one complication often occurred in one
woman. Therefore the number of women affected is less than the
number of complications.

use of forceps contraindicated (Seedat & Crichton 1962, Crichton & Seedat
1963, Gebbie 1966, Bird & Bal 1967).

Other fistulae and lacerations resulted, because the procedure had been
performed without inserting a urinary catheter.

PERINATAL MORTALITY

Perinatal mortality differed greatly in the different series (range 19–296 per
1000) with an overall rate of 112 (Table 9.1). Different levels of obstetrical
skills and technical support may explain this. Although comparison is
therefore difficult, fetal prognosis does not appear to have greatly improved
since the period between 1900 and 1960.

In some cases the fetus had already died before symphyseotomy was
undertaken. This should be a contraindication for the procedure and in
such cases destructive operation is an alternative.

OVERALL IMPRESSION—EXPERIMENTAL CONTROLS

All authors regarded symphyseotomy as a procedure with a definite place in
obstetric practice, at least in the circumstances they describe. Editorials in
the Lancet (1962, 1974) concluded that its urinary and orthopaedic complications have been exaggerated. Moreover, reports in the literature on the
ill-effects of symphyseotomy often lacked controls, and only three
controlled studies have been published (Lasbrey 1963, Hartfield 1973b,
Mola et al 1981). These studies, however, were not randomized, which
makes comparison with the control group difficult.

Lasbrey (1963) found minor symptoms at some time in the follow-up
period or in a subsequent pregnancy in 58% of 87 women who underwent
symphyseotomy, as compared with 60% of the 87 parous women in his
control group who had spontaneous deliveries.

The minor symptoms were:

— Pain in the symphysis.pubis;
— Groin, hip or thigh pain;

— Backache (including sacro-iliac pain); and
— Stress incontinence.

These symptoms did not interfere with day-to-day activity, except in one woman in the symphyseotomy group, who had severe sacro-iliac pain for 3 years. Generally the symptoms became less severe and resolved completely with the passage of time. A subsequent pregnancy tended to aggravate the symptoms.

SYMPHYSEOTOMY AS COMPARED WITH CAESAREAN SECTION

Denying symphyseotomy to the woman in need of it results in obstructed labour or makes caesarean section necessary as an emergency procedure in advanced labour. Therefore, a group of women who had caesarean section instead of symphyseotomy in order to relieve the obstruction could provide the best possible control group where randomization proved difficult.

Retrospective comparison of the results of symphyseotomy with those of caesarean section performed in advanced labour has been the subject of the other two controlled studies (Hartfield 1973b, Mola et al 1981). These studies confirmed that the long-term disabling sequelae of symphyseotomy have been overemphasized. There is also less mortality risk after symphyseotomy than after caesarean section, while maternal morbidity, although different in nature, did not differ much in frequency (Table 9.3).

PREGNANCY AFTER A PREVIOUS SYMPHYSEOTOMY

The pelvis often remains permanently enlarged after a symphyseotomy is performed. The procedure could therefore provide a cure for some cases of cephalopelvic disproportion. This is especially important when one is not sure that the woman will return to hospital in a subsequent pregnancy. Obviously caesarean section will not affect the pelvis and leaves the origin of disproportion untouched, thereby sending the woman home with a scarred uterus, which may then rupture in a subsequent unattended delivery at home.

Table 9.3 Comparison of outcome of symphyseotomy and Caesarean section for CPD in rural Tanzania (van Roosmalen 1987)

	Symphyseotomy ($n = 54$)	Caesarean section ($n = 100$)
Maternal mortality	0 (0%)	5 (5%)
Serious maternal morbidity*	4 (7%)	6 (6%)
Perinatal mortality**	11 (20%)***	13 (13%)

* Chi-square: 0.11 (NS).
** Chi-square: 1.45 (NS).
*** Included two deaths before symphyseotomy was started.

Table 9.4 Outcome of subsequent labour in women with a history of previous symphyseotomy in different communities

Author	SVD*	Oper. VD**	Caesarean section	Repeat symphys.
Gordon (1969) (n = 36)	29	3	4 (11%)	0
Hartfield (1973b) (n = 76)	58	8	5 (7%)	5
Norman (1978) (n = 28)	26	1	1 (4%)	0
Armon (1978) (n = 45)	32	7	6 (13%)	0
Mola et al (1981) (n = 19)	11	5	3 (16%)	0
Van Roosmalen (1987) (n = 25)	11	8	6 (24%)***	0
All cases (n = 229)	167 (73%)	32 (14%)	25 (11%)	5 (2%)

* SVD = spontaneous vertex delivery.
** Oper. VD = Vacuum extraction, forceps delivery.
*** Two cases of uterine rupture included.

The outcome of labour in women with a history of previous symphyseotomy is mentioned in Table 9.4.

Uncomplicated vaginal delivery occurred in 73%, while operative vaginal delivery took place in 14%. Caesarean birth occurred in 11%. Repeat symphyseotomy was performed in 2% of the cases: most authors consider this as contraindicated because of the fibrotic scarring in the symphysis pubis following the first operation.

The vaginal delivery rate after previous symphyseotomy is higher than after previous caesarean section for disproportion: 87% versus 44% (Van Roosmalen 1988). Nevertheless, a considerable percentage of women with previous symphyseotomy need an operative vaginal or abdominal delivery for subsequent births.

INDICATIONS AND TECHNIQUE

At present symphyseotomy is practised using Seedat & Crichton's method (1962, 1963), which is based upon Zarate's work (1955). The method differs from that of Zarate in that it advises against partial division of the symphysis, which is then completed by forceful abduction of the thighs. Seedat & Crichton fear that forceful abduction damages the sacro-iliac joints, possibly resulting in permanent pelvic instability and pain. They also stress the importance of avoiding the hyaline cartilage by strict adherence to the midline when dividing the symphysis pubis. Deviating from the midline may lead to osteitis pubis and subsequent difficulty in walking.

Symphyseotomy increases the pelvic diameters at all levels, although not

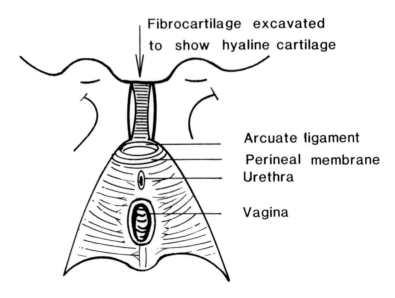

Fig. 9.1   Diagram of symphysis pubis.

to the same degree (Crichton & Clarke 1966). The transverse diameters particularly will be increased by the procedure. The bottom ends of the symphyseal joint separate more than the upper ends, which implicates that the outlet diameters increase more than the inlet ones. Because of this, some authors concluded falsely that symphyseotomy is only indicated in cases of outlet disproportion (Munro Kerr 1948).

Contrary to what has been taught in the past (Zarate 1955, Van der Linden 1961), the arcuate ligament beneath the symphysis is directly cut (Fig. 9.1). In order to avoid undue strain to the sacro-iliac joints, forceful abduction of the thighs should never be undertaken, and complete separation should be brought about by use of the scalpel only.

Indications

Symphyseotomy is mainly performed in cases of cephalopelvic disproportion with a vertex presentation and a living fetus. Whether symphyseotomy is indicated in such cases is mainly dependent on three interrelated factors:

— Descent of the fetal head;
— Degree of overlap as a result of fetal head moulding; and
— Dilatation of the cervix (Gebbie 1974).

One third or more of the fetal head should have entered the pelvic brim. The fetal head should not be felt prominent in front of the symphysis pubis, and cervical dilatation should be more than 7 cm in a primigravida, according to Gebbie's rules (1974). When symphyseotomy is performed in the second stage of labour, it often follows a failed trial of vacuum extraction. Another indication can be the pelvic entrapment of the after-coming head of a breech (Spencer 1987).

A SYMPHYSEOTOMY PROTOCOL

This protocol is adapted from Seedat & Crichton 1962, Crichton & Seedat 1963, Gebbie 1982.
   When the decision to perform a symphyseotomy has been made:

1.   Be sure that the bladder is empty at the start of the procedure.
2.   When a trial of vacuum extraction is indicated before proceeding to symphyseotomy, adhere to the rule of three pulls (dislodge–descent–delivery); when the head has not been born after the third pull, proceed to symphyseotomy.
3.   Inject 3–5 cm³ of lignocain at the site of the symphysis pubis and anaesthetize the perineum at the site of the intended episiotomy.
4.   Insert a conventional urinary catheter (sometimes the head has to be pushed up in order to achieve this).
5.   Place the woman in the lithotomy position not with the legs in stirrups, but instead supported on both sides by an assistant, the angle between the legs never being more than 80°; refrain from abduction of the legs during any stage of and after symphyseotomy in order to prevent straining of the sacro-iliac joints.

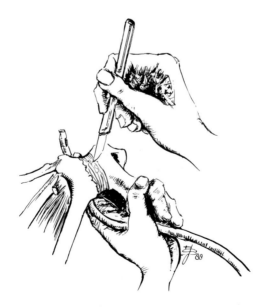

Fig. 9.2   Protection of uretha by left hand during the procedure of symphyseotomy.

6. Place your index and middle fingers of the left hand in the vagina and push the catheter (and thereby the urethra) aside (instead of the urethra your fingers now lie in the midline under the symphysis pubis) (Fig. 9.2)

7. Perform symphyseotomy preferably by the closed method, by which only a stab incision is made and the risk of infection reduced.

8. Incise in the midline in order to cut through the fibrocartilage of the joint (needling the joint and leaving the needle in situ can be an aid to finding the midline).

9. Enter the joint by a stab-incision with a solid-bladed scalpel in the midline at the junction of the upper and middle thirds; traverse the joint with the blade until the point is felt impinging on the vagina by the underlying finger of the left hand (Fig. 9.3). Use the upper third of the uncut symphysis as a fulcrum against which the scalpel is levered to incise the lower two-thirds of the symphysis. Take back and rotate the scalpel 180°. Cut the remaining upper third of the symphysis.

10. When the procedure is completed, it will be possible to insert a thumb into the divided joint. At this stage further descent of the head often occurs. This promotes further dilatation of the cervix, whereafter expulsion of the fetus can start.

11. As a result of symphyseotomy, the anterior vaginal wall with the urethra is now unsupported and any tension may produce extensive tearing which can include damage to the urethra. Never abduct the legs. Make a large episiotomy in order to relieve tension of the anterior vaginal wall. Adduct the legs at the crowning of the head and

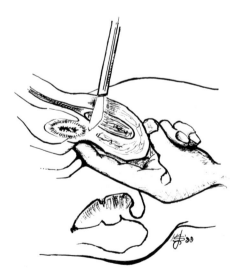

Fig. 9.3   Cutting through the fibrocartilage of the symphyseal joint.

if need be apply the vacuum extractor in order to pull the fetus downwards thereby relieving the anterior vaginal wall. Do not use the anterior wall as a fulcrum to deliver the head and the posterior shoulder as in normal delivery (forceps, manual rotation and Ritgen's manoeuvre all are contraindicated).

12.   After delivery of the newborn and the placenta, compress the symphysis by the thumb above and the index and middle fingers beneath for some minutes to express blood clots and promote haemostasis.

13.   Explore the uterus gently with the index and middle fingers to rule out uterine rupture. Exclude lacerations of the cervix and vagina by inspection. Close the skin incision at the symphyseal site before repair of the episiotomy.

14.   Postoperatively nurse the patient on her side as much as possible and strap the knees together. Insert a urinary catheter for three days. When there is frank haematuria or suspicion of fistula formation keep the catheter in place for at least ten days; a fistula needs continuous bladder drainage for six weeks.

15.   Administer a course of antibiotics, if possible to be started before the procedure. Usually penicillin/streptomycin or ampicillin/ metronidazol is given.

16.   Start mobilization when the catheter is removed, depending mainly on the ability of the woman herself; crutches or a stick can provide a sense of safety initially.

17.   On discharge, advise the woman to refrain from lifting heavy weights and from hard physical work during three months; hospital delivery is indicated in subsequent pregnancies.

CONCLUSIONS

The risk of maternal mortality after symphyseotomy nowadays has become negligible and is much lower than after caesarean section performed in advanced labour for the same indications.

Maternal morbidity can be effectively lowered by strict adherence to a protocol: the insertion of a urinary catheter, for instance, being mandatory when urological complications are to be avoided. Perinatal wastage is high, but often the fetus is already compromised on admission following a prolonged labour at home. Sepsis is another contributing factor. Strict adherence to the indications will lower perinatal mortality. Fetal death is a contraindication for the procedure.

One of the indications for symphyseotomy is a failed trial of vacuum extraction or forceps (Cox 1966, Gebbie 1966, Lammes 1969). This policy of trial first, however, may add to perinatal mortality, especially if one continues to pull too long. Some authors therefore advise against this policy (Gebbie 1974, Mola et al 1981). On the other hand, abandoning this trial will definitely lead to more symphyseotomies, which in some cases could have been easily prevented by a trial of vacuum extraction first (Armon & Philip 1978).

Previous symphyseotomy is said to cure cephalopelvic disproportion (Crichton & Clarke 1966). The outcome of subsequent pregnancy in our review supports this only to some extent, indicating the high risk of these women even after symphyseotomy. Symphyseotomy leaves the uterus unscarred. Yet, rupture of an unscarred uterus in a subsequent labour after symphyseotomy has been reported in the literature (Van Roosmalen 1987). The risk of caesarean birth after previous symphyseotomy (11%) is certainly higher than in the total obstetric population in developing countries.

The fact that in western countries at present symphyseotomy is not practised anymore does not make this operation second class or outdated in the greatly differing circumstances of developing countries, where caesarean birth is generally disliked and carries great maternal risks of mortality and serious morbidity, especially when performed in advanced labour.

Symphyseotomy, therefore, deserves a place in the management of cephalopelvic disproportion. It is an example of appropriate technology (Belsey 1985, Everett 1985). It is a relatively simple and rapid procedure to facilitate delivery in selected cases of obstructed labour. It diminishes the need for blood transfusion with its AIDS risk (Hermann et al 1988). It fulfils a cultural need to achieve vaginal delivery in difficult circumstances.

More research into the late sequelae of symphyseotomy should be undertaken in rural areas of developing countries, where the need for symphyseotomy still exists (Hartfield 1975). One such study is at present in progress in Zaïre (Hermann et al 1988).

Follow-up studies of those women living far from hospital often present great difficulty. It has been shown, however, that effective follow-up for other reasons can be feasible up to 100 km from a rural district hospital (Van Roosmalen-Wiebenga et al 1987).

ACKNOWLEDGEMENT

Figures 9.1, 9.2 and 9.3 were drawn by Mr J Stouten, 'Leerhuis', Department of Obstetrics and Gynaecology, Leiden State University, The Netherlands.

REFERENCES

Armon P J, Philip M 1978 Symphysiotomy and subsequent pregnancy in the Kilimanjaro Region of Tanzania, East Afr Med J 55: 306–313
Belsey M A 1985 Traditional birth attendants: a resource for the health of women. Int J Gynaecol Obstet 23: 247–248
Bird G C, Bal J S 1967 Subcutaneous symphysiotomy in association with the vacuum extractor. J Obstet Gynaecol Br Emp 74: 266–269

Cox M L 1966 Symphysiotomy in Nigeria. J Obstet Gynaecol Br Commwlth 73: 237–243
Crichton D, Clarke G C M 1966 Symphysiotomy—indications and contra-indications. S Afr
    J Obstet Gynaecol 4: 76–79
Crichton D, Seedat E K 1963 The technique of symphysiotomy. S Afr Med J 37: 227–231
Eastham N J 1948 Pelvic mensuration: a study in the perpetuation of error. Obstet Gynecol
    Surv 3: 301–329
Everett J 1985 Obstetric care. In: Appropriate technology, articles published in Br Med J
    London: Tavistock Square, pp 15–17
Fasbender H 1906 Geschichte der Geburtshulfe, Jena, p. 109, Varii Auctores de
    Symphysiotomia
Feyfer F M G de 1934 Ter inleiding. Opuscula Selecta Neerlandicorum de Arte Medica.
    Amsterdam, vol XII: XI–XII
Gebbie D A M 1966 Vacuum extraction and symphysiotomy in difficult vaginal delivery in a
    developing community. Br Med J 2: 1490–1493
Gebbie D A M 1974 Symphysiotomy. Trop Doct 4: 69–75
Gebbie D A M 1982 Symphysiotomy. Clin Obstet Gynaecol 9: 663–683
Giwa-Osagie O F, Azzan B B 1987 Destructive operations. In: Studd J (ed) Progress in
    Obstetrics & Gynaecology. Churchill Livingstone, Edinburgh, vol 6, pp 211–221
Gordon Y B 1969 An analysis of symphyseotomy at Baragwanath Hospital, 1964–1967. S Afr
    Med J 43: 659–662
Groshans G R F 1934 Waarneming eener operatie der doorsnede van de schaambeenderen.
    In: Varii Auctores de Symphysiotomia. Opuscula Selecta Neerlandicorum de Arte Medica.
    Amsterdam, vol XII, pp 65–69
Hartfield V J 1973a Subcutaneous symphysiotomy—time for a reappraisal? Aust N Z J
    Obstet Gynaecol 13: 147–152
Hartfield V J 1973b A comparison of the early and late effects of subcutaneous
    symphysiotomy and of lower segment caesarean section. J Obstet Gynaecol Br Commwlth
    80: 508–514
Hartfield V J 1975 Late effects of symphysiotomy. Trop Doct 5: 76–78
Hermann C B, Duale S, Petrick T, Stanback J, Nelson G, Potts M 1988 Comparative
    analysis of symphysiotomy, caesarean section and vacuum extraction for obstructed labor
    in a rural Zaïre referral hospital. Unpublished poster presentation, World Congress of
    Obstetrics and Gynaecology, Rio de Janeiro, Brazil
Kairuki H C M 1975 The place of symphysiotomy in the treatment of disproportion in
    Uganda. East Afr Med J 52: 686–693
Lammes F B 1969 Symphysiotomie in ontwikkelingslanden. Neth J Med 113: 1017–1020
Lancet Editorial 1962 Obstetrics in developing countries. Lancet i: 575
Lancet Editorial 1974 Symphysiotomy and vacuum extraction. Lancet i: 396–397
Lasbrey A H 1963 The symptomatic sequelae of symphysiotomy. S Afr Med J 37: 231–234
Linden A J van der 1961 Symphysiotomy and pubiotomy. Thesis, Utrecht
Mola G, Lamang M, McGoldrick I A 1981 A retrospective study of matched
    symphysiotomies and caesarean sections at Port Moresby General Hospital. Papua New
    Guinea Med J 24: 103–112
Mottiar Y, Saria G 1970 Symphysiotomy for mild cephalopelvic disproportion. Med J
    Zambia 4: 15–23
Munro Kerr J M 1948 The investigation and treatment of borderline cases of contracted
    pelvis. J Obstet Gynaecol Br Emp 55: 401–417
Munro Kerr 1982 Munro Kerr's Operative Obstetrics, 10th edn, Myerscough P R (ed).
    London, Baillière Tindall, pp 320–325
Norman R J 1978 Six years' experience of symphysiotomy in a teaching hospital. S Afr Med J
    54: 1121–1125
Onsrud M 1976 Symphysiotomy—an out of date obstetric operation? Nord Med 91: 227–228
Pereira J S 1964 A sinfisiotomia na obstetrica moderna. Anais Inst Med Tropical 21: 153–159
Roosmalen J van 1987 Symphysiotomy as an alternative to caesarean section. Int J Gynaecol
    Obstet 25: 451–458
Roosmalen J van 1988 Maternal health care in the South Western Highlands of Tanzania.
    PhD thesis, Leiden
Roosmalen-Wiebenga M W van, Kusin J A, With C de 1987 Nutrition rehabilitation in
    hospital—a waste of time and money? Evaluation of nutrition rehabilitation in a rural
    district hospital in SW Tanzania. J Trop Pediatr 33: 24–28

Seedat E K, Crichton D 1962 Symphysiotomy: technique, indications, and limitations. Lancet i: 554–559

Shorter E 1982 A history of women's bodies. Penguin Books, Middlesex, p 163

Spencer J O A 1987 Symphysiotomy for vaginal breech delivery. Br J Obstet Gynaecol 94: 716–718

Thiery M 1985 Operative verwijding van het bekken: een historisch overzicht. Tijdsch Geneeskunde 41: 293–306

Wright St Clair R E 1963 The history of mutilation operations. N Z Med J 62: 468–470

Young J H 1944 Caesarean section. The history and development of the operation from earliest times. Lewis, London, pp 83, 242

Zarate E 1955 Subcutaneous partial symphysiotomy. TICA, Buenos Aires

10. Complications of Caesarean section

S. M. Creighton   J. M. Pearce   S. L. Stanton

The Caesarean section rate continues to rise and has almost doubled from 5·2% in 1970–72 to 10·1% in 1982–84 (Confidential Enquiry 1970–72, 1982–84). Logically there should also be an associated rise in the complications occurring as a result of the operation. The rising rate also means an increasing number of pregnancies following previous Caesarean section, thereby increasing the number of pregnancies at risk of scar rupture.

This chapter will review the current management of common complications associated with Caesarean section with particular reference to pregnancy following a previous Caesarean section.

SURGICAL TECHNIQUE

Uterine incisions

A lower segment uterine incision is widely used as it has a much lower risk of scar rupture than a classical incision (0·5% compared with 2·2%). Care must be taken to reflect the bladder downwards before incising the uterus and it is at this time that most bladder injuries occur. The lower uterine segment starts to expand at 28 weeks gestation and a lower segment incision may not be indicated for fetuses below that age.

The classical incision which employs a midline uterine incision is rarely used today. It may be indicated in a few situations such as in the presence of cervical carcinoma, and with a transverse lie with a prolapsed arm (Lees & Singer 1982). It has also been used in the delivery of preterm infants at less than 28 weeks gestation when the lower segment is not sufficiently formed to allow passage of the fetal head although a De Lee uterine incision may be preferable in this situation.

A modified classical (or De Lee) incision is also vertical but the incision is not taken up onto the fundus of the uterus thus decreasing the risk of subsequent rupture. The incision is made as long as necessary and usually finishes level with the insertion of the round ligaments. It has the advantages of allowing easier access than the lower segment incision and causes less bleeding than a classical incision. Most studies of scar rupture do not differentiate between a classical and a De Lee incision but the risk of

163

rupture of the latter incision is usually quoted as lying between that of the classical and lower segment incisions.

Peritoneal closure

At present it is usual to close the peritoneum at Caesarean section. It has been shown that for gynaecological procedures, omitting peritoneal closure does not increase the length of hospital stay or the subsequent development of adhesions (Tulandi et al 1988). The sutures used to close the peritoneum may cause more adhesions than leaving raw edges. It would therefore seem logical to apply this to Caesarean section as it would have the advantage of shortening the operating time.

HAEMORRHAGE

Haemorrhage accounts for 6% of deaths associated with Caesarean section (Confidential Enquiry 1982–84) and an unknown proportion of post-operative morbidity. Risk factors include placenta praevia, placental abruption and uterine atony in multiple pregnancy or multiparous patients. Prolonged labour with Syntocinon stimulation is also usually regarded as a risk factor for haemorrhage although there have been no recent studies to confirm this. Disseminated intravascular coagulation is a rare cause but must be considered in cases of continuing haemorrhage.

Haemorrhage may be primary, delayed primary or secondary. Bleeding may come from the placental bed or may be due to a tear or extended uterine incision into major vessels. A rapid first line of uterine sutures must be placed to close the uterine incision taking care to include the angles in the suture. This may be facilitated by delivering the uterus onto the abdomen. Bleeding tears should be repaired in two layers.

Uterine atony may be corrected by a bolus dose of 10 units of Syntocinon given intravenously followed by a continuous infusion of 40 units of Syntocinon in 500 ml of normal saline over 2 hours. If the uterus fails to contract, 0·5 micrograms of prostaglandin E2 may be injected directly into the uterine muscle.

If the patient is collapsed, resuscitation must be instigated swiftly. Initial management is usually with simple crystalloid such as Hartmans solution followed by artificial colloid such as hydroxyethyl starch (Hetastarch) or gelatin solutions such as Gelofusine or Haemaccel. Artificial colloid lasts from 1 to 3 hours in the circulation and has no effect on coagulation. There is a small risk of anaphylactic-type responses which may be severe. Albuminoids are less commonly associated with anaphylactic responses but are more expensive and often not available. All of these measures are temporary until blood is available. In Caesarean sections with a high risk of haemorrhage, e.g. elective surgery for placenta praevia, blood should be routinely cross matched. Whole fresh blood is no longer available because of the need to screen for transmissible diseases and so stored blood is usually used. Stored blood loses its labile coagulation factors and platelets become denatured and so it is usual to give 2 units of fresh frozen plasma with each 6 units of stored blood. Platelets are not usually necessary and may be best avoided as denatured platelets may themselves trigger an intravascular coagulation.

More recently the cell saver has been used to prepare spilt red cells for autotransfusion. With the cell saver system it is possible to remove the plasma and recover 70–80% of intact red cells (Von Finck et al 1986). The disadvantage of this system is that as it returns washed red cells to the circulation; prolonged use therefore results in a loss of clotting factors and these need to be replaced with, for example, fresh frozen plasma.

If haemorrhage continues, more radical surgical intervention is required. Initially tying off the uterine arteries is performed and if this does not achieve haemostasis, the internal iliac arteries should also be ligated. The long term blood supply to the uterus is not compromised as an adequate collateral circulation is already present and takes effect immediately (Burchell & Olson 1966). It has been demonstrated that radio-opaque dye reaches all arteries of the pelvis immediately even after ligation of the internal iliac artery (Burchell 1968). These collateral vessels consist of three pairs of vessels; the lumbar-iliolumbar, the middle sacral-lateral sacral and the superior haemorrhoidal-middle haemorrhoidal vessels and reverse flow occurs in each of these to maintain pelvic blood supply. The pelvic blood supply is therefore so large that there is no compromise of the pelvic tissues following internal artery ligation, and subsequent normal pregnancies have been reported.

CAESAREAN HYSTERECTOMY

The most common indication for Caesarean hysterectomy is uncontrollable maternal haemorrhage especially associated with a morbidly adherent placenta. It may also be performed for co-existing cervical or uterine carcinoma, uterine rupture or as a sterilizing procedure (Britton 1980). The incidence of this procedure is lower in the United Kingdom than the United States as elective hysterectomy is usually postponed until after the puerperium when it is less hazardous. The maternal death rate associated with Caesarean hysterectomy from all causes is 0·7% (Park & Duff 1980) compared to 0·05% for all Caesarean sections (Confidential Enquiry 1982–84).

Caesarean hysterectomy should not be left too late as the risk of uncontrollable haemorrhage is increased. Pelvic tissue in pregnancy is lax with increased oedema and vascularity therefore care is needed especially in tying pedicles and the uterine side of the pedicle may also need to be ligated as back bleeding may be considerable (Sturdee & Rushton 1986). There may be difficulty in identifying the lower margin of the cervix and a subtotal hysterectomy may be performed either deliberately or in error. This can be corrected either at the time of hysterectomy or as a second procedure.

PREVENTION OF GENERAL POSTOPERATIVE PROBLEMS

Deep venous thrombosis and pulmonary thrombosis

Pulmonary embolism is the major cause of maternal mortality following Caesarean section accounting for 17% of direct deaths. It is difficult to assess the incidence of non-fatal pulmonary embolus and deep venous thrombosis occurring following Caesarean section. Only 50% of cases of pulmonary embolus are preceded by a clinically recognizable deep venous thrombosis and therefore clinical suspicion must be high. The patient may present with a pyrexia, cough, shortness of breath or acutely collapsed. Prophylaxis for all patients comprises care when positioning the patient's legs in theatre and early postoperative mobilization. Subcutaneous heparin (5000 units b.d.) can be used for elective procedures in patients considered to be at risk.

The risk of a thrombosis in a woman with a past history of a pulmonary embolus or deep venous thrombosis is 12% (Badaracco & Vessey 1974). It has been the practice to fully anticoagulate all women with a past history throughout pregnancy and the puerperium. This was done with the Hirsch regime of heparin in the first and third trimesters and warfarin in the second trimester, but the risks of congenital abnormality to the fetus and of uncontrollable haemorrhage should the mother bleed have suggested a revision of policy. Initially the change was made to subcutaneous heparin throughout pregnancy but as the risk of embolism is greatest in the puerperium, anticoagulation can be restricted to that time as long as the woman has close antenatal supervision to look for the signs and symptoms of thrombosis (Letsky & de Swiet 1984). Other patients at higher risk include patients who are obese and multiparae. At present epidural anaesthesia is contraindicated in women on subcutaneous heparin (Moir & Thorburn 1986) although epidural analgesia has been widely used with few problems in non-obstetric patients on anticoagulants (Odoon & Sin 1983).

Dextran administered intravenously during surgery has been advocated in women at a high risk and has the added advantage that an epidural is not contraindicated (Gruber 1980).

Urinary tract infection

Urinary tract infection is a risk of Caesarean section as most women are catheterized preoperatively and many units use an indwelling catheter. The risk of infection from a single catheterization has been quoted as less than 2% (Walter & Vejlsgaard 1978) although Cardozo et al (1989) found that in/out catheterization did not significantly increase the incidence of post-partum urinary tract infection providing care is taken with aseptic technique. In most units, all patients undergoing Caesarean section (routine or elective) are catheterized with an indwelling Foley catheter. This would seem sensible as voiding difficulties have been reported in 20% of women following Caesarean section with 11% having a significant postmicturition residual urine (Cardozo et al 1989). If a significant postmicturition residual is detected this can be managed most simply by instructing the patient to double void but if it persists clean intermittent self catheterization may be indicated.

Care must be taken in patients with epidural anaesthesia to ensure they void within 6 hours and the bladder may become overdistended for one or two days.

Chest infection

Postoperative chest infection occurs in up to 10% of patients following abdominal surgery. There are no figures for the risk of infection following Caesarean section but it is probably considerably lower than this. Predisposing factors include obesity, smoking and pre-existing upper respiratory tract infection (Marshall 1987). It is more common following general anaesthesia than epidural anaesthesia. Clinically the patient may present with a pyrexia and purulent sputum. There may be localized chest signs and it may progress to bronchopneumonia. A chest x-ray may reveal segmental atelectasis with patchy infiltration or lobar shadowing usually confined to the lower lobes. In high risk cases prophylactic physiotherapy and epidural anaesthesia are recommended. Postoperative pain may cause the patient to reduce inspiration and adequate postoperative analgesia is important to prevent this. Treatment of postoperative chest infection includes physiotherapy and antibiotics.

Endometritis

The incidence of endometritis is said to be 10 to 20 times higher for Caesarean section than vaginal delivery (Charles & Larsen 1989), with the commonest organisms being group B streptococcus, *Escherichia coli* and anaerobes. The risk of endometritis is increased with the length of labour, the number of vaginal examinations performed in labour (Apuzzio et al 1982) and the presence of chorioamnionitis (Koh et al 1979).

The diagnosis of endometritis is made on clinical history and examination. Ultrasound scan will exclude the presence of retained products and may show the presence of a phlegmon (Lavery et al 1985). A phlegmon is a firm non-fluctuant, indurated mass due to intense cellulitis usually located in the parametria. This must be distinguished from an infected haematoma or an abscess, as a phlegmon will resolve with antibiotics and conservative treatment, whereas an abscess needs surgical drainage usually by laparotomy.

Management of endometritis is conservative with antibiotic therapy. Isolation of the infecting organism is usually not possible as endometrial aspirates usually contain bacteria not relevant to the infection. Combination treatment is best with a broad spectrum antibiotic such as a cephalosporin and metronidazole.

Wound infection

The incidence of wound infection after Caesarean section has been quoted from 1 to 9%. The risk is higher with prolonged rupture of membranes, prolonged labour and with an inexperienced surgeon (Rehu & Nielsson 1980). The risk is also directly proportional to the number of vaginal examinations performed (Hawrylyshyn et al 1981) and is also more common in obese women probably as a result of an increase in wound haematoma.

The use of prophylactic antibiotics is controversial but probably cost effective (Mugford et al 1989). They have been shown to reduce conclusively the incidence of serious postoperative infection (Stiver et al 1984), endometritis (Gall 1979) and wound infection (Saltzman et al 1985). The best antibiotics to use are broad spectrum penicillins or cephalosporins. The lowest infection rate is with a combination of a broad spectrum penicillin with an aminoglycoside but this is outweighed by the risk of serious adverse side effects such as neprho- and oto-toxicity (Goodman et al 1980). There is no evidence of a reduced infection rate with metronidazole. It has also been shown that although there is no evidence of any advantage of high dose treatment over low does treatment, short courses are less effective than long courses of antibiotics (Scarpignato et al 1982). Prophylactic antibiotics are often not used because of the potential disadvantages. These include the theoretical risk of adverse drug reactions (Duff et al 1987) and the masking of neonatal sepsis (Cunningham et al 1983). This can be minimized by delaying first administration until after clamping the cord but this does reduce the effectiveness of the prophylaxis. The production of resistant strains of organisms is not a problem with single dose antibiotics but can be a problem with relatively few doses of some antibiotics particularly the cephalosporins. This may therefore be a problem with the longer (more than 72 hours) but more effective administration regimes. The extra cost of prophylaxis has also been quoted as a disadvantage but a recent study showed the cost was balanced by a reduction of length of admission with wound infections (Mugford et al 1989). At present however, despite evidence of the benefit of prophylactic antibiotics, they are usually reserved for those women at high risk such as the immunocompromised and those with valvular heart disease. They are usually given in a single dose 1 hour preoperatively as this achieves adequate blood levels while minimizing complications.

Appropriate treatment of wound infections depends upon isolation of the relevant organisms and sensitivity testing. The most common organisms involved are *Staphylococcus aureus*, anaerobes and Gram negative organisms such as *Streptococcus faecalis*. Staphylococci are sensitive to cloxacillin or flucloxacillin. If a streptococcal infection or a mixed infection of anaerobes and coliforms is present, a second generation cephalosporin is more appropriate. Cephalosporins are as effective as the penicillins and have a lower risk of sensitivity reactions but are expensive and are associated with a higher risk of pseudomembranous colitis. If the infection is unresponsive the wound may need opening, packing and draining.

It has been said that infection increases the possibility of uterine scar rupture in future pregnancies (Case et al 1971), however there is no evidence to support this unless the uterine wound is involved and a past history of a wound infection is not an indication for a repeat Caesarean section (Lavin et al 1982, Nielsen et al 1989).

Urinary complications

The risk of bladder or ureteric injury at Caesarean section is less than 1% (Evrad et al 1980). The bladder is most commonly injured during downward dissection before entry to the uterus particularly in a repeat Caesarean section. The ureters may be damaged if the uterine excision extends laterally. This is particularly likely if uterine closure is difficult and entails blind suturing. Ectopic ureters are rare (about 1 in 1900) and 80% of cases are associated with duplex collecting systems (Perlmutter et al 1986). Because of their abnormal position, they are more likely to be damaged. Pressure necrosis of the bladder following obstructed labour is rare in this country.

Management of damage to the urinary tract depends on the type of injury and when recognized. If the bladder is noted to be injured at the time of operation, it should be repaired in two layers with a suture such as plain catgut and the bladder should be drained continuously with a catheter for 7 to 10 days. Many clinicians give antibiotic cover with a broad spectrum drug such as a cephalosporin until the catheter is removed (Mundy 1987). Ureteric injuries are usually safest managed with the assistance of a urologist and treatment depends on the site and type of the lesion. If the ureter has been tied but not cut it is usually sufficient to remove the ligature, pass a ureteric catheter and drain the site of injury. If the ureter has been cut or crushed, ureteric anastomosis is required. A low ureteric injury may require reimplantation. To obtain more ureteric length and prevent tension on the repair procedures such as a psoas hitch or Boari flap may be utilized (Hendry 1985).

A bladder or ureteric injury which is missed at the time of operation may present as urine draining vaginally or through the incision. Once this is suspected, the bladder should be drained with a catheter and an intravenous urogram performed to look for a ureteric fistula. Surgical repair is usually needed and is performed immediately for ureteric injuries and up to 3 months postoperatively for vesical injuries. A successful repair is usually an indication for subsequent Caesarean section.

Bowel injury

Bowel injury is rare at Caesarean section but may occur particularly during a repeat procedure or if adhesions from previous surgery are present. Damage may be recognized by smell or faecal soiling. Management depends on the site of injury and is often best dealt with in conjunction with a general surgeon. Repair of small bowel is performed with a two layer closure using chromic cat gut in such a way as to preserve the lumen. If the injury is in the large bowel, the addition of a temporary defunctioning colostomy may be indicated. All such patients should receive intra-operative metronidazole and a cephalosporin which should be continued postoperatively.

Anaesthetic complications

Anaesthetic complications at present account for 8% of all direct deaths associated with Caesarean section. Almost all of these are associated with general anaesthesia. The primary causes are failure of endotracheal intubation and inhalation of acidic stomach contents resulting in adult respiratory distress syndrome (Mendelson's syndrome). Failure of intubation may be due to anatomical variations in the patient's neck or jaw or an abnormally small larynx or trachea. Technical problems include over inflation of the cuff, kinking of the tube and failure of ventilator connections. These problems may be worsened if they occur with an inexperienced junior anaesthetist. An anaesthetist of at least registrar grade should cover a labour ward and a fully trained assistant (ODA) should be present. A previously worked out drill must be learnt for all cases of failed intubation.

Aspiration effects may be decreased by keeping the mother nil by mouth during labour and the use of antacids prior to Caesarean section to raise the pH of gastric contents. Sodium citrate is the antacid of choice as magnesium trisilicate has been associated in a higher risk of lung parenchymal damage (Gibbs et al 1982). H2 antagonists such as cimetidine and ranitidine also decrease gastric acidity (Johnson et al 1983). To be effective cimetidine must be given 90–150 minutes preoperatively if given intramuscularly and 45 minutes preoperatively if intravenous; these are indicated in all high risk patients in labour (Pearce & Steel 1987).

For a full account of anaesthetic complications associated with Caesarean section see Moir & Thorburn (1986b).

Psychological complications

The psychological implications of Caesarean section are not well documented. Women who undergo Caesarean section are less likely to breast feed their baby and are reported to be less confident with themselves and their baby even a year after delivery (Biggs 1984). Caesarean section has also been shown to be associated with a higher incidence of longer lasting depression (US Dept Health and Human Services 1981) but not with a higher risk of puerperal psychosis. Studies assessing the effect of Caesarean section are rare but many studies have looked at the effects of restricted contact in the immediate postnatal period (inherent in Caesarean section). Restricted contact is associated with less affectionate maternal behaviour (Kontos 1978) and also with feelings of maternal incompetence and lack of confidence (Greenberg et al 1973). The mothers with restricted early neonatal contact are also more likely to discontinue breast feeding and there has also been demonstrated a higher incidence of child abuse and neglect in later life (O'Connor et al 1980). Further well conducted, controlled trials need to be carried out to identify women at particular risk.

MANAGEMENT OF A PREVIOUS CAESARIAN SECTION SCAR

The management of a patient with a previous Caesarean section scar is primarily a decision on mode of delivery. This depends to a great extent on whether the reason for the previous Caesarean section is recurrent or not. For example pelvic contracture is a recurrent cause but some situations are not as clear cut. For example, although placenta praevia is usually considered a non-recurring cause, there is a higher risk of placenta praevia in a subsequent pregnancy due to scar implantation (Singh et al 1981). The decision to allow a trial of labour also depends on other features of the pregnancy such as a breech presentation or the presence of pre-eclampsia.

In Britain the majority of patients are allowed a trial of labour including those with cephalopelvic disproportion as other factors such as fetal weight and position will influence the outcome. In the United States however a trial of labour is less common. Thirty per cent of Caesarean sections are elective repeat procedures thus forming a self propagating circle.

The role of pelvimetry

Lateral x-ray pelvimetry has been widely used in the diagnosis of cephalopelvic disproportion although its validity in a primigravid vertex presentation is disputed (Barton et al 1982). However in the case of a previous Caesarean section it is heavily relied upon to assess pelvic size for a subsequent trial of scar. Cephalopelvic disproportion is however a relative condition and it should be remembered that subsequent babies tend to be larger than the first. However Paul et al (1985) found that 77% of patients with a diagnosis of cephalopelvic disproportion achieved vaginal delivery in the subsequent pregnancy.

Recently both computerized axial tomography (CAT scanning) and magnetic resonance scanning (MRI) have been proposed as an alternative to conventional x-ray pelvimetry. CAT scanning involves one twentieth of the radiation of a conventional x-ray and provides detailed information including the sacrospinous diameters (Hibberd & Lyons 1989). MRI scanning also gives detailed results without the use of ionizing radiation. Both are at present expensive and not widely available.

Risks of scar rupture

The risk of scar rupture varies with the type of uterine scar. The commonest used estimated risk is of an overall risk of 2·2% for a classical scar and 0·5% for a lower uterine scar (Dewhurst 1957). More recent studies show similar risks (Molloy et al 1987, Phelan et al 1987). The maternal mortality associated with classical scar rupture is in the order of 5% with a fetal mortality of 73%. There is no significant maternal mortality associated with a lower segment scar but there is a fetal mortality of 12·5%. The risk of scar rupture with a De Lee's incision (low vertical incision) is estimated to lie somewhere between the two, but with the increasing use of this incision to deliver preterm infants, further evalution is needed of the exact risks (Paul et al 1985).

Management of a trial of scar

Women undergoing a trial of scar should always be looked after in a fully equipped labour ward with facilities for Caesarean section. Ideally the onset of labour should be spontaneous as the use of prostaglandin for induction of labour may entail a higher risk of uterine rupture and also spontaneous onset of labour is associated with a higher incidence of vaginal delivery.

Once in labour, continuous fetal monitoring should be carried out. Epidural analgesia is not contraindicated in trial of scar patients as although it was previously suggested that a good epidural block would mask the signs of uterine rupture (Gibbs 1980) there is no evidence to support this (Stoval et al 1987, Phelan 1987).

The use of Syntocinon in trial of scars is also controversial and in the past has been discouraged both to induce and augment labour. Recent studies have found no increased risk of uterine scar rupture with the use of Syntocinon (Flamm et al 1988). Syntocinon may however be used with more confidence in the presence of intra-uterine pressure catheters and these are advocated to allow augmentation of labour to achieve optimum uterine activity (Gibb & Arulkumaran 1987). Once this optimum activity is achieved (on the 50th centile), a cervical dilatation rate of less than 1 cm per hour should be taken as a sign of cephalopelvic disproportion and a Caesarean section performed.

Recognition of the ruptured uterus

Uterine rupture can be divided into scar dehiscence and scar rupture. Rupture is usually defined as complete separation of the uterine scar with rupture of the membranes and communication between the uterine and peritoneal cavities whereas dehiscence is the separation of the scar with intact peritoneum. Scar dehiscence may be noted on ultrasound scan as a 'window' in the scar or may be felt during examination under epidural. It is also found at Caesarean section although there may have been no clinical signs of uterine rupture. The incidence of scar dehiscence (as opposed to scar rupture) in repeat Caesarean section is 4% (Nielsen et al 1989).

Scar rupture is classically associated with an acute onset of abdominal pain which is continuous and does not remit between contractions. However this may not be the case with lower uterine scars which, as they are fibrous, usually rupture painlessly. Scar rupture may also present as acute fetal distress as shown on the cardiotocograph or as an acute cessation of labour. Once the diagnosis is made, resuscitation of the mother must be commenced and preparation made for immediate laparotomy and delivery of the fetus. Full resuscitation may not be possible until the fetus is delivered and the bleeding margins of the tear can be sutured or clamped.

Once delivered, the decision is made as to whether repair of the rupture or a Caesarean hysterectomy is more appropriate. This choice depends upon the type and extent of the rupture, the patient's general condition, in particular the presence of uncontrollable haemorrhage, and to some extent on a woman's previous obstetric history. If the patient is in a poor condition, repair of the tear has been advocated as less traumatic to the patient than hysterectomy (Sheth 1969). Tears in the upper part of the uterus are more difficult to repair and hysterectomy is usually the operation of choice. Repair of the tear (if feasible) along with sterilization has been proposed for women with large families who for cultural reasons, wish to retain a uterus (Sheth 1969). It would be expected that the risk of rupture in a subsequent pregnancy following repair of a tear would be high. However, no maternal morbidity was associated with this in patients delivered by elective Caesarean section at 38 weeks (Reyes-Ceja et al 1969) and a previous ruptured uterus is therefore an indication for an elective Caesarean section.

Some clinicians advocate postpartum transcervical palpation of the uterine scar (Gibbs 1980), but there appears to be no clinical benefit in treating asymptomatic scars and scars may even be extended by the examining finger (Nielsen et al 1989).

CONCLUSION

With the rising incidence of Caesarean section, there is a tendency to regard it as an uncomplicated and straightforward procedure. Complications do occur causing a significant morbidity and mortality. Care must be taken with every patient to look out for these complications and instigate immediate treatment.

At present, management of women with a previous Caesarean section is controversial. It is accepted that a trial of labour can be attempted in most cases and that there is no place for use of a uterine scar as a sole indication for a repeat Caesarean section. There is, however, no widespread policy for the use of Syntocinon and epidurals in these women. Careful observation throughout labour in a well equipped unit is necessary and prompt management if scar rupture does occur are basic principles.

REFERENCES

Apuzzio J J, Reyelt C, Pelosi M, Sen P, Louria D B 1982 Prophylactic antibiotics for Cesarean section: comparison of high risk and low risk patients for endometritis. Obstet Gynecol 59: 693–698

Badaracco M A, Vessey M 1974 Recurrence of venous thromboembolic disease and the use of oral contraceptives. Br Med J i: 215–217

Barton J J, Garbaciak J A Jr, Ryan G M Jr 1982 The efficacy of x-ray pelvimetry. Am J Obstet Gynecol 143(3): 304–311

Biggs J S 1984 The rise of the caesarean section: a review. Aust NZ J Obstet Gynaecol 24 (2): 68–71

Britton J J 1980 Sterilisation by caesarean hysterectomy. Am J Obstet Gynecol 137: 887–890

Burchell C R 1968 The physiology of internal iliac ligation. J Obstet Gynaecol Br Commwlth 75: 642–651

Burchell C R, Olson G 1966 Internal iliac ligation; aortograms. Am J Obstet Gynecol 94: 117–124

Cardozo L D, Barnick C, Beness C 1989 Post-partum voiding dysfunction. Int Urogynaecol J 1: 2

Case B D, Corcoran R, Jeffcote N, Randle G H 1971 Cesarean section and its place in modern obstetric practice. J Obstet Gynaecol Commwlth 78: 203–214

Charles D, Larsen B 1989 Puerperal sepsis. In: Turnbull A, Chamberlain G (eds) Obstetrics. Churchill Livingstone, Edinburgh, pp 917–932

Cunningham F G, Leveno K J, DePalma R T, Roark M, Rosenfeld C R 1983 Perioperative antimicrobials for cesarean delivery: before or after cord clamping? Obstet Gynecol 62: 151–154

Dewhurst C J 1957 The ruptured caesarean section scar. J Obstet Gynaecol British Empire 64: 113–118

Duff P, Robertson A W, Read J A 1987 Single dose cefazolin vs cefonicid for antibiotic prophylaxis in cesarean delivery. Obstet Gynecol 70: 718–721

Evrad J R, Gold E M, Cahill T F 1980 Cesarean section: a contemporary assessment. J Reprod Med 24: 147–149

Flamm B L, Lim O W, Jones C, Fallon D, Newman L A, Mantis J K 1988 Vaginal birth after cesarean section: Results of a multicenter study. Am J Obstet Gynecol 158: 1079–1084

Gall S A 1979 The efficacy of prophylactic antibiotics in Cesarean section. Am J Obstet Gynecol 137: 506

Gibb D M F, Arulkumaran S 1987 Uterine contractions and the fetus. In: Studd J (ed) Progress in obstetrics and gynaecology, vol 6. Churchill Livingstone, Edinburgh, pp 133–154

Gibbs C E 1980 Planned vaginal delivery following cesarean section. Clin Obstet Gynecol 23: 507–515

Gibbs C B, Spohr L, Schmidt D 1982 The effectiveness of sodium citrate as an antacid. Anaesthesiology 57: 44

Goodman A G, Goodman L S, Gilman A 1980 The pharmacological basis of therapeutics, 6th edn. Macmillan, New York

Greenberg M, Rosenberg I, Lind J 1973 First mothers rooming-in with their new borns: its impact upon the mother. Am J Orthopsychiatry 43: 783–788

Gruber H F 1980 Incidence of fatal post-operative pulmonary embolus after prophylaxis with Dextran-70 and low dose heparin—an international multicentre study. Br Med J 280: 69–72

Hawrylyshyn P A, Bernstein P, Papsin F R 1981 Risk factors associated with infection following caesarean section. Am J Obstet Gynecol 139: 294

Hendry W F 1985 Urinary tract injuries during gynaecological surgery. In: Studd J (ed) Progress in obstetrics and gynaecology, vol 5. Churchill Livingstone, Edinburgh, pp 362–377

Hibberd B M, Lyons K 1989 Digital radiological pelvimetry—a new dimension for pelvic assessment. Proc British Congress Obstetrics and Gynaecology, London

Johnson J R, Moore J, McCaughey W 1983 Use of cimetidine as an oral antacid in obstetric anaesthesia. Anaesth Analg 62: 720–722

Koh K S, Chan F H, Monfored A H, Ledger W J, Paul R H 1979 The changing perinatal and maternal outcome in chorioamnionitis. Obstet Gynecol 53: 730–734

Kontos D 1978 A study of the effects of extended mother-infant contact on maternal behaviour at one and three months. Birth Family J 5: 133–140

Lavery J P, Howell R S, Shaw L 1985 Ultrasonic demonstration of a phlegmon following Cesarean section. JCU 13(2): 134–136

Lavin J P, Stephens R J, Miodovnik M, Barden T P 1982 Vaginal delivery in patients with a prior cesarean section. Obstet Gynecol 59: 135–148

Lees D H, Singer A 1982 Caesarian section. In: Surgery of conditions complicating pregnancy. Wolfe Medical, London, pp 111–130

Letsky E A, De Swiet M 1984 Thromboembolism in pregnancy and it's management. B J Haematol 57: 4

Marshall A 1987 Post-operative respiratory problems. In: Taylor T H, Major E (eds) Hazards and complications of anaesthesia. Churchill Livingstone, Edinburgh, pp 188–196

Moir D D, Thorburn J 1986a Regional analgesia in obstetrics. In: Obstetric anaesthesia and analgesia, 3rd edn. Baillière Tindall, London

Moir D D, Thorburn J 1986b Obstetric anaesthesia and analgesia, 3rd edn. Baillière Tindall, London

Molloy B G, Shiel O, Duignan N M 1987 Delivery after caesarean section: a review of 2176 consecutive cases. Br Med J 294: 1645–1647

Mugford M, Kingston J, Chalmers I 1989 Reducing the incidence of infection after caesarean section: implication of prophylaxis with antibiotics for hospital resources. Br Med J 299: 1003–1006

Mundy A R 1987 Urological injuries and how to cope. In: Stanton S L (ed) Principles of gynaecological surgery. Springer Verlag, London, pp 175–246

Nielsen T F, Ljungblad U, Hagberg H 1989 Rupture and dehiscence of cesarean section scar during pregnancy and delivery. Am J Obstet Gynecol 160 (3): 569–573

O'Connor S, Vietze P M, Sherrod K B, Sandler H M, Altemeier W A 1980 Reduced incidence of parenting inadequacy following rooming-in. Pediatrics 66: 176–182

Odoon J A, Sih I L 1983 Epidural analgesia and anticoagulant therapy. Experience with 1000 cases of continuous epidural. Anaesthesia 38: 254

Park R C, Duff W P 1980 Role of caesarean hysterectomy in modern obstetric practice. Clin Obstet Gynecol 23: 601–620

Paul R H, Phelan J P, Yeh S Y 1985 Trial of labour in the patient with a prior Cesarean birth. Am J Obstet Gynecol 151: 297–304

Pearce J M P, Steel S A 1987 A manual of labour ward practice. Wiley, London, p 39

Perlmutter A D, Retik A B, Bauer S B 1986 Ectopic ureter. In: Walsh P C, Gittes R F, Perlmutter A D, Stamey T A (eds) Cambell's Urology. Saunders, Philadelphia, pp 1735–1739

Phelan J P, Clark S L, Diaz M A, Paul R H 1987 Vaginal birth after cesarean. Am J Obstet Gynecol 157 (6): 1510–1515

Rehu M, Nilsson C G 1980 Risk factors for febrile mobidity associated with caesarean section. Obstet Gynecol 56: 259–264

Report on Confidential Enquiry into Maternal Deaths in England and Wales, 1970–72, 1982–84. HMSO, London

Reyes-Ceja L, Cabrera R, Insfran E, Herrera-Lasso F 1969 Pregnancy following previous uterine rupture. Study of 19 patients. Obstet Gynecol 34(3): 387–389

Saltzman D H, Eron L J, Kay H H, Sites J G 1985 Single dose antibiotic prophylaxis in high risk patients undergoing cesarean section; a comparative trial. J Reprod Med 31: 709–712

Scarpignato C, Caltabiano M, Condemi V, Mansani F E 1982 Short term vs long term cefuroxime prophylaxis in patients undergoing emergency cesarean section. Clin Ther 5: 186–192

Sheth S S 1969 Suturing of the tear as treatment in uterine rupture. Am J Obstet Gynecol 105(3): 440–443

Singh P M, Rodrigues L, Gupta A N 1981 Placenta previa and previous Cesarean section. Acta Obstet Gynecol Scand 60: 367

Stiver H G, Forward K R, Livingston R A et al 1983 Multicenter comparison of cefoxitin vs cefazolin for prevention of infectious morbidity after non-elective cesarean section. Am J Obstet Gynecol 145: 158–163

Stiver H G, Tyrrell D L, Livingston R A, Lemay M, Hunter J D W, Beresford P 1984 Comparative cervical microflors shifts after cefoxitin or cefazolin prophylaxis against infection following cesarean section. Am J Obstet Gynecol 149: 718–721

Stoval T G, Shaver D C, Solomon S K, Anderson G A 1987 Trial of labor in previous cesarean section patients, excluding classical cesarean sections. Obstet Gynecol 70: 713–717

Sturdee D W, Rushton D I 1986 Caesarean and post-partum hysterectomy 1968–83. B J Obstet Gynaecol 93: 270–274

Tulandi T, Hum H S, Gelfand M M 1988 Closure of laparotomy incisions with or without peritoneal suturing and second look laparoscopy. Am J Obstet Gynecol 158: 536–537

US Dept of Health and Human Services 1981 Cesarean childbirth: report of a consensus conference. NIH publications no. 82–2067

Von Finck M, Schnidt R, Schneider W, Feine U 1986 The quality of washed autotransfused erythrocytes. The elimination of plasma hemoglobin, osmotic fragility and survival rate of retransfused erythrocytes. Anaesthetist 35(ii): 686–692

Walter S, Vejlsgaard R 1978 Diagnostic catheterisation and bacteriuria in women with urinary incontinence. Br J Urol 50: 106–108

11. Birth asphyxia and neonatal resuscitation

G. Constantine   J. B. Weaver

WHAT IS BIRTH ASPHYXIA?

Although the clinical picture of a pale, hypotonic baby that fails to breathe spontaneously may appear characteristic, there is not a single accepted definition of birth asphyxia. Definitions used are based on Apgar scores, umbilical cord acid/base status, time to spontaneous breathing, and the neurological/behavioural condition of the infant. Using these definitions, the reported incidence of birth asphyxia lies between 2·9 and 9·0/1000 deliveries (Levene 1988a). Each of these has a variable degree of correlation with subsequent outcome. In the following discussion, unless stated otherwise, sensitivity refers to the % of handicapped/dead infants predicted by an abnormal test and specificity to the % of normal infants predicted by a normal test.

Apgar scores

The most widely used indicator of fetal condition at birth is the Apgar score (Apgar 1953). The International Classification of Disease defines mild asphyxia as a 1 min score of $\leqslant 6$ and severe asphyxia as a 1 min score $\leqslant 3$. The Apgar score was however designed to give an overview of fetal condition at set times following delivery, and to highlight those babies in need of resuscitation, not to define those babies with hypoxia. It is affected by other variables such as maternal opiate use, prematurity (Catlin et al 1986), aspiration of mucous/meconium, cardiac, respiratory, muscle and CNS problems, and even in the hypoxic newborn does not give an indication of the time or duration of insult.

The National Collaborative Perinatal Project (NCPP) followed up 41 018 children of 51 285 delivered between 1959 and 1966 and correlated Apgar scores at 1, 5, 10, 15 and 20 minutes with subsequent outcome (Nelson & Ellenberg 1981). Very low late Apgar scores (0–3 at 20 min) were significantly related to mortality during the first year of life (96% in those < 2500 g, 59% > 2500 g). Low Apgar scores were only weakly related to morbidity as 80% of infants with a score $\leqslant 3$ at 10, 15 and 20 min that survived were without major handicap. Conversely, of those babies developing cerebral palsy 55% had scores >7 at 1 min, and 73% >7 at 5 min.

Using a 5 min score of ≤7, Ruth & Raivio found the Apgar score to have a sensitivity of 12% and a positive predictive value of 19% for abnormal neurodevelopment at 12 months of age (Ruth & Raivio 1988).

In another study of 20 975 full term births, a 10 min Apgar score ≤5 was the most sensitive of six different Apgar ratings in predicting adverse outcome at 2·5 years. Although having a specificity of 95%, the sensitivity was still only 43% (Levene et al 1986).

The correlation between Apgar score and acid/base balance in the umbilical cord has also been assessed (James et al 1958, Sykes et al 1982, Fields et al 1983, Lauener et al 1983, Suidan & Young 1985, Silverman et al 1985, Dijxhoorn et al 1986, Marrin & Paes 1988, Gilstrap et al 1989, Thorp et al 1989). Except at the extremes of acidosis this was weak.

Apgar scores may therefore alert the birth attendants to the need for neonatal resuscitation, but the traditional 1 and 5 min scores have little prognostic value. Very late low Apgar scores that fail to rise, appear of some prognostic value, but even so many such infants will be neurologically normal whilst most cases of subsequent disability will be missed.

Cord acid/base status

Birth asphyxia suggests a lack of oxygen, retention of carbon dioxide and acidosis in the newborn infant. The measurement of acid/base status in the umbilical cord would therefore appear an attractive way of defining an asphyxiated group of babies (Sykes et al 1982, Silverman et al 1985, Dijxhoorn et al 1986, Gilstrap et al 1989, Thorp et al 1989). Most studies consider an umbilical artery $pH < 7.1$ to indicate severe asphyxia, and a $pH < 7.2$ to indicate some degree of asphyxia, although there is variation.

Some degree of hypoxia during labour is very common however, and most hypoxic/acidaemic infants appear and behave normally, needing no resuscitation (Suidan & Young 1985, Gilstrap et al 1989, Thorp et al 1989). One study defined a pathological acidosis as a $pH \leqslant 7.10$, base deficit > 12 (Sykes et al 1982). Using this definition 81% of babies with a 5 min Apgar score of <7 were not acidotic, whilst 73% of those who were acidotic had normal Apgar scores and needed no resuscitation. This same population was followed up for neurodevelopmental outcome at 4·5 years of age (Dennis et al 1989). No significant associations between acidosis and developmental outcome were found.

Other studies in high risk groups with growth retardation and/or prematurity, have shown some evidence that acidaemia at birth is associated with neonatal neurological signs (Huisjes et al 1980), and degrees of major deficit at 12 months (Low et al 1984). In low risk acidaemic fetuses, an association with neonatal signs is less clear (Dijxhoorn et al 1986), whilst there is no correlation with abnormal development at 1–5 years (Low et al 1983, Touwen & Huisjes 1984, Ruth & Raivio 1988). Surprisingly babies with low Apgar scores and severe acidaemia appear to have a better outcome than those with low scores who are not acidotic (Dijxhoorn et al 1986, Ruth & Raivio 1988, Dennis et al 1989). Combining Apgar scores and cord arterial pH, suggests that severe depression ($\leqslant 3$ at 1 and 5 min, pH $< 7{\cdot}00$) is needed before significant birth asphyxia can be confidently diagnosed (Gilstrap et al 1989).

In low risk groups, acidosis at birth as defined by cord pH values of $< 7{\cdot}1$ together with a base deficit of > 12, does not have a strong correlation with the need for resuscitation or neonatal neurological signs, and has no correlation with subsequent neurological development. Where umbilical cord arterial pH is of value is in demonstrating that 80% of depressed newborns will have a totally normal pH (Sykes et al 1982, Thorp et al 1989). Also since 90% of cerebral palsy is not caused by birth asphyxia (Nelson 1988) a normal pH at birth will exclude this as a cause if disability subsequently develops.

Time to spontaneous respiration

Failure to commence spontaneous respiration within 1 min of birth has been used as one definition of birth asphyxia. There are however many causes of delayed respiration beside hypoxia. In support of this, one study showed that 57% of babies requiring endotracheal intubation, had a normal umbilical cord pH at birth (Lissauer & Steer 1986).

Using a definition of positive pressure ventilation for over 1 min, the overall incidence of birth asphyxia was found to be 1·2%, with an incidence of 9% at $\leqslant 36$ weeks, and 0·5% at $\geqslant 37$ weeks (MacDonald et al 1980). This was related strongly to gestational age and birthweight. Follow up of a cohort of these babies showed a similar incidence of neurodevelopmental disability to other studies using different criteria (Mulligan et al 1980).

As a definition of birth asphyxia it would appear to have little to recommend it. What is certain however is that it defines a group in need of resuscitation whatever the aetiology.

Hypoxic-ischaemic encephalopathy

Observation of the neurological condition of the baby during the neonatal period has been shown to have a useful prognostic value, encephalopathy being associated with birth asphyxia.

Simple 3 stage grading systems of postasphyxial encephalopathy have been reported and are in wide use (Sarnat & Sarnat 1976, Fenichel 1983, Levene et al 1985, Amiel-Tison & Ellison 1986).

Grade 1:   no alteration in level of consciousness, but appear hyperalert
(mild)   with hyper-reflexia, tachycardia, jitteriness and dilated
               pupils. No fits.
Grade 2:   lethargy, miosis, bradycardia, hypotonia, weak suck, poor
(moderate)   Moro reflex. Not comatose. Fits occur.
Grade 3:   stupor, flaccidity, small midposition pupils reacting poorly
(severe)   to light, hypotonia, absent suck and Moro reflexes.
               Prolonged fits.

Using these criteria an incidence of 6/1000 births has been reported, with moderate and severe encephalopathy occurring in 1·1 and 1·0/1000 births respectively (Levene et al 1985).

Mild encephalopathy should resolve within 48 h, whilst moderate and severe encephalopathy follow a progression of signs leading to death or recovery (often with handicap) over a period of weeks (Levene 1988a).

The outcome of babies with grade 1, 2 and 3 encephalopathy is shown in Table 11.1. Likelihood of a handicap (sensitivity) appears to be predicted with almost complete accuracy (96%) by moderate or severe encephalopathy, compared to 43% for a 10 min Apgar score ≤5 (Levene et al 1986). Using an extended postasphyxial score based on 17 items, a score ≤6 predicted death or severe handicap at 12 months with a sensitivity of 95% and specificity of 83% (Lipper et al 1986).

Whilst appearing a reliable indicator of future handicap, encephalopathy does not appear to be specifically related to hypoxia. In high risk neonates, using umbilical artery base deficit as a measure, 12% of babies with mild to moderate and 22% with severe encephalopathy were acidotic at birth (Low et al 1985). In the same study 56% of severely acidotic infants had some degree of encephalopathy.

Neonatal seizures have been studied independently, but have many other causes besides birth asphyxia, including infection, metabolic abnormalities, trauma and cerebral abnormalities (Lancet 1989a). When secondary to birth asphyxia, they begin during the first 48–72 h of life (Brown et al 1974, Minchom et al 1987) and are a risk factor for subsequent development of cerebral palsy (Nelson & Ellenberg 1986). Using NCPP data for babies

Table 11.1   % severely abnormal or dead infants at time of follow up in years

| Authors | n | Grade of encephalopathy | | | Follow up (y) |
		1	2	3	
Sarnat & Sarnat (1976)	21	—	25	100	1
Finer et al (1981)	89	0	15	92	3·5
Robertson & Finer (1985)	200	0	27	100	3·5
Low et al (1985)	42	—[a]	27	50	1
Levene et al (1986)	122	1[b]	25	75	2·5

[a] Grade 1 and 2 combined
[b] Death from congenital myopathy

weighing more than 2500 g, the combination of a low Apgar score, seizures and encephalopathy defined a group of infants with a risk for chronic motor disability of 55% and for death or disability of 70% (Ellenberg & Nelson 1988).

What then are we to conclude? Whilst it is possible to define birth asphyxia using any of the criteria outlined above, none is specific for hypoxia during birth except umbilical artery pH and base deficit levels. Using these however, numbers of clinically normal babies will be labelled asphyxiated, whilst significant neurodevelopmental abnormality cannot be accurately predicted. It is however possible to conclude that significant birth asphyxia did not exist if the umbilical artery pH is normal, and/or encephalopathy does not occur. If a neurodevelopmental handicap subsequently becomes manifest, it is unlikely to be related to birth asphyxia (irrespective of Apgar score or cord pH) unless moderate to severe encephalopathy occurred.

WHAT DAMAGE DOES BIRTH ASPHYXIA CAUSE AND HOW CAN IT BE DETECTED?

Severe asphyxia during labour may lead to a stillbirth or neonatal death. It is unclear however why hypoxia, sufficient to kill 50% of term newborn infants, should leave 75% of survivors without handicap (Nelson & Ellenberg 1981). Mechanisms that lead to brain damage in birth asphyxia are not fully understood. Both oxygenation and perfusion abnormalities appear to play a role, the insult sustained and subsequent outcome being dependent on the degree of asphyxia, its duration and the gestational age and birthweight of the fetus (Levene 1987).

During asphyxia cerebral blood flow is selectively maintained to vital brainstem structures at the expense of the cerebral cortex. With restoration of the systemic circulation reactive hyperaemia occurs and cerebral blood flow increases to above pre-ischaemic levels. After this period of initial hyperaemia, the cerebral blood flow rapidly falls in some cases and this has been described as the no-reflow phenomenon (Archer et al 1986). In preterm infants with asphyxia, cerebral autoregulation mechanisms also become defective allowing fluctuations in systemic blood pressure to be transmitted directly to the brain (Lou et al 1979) with subsequent haemorrhage.

Whilst blood flow to the fetal brain, heart and adrenals increases with increasing hypoxia, that to the kidneys, liver and gastrointestinal tract decreases. Subsequent to severe birth asphyxia, renal failure and necrotizing enterocolitis are not uncommon, together with heart failure, meconium aspiration, metabolic problems and DIC (Levene 1988a, Perlman 1989).

In the preterm infant specific forms of cerebral injury are found although some controversy exists over their pathogenesis and nomenclature. These are haemorrhage into the germinal matrix (GMH), ventricles (IVH) and periventricular tissue (PVH) secondary hyperfusion, and periventricular leukomalacia (PVL) followed by cystic degeneration secondary to hypoperfusion (Levene 1987, de Vries et al 1988). These occur in the periventricular white matter which, in the preterm neonate, is the borderzone between the centripetal and centrifugal arterial arcades, and thus has a relatively precarious blood supply. Both PVH and PVL can be demonstrated and their development followed by neonatal ultrasound of the infant brain using a 7·5 Hz transducer imaging through the anterior fontanelle (Trounce & Levene 1988). This is important as follow up studies have shown IVH, PVH and PVL to have different aetiologies and prognoses. In particular there is little evidence linking GMH, IVH or PVH with intrapartum events or asphyxia (Beverley & Chance 1984, de Vries et al 1988), most cases being postnatal in origin.

In one study, all survivors with extensive PVL developed severe cerebral palsy and mental retardation, whilst 50% of survivors with extensive PVH were normal, and only 11% had a severe handicap (de Vries et al 1985). In this study, 2 cases were found on scans shortly after birth suggesting a prenatal insult.

In babies of ⩽1500 g or <34 weeks gestation, Weindling et al found 34/86 developed PVH, whilst 7/86 developed cystic PVL (Weindling et al 1985). The development of PVH was associated with perinatal hypoxia, but more so with postnatal acidosis, hypercapnia and hypoxia. PVL showed a stronger association with perinatal hypoxia defined as a 5 min Apgar score of ⩽6 and/or umbilical artery pH⩽7·15, 4/7 cases having shown evidence of an antepartum haemorrhage. A similar association with maternal antepartum haemorrhage together with intrapartum asphyxia, multiple births and pre-eclampsia has been reported elsewhere (Sinha et al 1985, Calvert et al 1986, de Vries et al 1988). Whilst birth asphyxia in preterm babies may certainly lead to subsequent brain damage detectable by ultrasound, antenatal, and particularly postnatal insults appear more closely related.

During asphyxia, three types of brain damaging mechanisms occur; acidosis, the accumulation of cytotoxic amino acids and generation of oxygen derived free radicals together with calcium ion intoxication (Kjellmer 1988). In the term asphyxiated neonate, the accumulation of these products of anaerobic metabolism leads to neuronal damage, oedema and the clinical signs of encephalopathy. The ultrasound features that accompany encephalopathy are not easy to assess, taking the form of a generalized increase in echodensity throughout the brain or confined to the basal ganglia (Levene 1988a, Hill & Volpe 1989). Other methods including computed tomography (CT) and magnetic resonance (MRI) scanning have been reviewed elsewhere (Flodmark 1988, Hill & Volpe 1989). CT scanning in such cases may show a diffuse decrease in tissue attenuation maximal at 2–4 days following the hypoxic episode and correlating well with a poor neurological outcome (Lupton et al 1988). Other studies have shown CT appearances to be more prognostic after the first week of life

(Adsett et al 1985, Lipp-Zwahlen et al 1985, Lipper et al 1986). In addition a minority may develop subcortical leukomalacia, parasagittal injury, or damage to the basal ganglia (Levene 1988a).

Ultrasound is also useful in the eary assessment of asphyxiated neonates. As most cerebral lesions develop over a finite time scale, it is possible to show abnormalities suggesting damage caused by antenatal insults, thus ruling out intrapartum factors.

Other studies have used neonatal cerebral Doppler studies, electro-encephalography, intracranial pressure measuring and biochemical markers of brain damage to predict outcome following birth asphyxia. Those with most application and promise appear to be Doppler studies and bio-chemical markers.

In asphyxiated neonates during the first 5 days of life, Doppler studies of the anterior cerebral arteries show a close correlation with outcome (Archer et al 1986). No infants with a normal resistance index were handicapped when followed up between 6 and 36 months, whilst the accuracy in predicting outcome was 86%, a low resistance index of <0.55 having a sensitivity of 100% and a specificity of 81% for adverse outcome. Other studies have shown a similar sensitivity but a lower specificity (Den Ouden et al 1987). The same group have also studied cerebral blood flow velocity (CBFV). In 34 neonates with severe encephalopathy (Levene et al 1989), a CBFV < 3 s.d. or > 2 s.d. from the mean had a positive predictive value for a poor outcome of 94%.

Birth asphyxia leads to the accumulation of metabolites of anaerobic metabolism and products of cerebral damage (Lancet 1988). Metabolites of anaerobic metabolism such as lactate and hypoxanthine have been studied in blood, urine and CSF, but suffer from the same drawbacks as measures of acid/base balance, and have no better predictive power for subsequent outcome. Enzyme indicators of neuronal cell damage such as levels of hydroxybutyrate, lactate dehydrogenase and brain specific creatine phosphokinase (CPK-BB) (Walsh et al 1982, Fernandez et al 1987) have been assessed in serum and CSF. Fernandez et al measured CPK-BB at 4 h of age in 53 neonates including 33 with birth asphyxia, and followed them up for between 9 and 23 months (Fernandez et al 1987). A normal CPK-BB at 4 h successfully predicted a favourable outcome in 96% of cases. On the other hand an elevated level was only 50% reliable as a predictor of poor neurodevelopmental outcome.

Recently ^{31}P magnetic resonance spectrometry has been used to quantify impaired oxidative phosphorylation secondary to birth asphyxia (Hamilton et al 1988). Sixty-one asphyxiated neonates between 27 and 42 weeks gestation were studied with this technique, of which 23 died and 38 were assessed at 12 months of age (Azzopardi et al 1989). Of the 28 with a low phosphocreatine:inorganic phosphate ratio, 19 died and 9 survived, 7 with a serious impairment. This shows a 74% sensitivity and 92% specificity with a positive predictive value for a poor outcome of 93%. Of the 12 infants with a low ATP:total phosphate ratio 11 died, the survivor being severely handicapped; a sensitivity of 47%, specificity of 97% and a positive predictive value for a poor outcome of 91%.

WHAT PROPORTION OF HANDICAP CAN BE ASCRIBED TO BIRTH ASPHYXIA?

That birth asphyxia may lead to neurodevelopmental handicap is not in doubt. As long ago as 1897 however Freud challenged the conventional wisdom that cerebral palsy was always a direct result of birth asphyxia when he stated 'Difficult birth is merely a symptom of deeper effects that influenced the development of the fetus' (Freud 1897), a view that did not find greater acceptance until recent years. Two large population studies have attempted to assess what proportion of handicap can be attributed to birth asphyxia.

Out of the 41 018 children followed up in the NCPP study, there were 189 children with cerebral palsy, 21% of whom had at least one marker of perinatal asphyxia (Nelson & Ellenberg 1986). However a third of these children had other major malformations outside the CNS, and more than 50% of children with evidence of serious asphyxia had an indicator that the cerebral palsy may have stemmed from prelabour problems. In a summary based on this data the proportion of cerebral palsy arising from intrapartum asphyxia was in the range 3–13%, and statistically could not exceed 21%.

In the second study all children with cerebral palsy born in Western Australia between 1975–1980 were studied and compared with matched controls (Blair & Stanley 1988). Only about 8% were thought to be related to birth asphyxia, a figure consistent with that from the NCPP study. These estimates may explain why the incidence of cerebral palsy (2–2·5/1000) has not changed in Western countries since the early 1950s despite a substantial fall in the perinatal mortality rate and obstetric interventions aimed at reducing birth asphyxia (Nelson 1988, Freeman & Nelson 1988). Only 15% of severe mental retardation can be accounted for by birth asphyxia, and then only when associated with neurological deficit, the majority of severely asphyxiated babies that survive do so without mental retardation (Paneth & Stark 1983).

Cerebral palsy and mental retardation are therefore not usually associated with birth asphyxia, but with other prenatal (de Vries et al 1988), postnatal and idiopathic factors. This fact has important medicolegal implications (Freeman & Nelson 1988, Nelson 1988, Lancet 1989b, Hall 1989).

WHAT CONDITIONS LEAD TO BIRTH ASPHYXIA?

There is a strong relationship between prematurity, IUGR and cerebral palsy (Ellenberg & Nelson 1979), but determining how much handicap in these groups is specifically related to birth asphyxia is difficult. Cordocentesis has demonstrated hypoxia and acidosis to be present antenatally in some growth retarded fetuses (Pearce & Chamberlain 1987, Nicolaides & Soothill 1989). Such fetuses will enter labour in a state of chronic hypoxia and may be unable to withstand the hypoxic stress of normal labour. Hypoxic insults in labour insufficient to affect the uncompromised fetus may thus severely affect the already compromised fetus and lead to significant clinical birth asphyxia. Studies of the incidence of postasphyxial encephalopathy show that around 25–29% of cases occur in growth retarded fetuses (Finer et al 1981, Levene et al 1985), whilst in growth retarded fetuses neonatal neurological signs show an association with acidosis not present in those of normal weight for gestation (Huisjes et al 1980). Other studies however have failed to show an association between acidosis and IUGR or prematurity (Ruth & Raivio 1988).

The influence of prematurity on the incidence and outcome of birth asphyxia is difficult to assess, being influenced both by the cause of the prematurity, and any concomitant IUGR. In addition premature fetuses often have a poor respiratory effort associated purely with prematurity, and may falsely be labelled 'asphyxiated'. In the preterm infant severe hypoxia causes specific lesions (GMH, IVH, PVH and PVL) which whilst common, are related to delays in resuscitation and postnatal problems more frequently than birth asphyxia. Determining therefore whether premature infants are at increased risk of birth asphyxia, and the proportion of handicap due to this cause, is difficult.

The combination of prematurity with IUGR does however appear to place neonates at a significantly higher risk of birth asphyxia and subsequent handicap (Huisjes et al 1980, Visser & Dijxhoorn 1987).

These two groups appear to have less reserve to combat the effects of hypoxia, acidosis may increase rapidly (Westgren et al 1984) and there is some additional risk of significant birth asphyxia. This should be borne in mind when assessing the need to expedite delivery in such patients.

Birth asphyxia may be secondary to chronic partial asphyxia or acute asphyxia from events such as abruption or cord prolapse. Possible specific aetiologies of birth asphyxia therefore include:

Chronic placental insufficiency secondary to any cause
Hypertonic uterine action
Shoulder dystocia
Delay in delivering the aftercoming head of a breech
Abruption
Cord prolapse
Cord compression.

Other causes of a 'flat' baby which fails to breathe spontaneously and effectively at birth are not related to birth asphyxia. These include maternal opiate use, prematurity, aspiration of mucous/meconium, cardiac, respiratory, muscle and CNS problems, birth trauma, Jeune's syndrome and lung hypoplasia secondary to prolonged ruptured membranes. All may however lead to postnatal asphyxia if timely resuscitation is not commenced.

HOW SHOULD THE ASPHYXIATED NEONATE BE RESUSCITATED?

When animal neonates are subject to experimental asphyxia, there is an early period of gasping followed by a period of primary apnoea lasting 1–2 min. Following this there commences a period of irregular gasping for around 3 min during which the heart rate and blood pressure begin to fall. Finally terminal apnoea intervenes, and if not resuscitated the animal dies. These phases are associated with increasing acidosis, such that in terminal apnoea the pH is $< 7{\cdot}00$.

Whatever its failings as a predictive tool, the Apgar score achieves the end of encouraging assessment of the newborn, and in particular heart rate and respiration. At its simplest, if the baby does not breathe and has a heart rate of > 100, the apnoea is primary and breathing will start spontaneously or after sensory stimulation. If the heart rate is < 100, the apnoea is terminal and active measures must be taken (Kjellmer 1988).

Techniques of neonatal resuscitation are covered in most neonatology and obstetric texts (Robertson 1986, Kjellmer 1988), and there is little controversy over basic measures. Problems have arisen however over the practical implementation of these measures and the availability of suitably trained key personnel. Around 70% of neonates needing resuscitation come from predictably high risk groups, whilst 30% are unexpected (Gupta & Tizard 1967). Thus whilst a paediatrician should be present at any high risk delivery, any delivery may unexpectedly result in the birth of a baby in urgent need of resuscitation. Immediate resuscitation of a 'flat' neonate is therefore a skill with which every practising obstetrician and midwife should be familiar.

In an effort to establish basic and workable guidelines for all units, a working party with representatives from the British Paediatric Association, College of Anaesthetists, Royal College of Midwives and Royal College of Obstetricians and Gynaecologists was formed. This reported in 1989, and produced two booklets; Resuscitation of the Newborn parts 1 and 2, basic and advanced resuscitation respectively, detailing a suitable training programme for doctors and midwives. It is recommended that a consultant paediatrician in each district should be nominated to ensure that all midwives and doctors dealing with neonates at birth are capable of basic resuscitation of the newborn (BRNB). This emphasizes the need to keep babies warm and dry, the potential dangers of unnecessary oropharyngeal suction, ventilation with a bag and mask and cardiac massage, and gives practical, illustrated and coherent advice. The BRNB plan is summarized in Figure 11.1.

Every obstetric unit should also have at least one person (usually a paediatrician) available at all times on the premises who has been trained in,

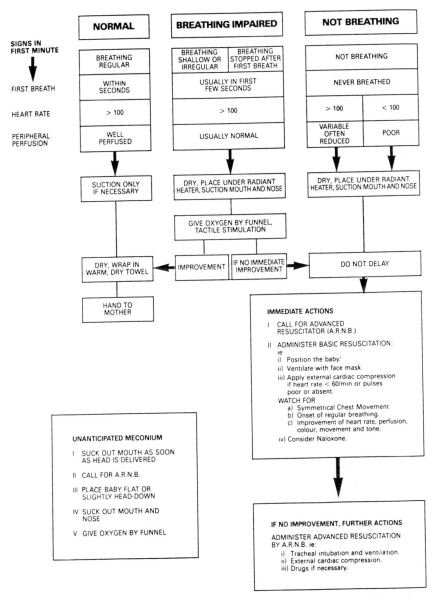

Fig. 11.1 Basic resuscitation of the newborn. Reproduced from *Resuscitation of the newborn* with permission from the Royal College of Obstetricians & Gynaecologists and the British Paediatric Association.

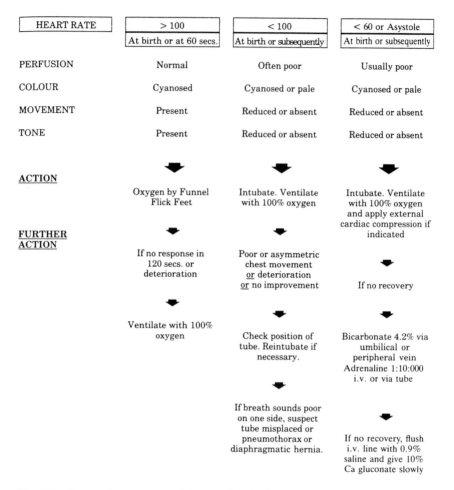

HEART RATE	> 100	< 100	< 60 or Asystole
	At birth or at 60 secs.	At birth or subsequently	At birth or subsequently
PERFUSION	Normal	Often poor	Usually poor
COLOUR	Cyanosed	Cyanosed or pale	Cyanosed or pale
MOVEMENT	Present	Reduced or absent	Reduced or absent
TONE	Present	Reduced or absent	Reduced or absent

ACTION

Oxygen by Funnel
Flick Feet

Intubate. Ventilate
with 100% oxygen

Intubate. Ventilate
with 100% oxygen
and apply external
cardiac compression if
indicated

**FURTHER
ACTION**

If no response in
120 secs. or
deterioration

Poor or asymmetric
chest movement
or deterioration
or no improvement

If no recovery

Ventilate with 100%
oxygen

Check position of
tube. Reintubate if
necessary.

Bicarbonate 4.2% via
umbilical or
peripheral vein
Adrenaline 1:10:000
i.v. or via tube

If breath sounds poor
on one side, suspect
tube misplaced or
pneumothorax or
diaphragmatic hernia.

If no recovery, flush
i.v. line with 0.9%
saline and give 10%
Ca gluconate slowly

Fig. 11.2 Suggested management of the apnoeic baby. Reproduced from *Resuscitation of the newborn* with permission from the Royal College of Obstetricians & Gynaecologists and the British Paediatric Association.

and can administer, advanced resuscitation of the newborn (ARNB). This includes intubation and ventilation, umbilical vein catheterization and the administration of sodium bicarbonate, adrenalin and calcium gluconate. The suggested management of apnoea is shown in Figure 11.2. Other aspects covered include the management of meconium aspiration (Fig. 11.3), hydrops fetalis, diaphragmatic herniae, pneumothorax and acute blood loss. These manuals should be available on all delivery suites and be required reading for all doctors and midwives.

Most asphyxiated neonates respond well to immediate resuscitation, 93% of infants with Apgar scores of 0 at 1 min and/or 0–3 at 5 min being normal at follow up (Thomson et al 1977). If a baby fails to respond,

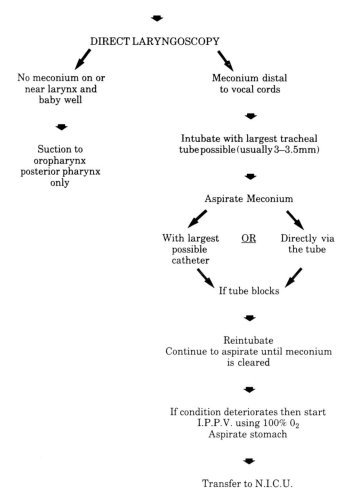

Fig. 11.3   Management of meconium aspiration. Reproduced from *Resuscitation of the newborn* with permission from the Royal College of Obstetricians & Gynaecologists and the British Paediatric Association.

however, how long should resuscitative efforts continue? Studies of severely asphyxiated term neonates have shown babies who do not breathe spontaneously within 30 min of birth or the return of cardiac output to have a very poor prognosis, either dying or developing quadriplegia (Steiner & Nelligan 1975, Koppe & Kleiverda 1984). Other studies have shown an Apgar score of 0–3 at 20 min (Nelson & Ellenberg 1981) and no spontaneous respiration by 20 min (Ergander et al 1983) to correlate well with death and also severe handicap in survivors. Resuscitation should therefore be abandoned if an infant has no cardiac output after 10 min or does not breathe spontaneously by 30 min (Levene 1988b).

Ongoing management of neonates with hypoxic-ischaemic encephalopathy is reviewed in specialist paediatric texts (Levene 1987, Levene 1988b, Hill & Volpe 1989).

The fact that only a small proportion of neurodevelopmental handicap can be attributed to birth asphyxia should not be taken to imply that a *laissez-faire* attitude towards labour and delivery is justified. As long as any fresh stillbirth, neonatal death or handicap is related to asphyxia, close and prompt attention to labour, delivery and presumed fetal distress, however imprecise our monitoring techniques, is mandatory.

REFERENCES

Adsett D B, Fitz C R, Hill A 1985 Hypoxic ischaemic cerebral injury in the term newborn: correlation of CT findings with neurological outcome. Dev Med Child Neurol 27: 155–160

Amiel-Tison C, Ellison P 1986 Birth asphyxia in the full term newborn: early assessment and outcome. Dev Med Child Neurol 28: 671–682

Apgar V 1953 A proposal for a new method of evaluation of the newborn infant. Curr Res Anesth Analg 32: 260–267

Archer L N J, Levene M I, Evans D H 1986 Cerebral artery doppler ultrasonography for prediction of outcome after perinatal asphyxia. Lancet 2: 1116–1118

Azzopardi D, Wyatt J S, Cady E B et al 1989 Prognosis of newborn infants with hypoxic ischaemic brain injury assessed by phosphorous magnetic resonance spectrometry. Paediatr Res 25: 445–451

Beverley D W, Chance G 1984 Cord blood gases, birth asphyxia and intraventricular haemorrhage. Arch Dis Child 59: 884–897

Blair E, Stanley F J 1988 Intrapartum asphyxia: a rare cause of cerebral palsy. J Paediatr 112: 515–519

Brown J K, Purvis R J, Forfar J O, Cockburn F 1974 Neurological aspects of perinatal asphyxia. Dev Med Child Neurol 16: 567–580

Calvert S A, Hoskins E M, Fong K W, Forsyth S C 1986 Periventricular leukomalacia; ultrasonic diagnosis and neurological outcome. Acta Paediatr Scand 75: 489–496

Catlin E A, Carpenter M W, Brann B S et al 1986 The Apgar score revisited: influence of gestational age. J Pediatr 109: 865–868

Dennis J, Johnson A, Mutch L, Yudkin P, Johnson P 1989 Acid-base status at birth and neurodevelopmental outcome at 4½ years. Am J Obstet Gynecol 161: 213–220

Den Ouden L, van Bel F, van de Bor M, Stijnen T, Ruys J 1987 Doppler flow velocity in anterior cerebral artery for prediction of outcome following birth asphyxia. Lancet 1: 562

de Vries L S, Dubowitz L M S, Dubowitz V et al 1985 Predictive value of cranial ultrasound in the newborn baby: a reappraisal. Lancet 2: 137–140

de Vries L S, Larroche J C, Levene M I 1988 Germinal matrix haemorrhage and intraventricular haemorrhage/cerebral ischaemic lesions. In: Levene M I, Bennett M J, Punt J (eds) Fetal and neonatal neurology and neurosurgery. Churchill Livingstone, Edinburgh, pp 312–338

Dijxhoorn M J, Visser G H A, Fidler V J, Touwen B C L, Huisjes H J 1986 Apgar score, meconium and acidemia at birth in relation to neonatal neurological morbidity in term infants. Br J Obstet Gynaecol 93: 217–222

Ellenberg J H, Nelson K B 1979 Birth weight and gestational age in children with cerebral palsy or seizure disorders. Am J Dis Child 133: 1044

Ellenberg J H, Nelson K B 1988 Cluster of perinatal events identifying infants at high risk for death or disability. J Pediatr 113: 546–552

Ergander U, Eriksson M, Zetterstrom R 1983 Severe neonatal asphyxia: incidence and prediction of outcome in the Stockholm area. Acta Paediatr Scand 72: 321–325

Fenichel G M 1983 Hypoxic-ischemic encephalopathy in the newborn. Arch Neurol 40: 261–266

Fernandez F, Verdu A, Quero J, Perez-Higueras A 1987 Serum CPK-BB isoenzyme in the assessment of brain damage in asphyctic term infants. Acta Paediatr Scand 76: 914–918

Fields L M, Entman S S, Boehm F H 1983 Correlation of the one minute Apgar score and the pH value of umbilical arterial blood. South Med J 76: 1477–1479

Finer N N, Robertson C M, Richards R T, Pinnell L E, Peters K L 1981 Hypoxic ischemic encephalopathy in term neonates: perinatal factors and outcome. J Pediatr 98: 112–117

Finer N N, Robertson C M, Peters K L, Coward J H 1983 Factors affecting outcome in hypoxic ischaemic encephalopathy in term infants. Am J Dis Child 137: 21–25

Flodmark O 1988 Computed tomography and magnetic resonance imaging of the neonatal central nervous system. In: Levene M I, Bennett M J, Punt J (eds) Fetal and neonatal neurology and neurosurgery. Churchill Livingstone, Edinburgh, pp 122–138

Freeman J M, Nelson K B 1988 Intrapartum asphyxia and cerebral palsy. Pediatrics 82: 240–249

Freud S 1897 Die Infantile Cerebrallahmung, A Holder, Wien

Gilstrap L C, Leveno K J, Burris J, Williams M L, Little B B 1989 Diagnosis of birth asphyxia on the basis of fetal pH, Apgar score, and newborn cerebral dysfunction. Am J Obstet Gynecol 161: 825–830

Gupta J M, Tizard J P M 1967 The sequence of events in neonatal apnoea. Lancet i: 55–59

Hall D M B 1989 Birth asphyxia and cerebral palsy. Br Med J 299: 279–282

Hamilton P A, Hope P, Reynolds E O R 1988 Magnetic resonance spectroscopy. In: Levene M I, Bennett M J, Punt J (eds) Fetal and neonatal neurology and neurosurgery. Churchill Livingstone, Edinburgh, pp 219–228

Hill A, Volpe J J 1989 Perinatal asphyxia: clinical aspects. Clin Perinatol 16: 435–458

Huisjes H J, Touwen B C L, Hoekstra J et al 1980 Obstetrical-neonatal neurological relationships. A replication study. Eur J Obstet Gynaecol Reprod Biol 10: 247–256

International Classification of Diseases 1980 9th rev, Clinical modifications, 2nd edn Washington DC, DHSS publication no (PHS) 80, 1260

James L S, Weisbrot I M, Prince C E, Holaday D A, Apgar V 1958 The acid base status of human infants in relation to birth asphyxia and the onset of respiration. J Pediatr 52: 379–384

Kjellmer I 1988 Prenatal and intrapartum asphyxia. In: Levene M I, Bennett M J, Punt J (eds) Fetal and neonatal neurology and neurosurgery. Churchill Livingstone, Edinburgh, pp 357–369

Koppe J G, Kleiverda G 1984 Severe asphyxia and outcome of survivors. Resuscitation 12: 193–206

Lancet 1988 Biochemical assessment of birth asphyxia. Lancet 2: 548–549

Lancet 1989a Neonatal seizures. Lancet 2: 135–137

Lancet 1989b Cerebral palsy, intrapartum care and a shot in the foot. Lancet 2: 1251–1252

Lauener P A, Calame A, Janecek P, Bossart H, Monod J F 1983 Systematic pH measurements in the umbilical artery: causes and predictive value of neonatal acidosis. J Perinat Med 11: 278–285

Levene M I 1987 Neonatal neurology. Current Reviews in Paediatrics 3. Churchill Livingstone, Edinburgh

Levene M I 1988a The asphyxiated newborn infant. In: Levene M I, Bennett M J, Punt J (eds) Fetal and neonatal neurology and neurosurgery. Churchill Livingstone, Edinburgh, pp 370–382

Levene M I 1988b Management and outcome of birth asphyxia. In: Levene M I, Bennett M J, Punt J (eds) Fetal and neonatal neurosurgery. Churchill Livingstone, Edinburgh, pp 383–392

Levene M I, Kornberg J, Williams T H C 1985 The incidence and severity of post-asphyxial encephalopathy in full term infants. Early Hum Dev 11: 21–26

Levene M I, Sands C, Grindulis H, Moore J R 1986 Comparison of two methods of predicting outcome in perinatal asphyxia. Lancet 1: 67–68

Levene M I, Fenton A C, Evans D H, Archer L N J, Shortland D B, Gibson N A 1989 Severe birth asphyxia and abnormal cerebral blood flow velocity. Dev Med Child Neurol 31: 427–434

Lipper E G, Voorhies T M, Ross G, Vannucci R C, Auld P 1986 Early predictors of 1 year outcome for infants asphyxiated at birth. Dev Med Child Neurol 28: 303–309

Lipp-Zwahlen A E, Deonna T, Micheli J L, Calame A, Chrzanowski R, Cetre E 1985 Prognostic value of neonatal CT scans in asphyxiated term babies: low density score compared with neonatal neurological signs. Neuropediatrics 16: 209–217

Lissauer T J, Steer P J 1986 The relation between the need for intubation at birth, abnormal cardiotocograms in labour and cord artery blood gas and pH values. Br J Obstet Gynaecol 93: 1060–1066

Lou H C, Lassen N A, Friis-Hansen B 1979 Impaired autoregulation of cerebral blood flow in the distressed newborn infant. J Pediatr 94: 118–121

Low J A, Galbraith R S, Muir D W, Killen H L, Pater E A, Karchmar E J 1983 Intrapartum fetal hypoxia: a study of long term morbidity. Am J Obstet Gynecol 145: 129–134

Low J A, Galbraith R S, Muir D W, Killen H L, Pater E A, Karchmar E J 1984 Factors associated with motor and cognitive deficits in children after intrapartum fetal hypoxia. Am J Obstet Gynecol 148: 533–539

Low J A, Galbraith R S, Muir D W, Killen H L, Pater E A, Karchmar E J 1985 The relationship between perinatal hypoxia and newborn encephalopathy. Am J Obstet Gynecol 152: 256–260

Lupton B A, Hill A, Roland E H et al 1988 Brain swelling in the asphyxiated term newborn: pathogenesis and outcome. Pediatrics 82: 139–146

MacDonald H M, Mulligan J C, Allen A C, Taylor P M 1980 Neonatal asphyxia 1. Relationship of obstetric and neonatal complications to neonatal mortality in 38 405 consecutive deliveries. J Pediatr 96: 898–902

Marrin M, Paes B A 1988 Birth asphyxia: does the Apgar score have prognostic value? Obstet Gynecol 72: 120–123

Minchom P, Niswander K, Chalmers I et al 1987 Antecedents and outcome of very early neonatal seizures in infants born at or after term. Br J Obstet Gynaecol 94: 431–439

Mulligan J C, Painter M J, O'Donoghue P A, MacDonald H M, Allen A C, Taylor P M 1980 Neonatal asphyxia 2: neonatal mortality and long-term sequelae. J Pediatr 96: 903–907

Nelson K B 1988 What proportion of cerebral palsy is related to birth asphyxia? J Pediatr 112: 572–574

Nelson K B, Ellenberg J H 1981 Apgar scores as predictors of chronic neurologic disability. Pediatrics 68: 36–44

Nelson K B, Ellenberg J H 1986 Antecedents of cerebral palsy: multivariate analysis of risk. N Engl J Med 315: 81–86

Nelson K B, Ellenberg J H 1987 The asymptomatic newborn and risk of cerebral palsy. Am J Dis Child 141: 1333–1335

Nicolaides K H, Soothill P W 1989 Cordocentesis. In: Studd J W (ed) Progress in obstetrics and gynaecology vol 7. Churchill Livingstone, Edinburgh, pp 123–144

Paneth N, Stark R I 1983 Cerebral palsy and mental retardation in relation to indicators of perinatal asphyxia. An epidemiologic overview. Am J Obstet Gynecol 147: 960–966

Pearce J M, Chamberlain G V P 1987 Ultrasonically guided percutaneous umbilical blood sampling in the management of intrauterine growth retardation. Br J Obstet Gynaecol 94: 318–321

Perlman J M 1989 Systemic abnormalities in term infants following perinatal asphyxia: relevance to long term neurologic outcome. Clin Perinatol 16: 475–484

Resuscitation of the Newborn Parts 1 & 2. Royal College of Obstetricians and Gynaecologists 1989

Robertson N R C 1986 Resuscitation of the newborn. In: Robertson N R C (ed) Textbook of neonatology. Churchill Livingstone, Edinburgh, pp 239–258

Robertson C, Finer N 1985 Term infants with hypoxic-ischemic encephalopathy: outcome at 3·5 years. Dev Med Child Neurol 27: 473–484

Ruth V J, Raivio K O 1988 Perinatal brain damage: predictive value of metabolic acidosis and the Apgar score. Br Med J 297: 24–27

Sarnat H B, Sarnat M S 1976 Neonatal encephalopathy following fetal distress. Arch Neurol 33: 696–705

Silverman F, Suidan J, Wasserman J, Antoine C, Young B K 1985 The Apgar score. Is it good enough? Obstet Gynecol 66: 331–336

Sinha S K, Davies J M, Sims D G, Chiswick M L 1985 Relation between periventricular haemorrhage and ischaemic brain lesions diagnosed by ultrasound in very preterm infants. Lancet 2: 1154–1155

Steiner H, Neligan G 1975 Perinatal cardiac arrest: quality of the survivors. Arch Dis Child 50: 696–702

Suidan J S, Young B K 1985 Acidosis in the vigorous newborn. Obstet Gynecol 65: 361–364

Sykes G S, Molloy P M, Johnson P et al 1982 Do Apgar scores indicate asphyxia? Lancet 1: 494–496

Thomson A J, Searle M, Russell G 1977 Quality of survival after severe birth asphyxia. Arch Dis Child 52: 620–626

Thorp J A, Sampson J E, Parisi V M, Creasy R K 1989 Routine umbilical cord gas determinations? Am J Obstet Gynecol 161: 600–605

Touwen B C L, Huisjes H J 1984 Acidaemia and its neurological effects. In: Clinch J, Mathews T (eds) Proceedings of IX European Congress of Perinatal Medicine. MTP Press, Dublin, Ireland, pp 99–103

Trounce J Q, Levene M I 1988 Ultrasound imaging of the neonatal brain. In: Levene M I, Bennett M J, Punt J (eds) Fetal and neonatal neurology and neurosurgery. Churchill Livingstone, Edinburgh, pp 139–148

Visser G H A, Dijxhoorn M J 1987 Intrapartum cardiotocogram, Apgar score and acidaemia at birth: relationship to neonatal neurological morbidity. In: Kubli F et al (eds) Perinatal events and brain damage in surviving children. Springer Verlag, Heidelberg, p 168

Walsh P, Jedeikin R, Ellis G, Primhak R, Makela S K 1982 Assessment of neurologic outcome in asphyxiated term infants by use of serial CK-BB isoenzyme measurement. J Pediatr 101: 988–992

Weindling A M, Wilkinson A R, Cook J, Calvert S A, Fok T F, Rochefort M J 1985 Perinatal events which precede periventricular haemorrhage and leukomalacia in the newborn. Br J Obstet Gynaecol 92: 1218–1223

Westgren M, Harmquist P, Ingemarsson I, Svenningsen N 1984 Intrapartum acidosis in preterm infants: fetal monitoring and longterm morbidity. Obstet Gynecol 63: 355–359

12. The lower urinary tract in pregnancy, labour and the puerperium

C. G. W. Barnick   L. Cardozo

During pregnancy the physiology and functional anatomy of the lower urinary tract change and as a result many women develop urinary symptoms. However a surprisingly small number develop urological complications other than urinary tract infection.

During and immediately after labour the lower urinary tract is particularly vulnerable to damage. For example urinary retention may occur in relation to epidural analgesia and forceps delivery, and prolonged labour may cause pressure necrosis and fistula formation. Many of these problems have been overcome by changes in obstetric practice such as the avoidance of prolonged labour and early catheterization.

In this chapter the problems that are encountered will be divided into complications of:

1. Pregnancy
2. Labour
3. Puerperium

COMPLICATIONS OF PREGNANCY

During pregnancy renal physiology is considerably altered. Effective renal plasma flow and glomerular filtration rate are substantially increased early in pregnancy. This occurs in response to a combination of factors: an increase in the cardiac output, the relatively hypervolaemic state of pregnancy and endocrine factors such as increased secretion of aldosterone, prolactin, cortisol and placental lactogen (Phillips & Kwart 1983). This leads to a significant increase in the mean 24 h urine output in the first trimester, and may also cause increased nocturnal urine production (Parboosingh & Doig 1973). Simultaneously the lower urinary tract undergoes considerable morphological changes as a result of mechanical and hormonal influences. The ureters may be compressed by the gravid uterus and fetus or possibly by the engorged ovarian veins (the right ureter is compressed more than the left as the sigmoid colon provides relative protection to the left ureter). Endocrine effects due mainly to increased levels of gonadotrophins and progesterone lead to hypertrophy of the ureteric muscle, tissue oedema and an alteration in the spatial relationship of cells within the ureteric wall, which ultimately cause the ureter to become hypotonic and dilated (Fainstat 1963).

Controversy exists as to the relative importance of these factors, hormonal or mechanical, but together they are responsible for the genesis of the ureteral and calyceal dilatation, which is seen in 81% to 93% of pregnancies (Fayad et al 1973).

The bladder and urethra are also affected, the epithelium becomes relatively hyperaemic and the high oestrogen levels influence the lining of the urethra to become more squamous-like.

URINARY SYMPTOMS

Symptoms of urinary frequency and stress incontinence are commonly encountered during pregnancy.

Urinary frequency

Frequency of micturition is so common that it has been described as one of the four cardinal symptoms of pregnancy. It occurs in approximately 81% of pregnancies, usually starts in the first trimester and once present it generally becomes progressively worse until term (Francis 1960a).

Several aetiological factors have been implicated including increased fluid intake and subsequent urine output, and mechanical factors such as the pressure exerted on the bladder by the pregnant uterus. The relative importance of these was studied in 100 normal pregnant women by Francis (1960a). She concluded that increased fluid intake is the single most important factor. In the third trimester a reduction in bladder capacity may further complicate the situation but this remains controversial and requires more detailed evaluation.

Stress incontinence

It is well known that the pelvic floor may be damaged during vaginal delivery, and that this increases the risk of stress incontinence developing in the future (Snooks et al 1986). But it has been noted that symptoms of stress incontinence may develop in the antenatal period in about 50% of primigravida and the majority of multigravida, suggesting that it is the whole pregnancy and not simply the delivery which is important in the genesis of this symptom (Francis 1960b). Stanton et al (1980) also showed pregnancy rather than delivery to be the important factor.

Pelvic floor exercises have previously been widely prescribed as a preventive measure for stress incontinence during pregnancy and the puerperium, despite the lack of any supportive scientific evidence. However a recent controlled study from Denmark shows that training of the pelvic floor using a simple regimen of 50 brief, maximal pelvic floor contractions morning and evening during the third trimester and puerperium, as compared to pelvic floor exercises in the puerperium alone, leads to a significant improvement in pelvic floor contractility at 8 weeks and 8 months postpartum (Nielsen et al 1988). This, together with previous evidence of the efficacy of pelvic floor exercises in the treatment of stress incontinence, would suggest that a simple regimen of pelvic floor exercises should be advocated during pregnancy as a useful preventive measure.

BACTERURIA IN PREGNANCY

Bacteruria in pregnancy can be divided into three main entities, asymptomatic bacteruria, acute cystitis and acute pyelonephritis.

Asymptomatic bacteruria

This is the most common medical complication of pregnancy. It occurs in 2–10% of pregnant women, which is similar to the prevalence seen in women who are not pregnant. Surprisingly there is little, if any, evidence to suggest that pregnancy is a significant risk factor in relation to this problem. Of greater importance is the outcome of asymptomatic urinary tract infection. In non-pregnant women bacteruria is often transient, has a high spontaneous cure rate and rarely leads to pyelonephritis (Williams 1986). During the third trimester of normal pregnancy, physiological changes in the urinary tract such as dilatation, relative obstruction of the ureters and reflux, which are present in 3–4% of women, predispose to symptomatic urinary tract infection. Consequently approximately 25% of women with untreated bacteruria during pregnancy will develop a symptomatic urinary tract infection.

In view of the high prevalence of asymptomatic bacteruria and the possible prevention of pyelonephritis most centres now routinely perform analysis of a midstream specimen of urine on a number of hospital visits. As this practice is both expensive and time consuming, several investigators have studied other possible screening techniques based on the concept of eliminating or reducing the need for culture of non-significant urine samples (Lenke & Van Dorsten 1981, Marquette et al 1985, Van Dorsten & Bannister 1986, McNeely et al 1987). These techniques incorporate microscopy and/or tests for nitrites or leucocyte esterase. The most encouraging report to date is a test looking for both nitrites and leucocyte esterase in the urine using a lab stick to give a sensitivity and specificity for urinary tract infection of greater than 90% (Robertson & Duff 1988). This might therefore offer a quicker and cheaper alternative to routine microscopy, culture and sensitivity which could be reserved for those patients who have a positive screening test result.

The treatment of asymptomatic bacteruria outside pregnancy remains controversial. In pregnancy, however, the increased risk of upper tract involvement represents a significant risk to both mother and fetus, therefore all women with asymptomatic bacteruria in pregnancy should be treated. Such a policy will prevent 80% of cases of antenatal pyelonephritis (McNeely 1988).

The choice of antibiotic and the duration of antibiotic treatment is the subject of some debate. In pregnancy the additional risks of the effect of antibiotic treatment on the mother and fetus must be carefully considered. The beta-lactam antibiotics (penicillins and cephalosporins) are probably the safest antimicrobials to use (Chow & Jewesson 1985), whilst sulphonomides, Septrin and aminoglycosides are relatively contraindicated as they are potentially harmful to the fetus. Most urinary pathogens contracted outside hospital are sensitive to penicillins or cephalosporins, but the ideal dose and duration of therapy are not yet clear. Single dose therapy has obvious advantages as compliance is ensured, toxicity is minimized and it is cost effective, but there is a higher risk of long-term recurrence. A recent study shows that single dose therapy with amoxycillin cures only 75% of women and suggests that the failure rate of 25% might be due to renal rather than bladder bacteruria (Jakobi et al 1987). Therefore, until larger prospective controlled studies comparing single dose treatment to standard short course antibiotic therapy (7–14 days) have been performed, the latter should continue to be the treatment of choice for asymptomatic bacteruria (McNeely 1988).

Whatever treatment is given for bacteruria in pregnancy following therapy, monthly urine culture should be performed because of the high risk of recurrence. Long-term antibiotic cover is only indicated in women who have recurrent infection (more than 2), or where there are other underlying features such as diabetes or neurological disease.

Acute cystitis

This occurs in approximately 1% of pregnant women. It is more common in the second trimester, is not usually proceeded by asymptomatic bacteruria and rarely proceeds to pyelonephritis (Harris et al 1982). Thus it is considered to be a separate entity although the treatment is the same as for asymptomatic bacteruria.

Acute pyelonephritis

The incidence is approximately 1–2% in pregnant women. It is one of the commonest causes of hospitalization during pregnancy. Pyelonephritis is usually a sequel to untreated asymptomatic bacteruria, and can therefore be prevented in at least 70% of cases by the prompt treatment of this condition (Little 1966, Gilstrap et al 1981). It classically presents with nausea, rigors, loin pain, frequency and dysuria. Treatment must be aggressive as it may be a life threatening condition. Bacteraemia occurs in about 7% and septic shock in about 1–2% of cases (Duff 1984). Patients should be admitted to hospital for rehydration and parenteral antibiotic therapy including a penicillin (ampicillin) together with an aminoglycoside (gentamicin) for 5 days, followed by a 10-day course of oral therapy. The recurrence rate following successful treatment of this type and duration is approximately 10%, and this does not appear to be greatly affected by long-term antibiotic prophylaxis (Lenke et al 1983), which is not recommended unless recurrent infection occurs.

There is some evidence to suggest that bacteruria, particularly if it is difficult to eradicate, serves as a marker for underlying renal tract abnormalities (Neaye 1979). Therefore all women with recurrent or relapsing infection during pregnancy need further investigation after the puerperium, but this should not be undertaken until at least 3 months postpartum, to allow all the pregnancy related anatomical and physiological changes to resolve.

URINARY RETENTION

Urinary retention is not commonly encountered during pregnancy. The usual urological, neurological and psychogenic causes may occur, but impaction of the retroverted gravid uterus at about 16 weeks gestation is the classic cause. Despite the fact that it was described as early as 1754 (Smellie) and has been studied in some detail, it is still not clear exactly why this should occur. The usual explanation is that the bladder is displaced into the lower abdomen thus stretching and narrowing the urethra. The validity of this theory has been investigated and disproved by radiological studies which showed that during pregnancy the urethro-vesical angle is at a normal level and the urethra is not elongated (Francis 1960a). She concluded that urinary retention is the result of the pelvic tumour (the enlarged uterus) interfering with the normal mechanism by which the internal urethral meatus opens, and is not due to anatomical repositioning of the bladder neck. Treatment of this problem is simple: catheterization to empty the bladder, and manual correction of the position of the uterus using a ring or Hodge pessary to maintain it in anteversion. Where the bladder has become grossly overdistended, voiding difficulties may ensue. Careful monitoring of fluid intake and output, together with an ultrasound scan to check for a residual urine are therefore recommended prior to discharge from hospital.

URINARY CALCULI

Physical and biochemical changes in pregnancy, e.g. stasis, obstruction, and infection make stone formation more likely in the pregnant patient.

Despite this, the overall rate probably varies little from the non-pregnant population of comparable age (Cumming & Taylor 1979). The incidence of urinary calculi in pregnancy is only approximately 0·3%, but they may cause significant pathology. Delay in diagnosis and definitive therapy may result in permanent renal damage (Harris & Dunnihoo 1967). Symptoms are atypical during pregnancy, particularly after the first trimester. Acute pyelonephritis is the commonest presentation whilst haematuria is not a reliable finding. The pyelonephritis in pregnant women with an underlying calculus may respond to antibiotic treatment supporting the need for a postpartum intravenous urogram in all women who develop acute pyelonephritis in pregnancy.

The stones are usually single, predominately of calcium composition and about 50% are passed spontaneously.

Criteria indicating the need for urological investigation during pregnancy include:

1. Symptoms suggestive of calculi, i.e. painful haematuria, renal colic or persistent flank pain
2. A previous history of calculi
3. Unusually severe pyelonephritis unresponsive to therapy
4. Recurrent symptomatic urinary tract infection (Harris & Dunnihoo 1967).

During the first or second trimester a calculus can be safely removed either by basket extraction or ureterolithotomy. In the first or second trimester treatment should be undertaken unless the calculus is asymptomatic and there is no evidence of obstruction. During the third trimester surgery should be as conservative as possible. In cases of obstruction or pyelonephrosis it may be beneficial to initially perform a nephrostomy and delay definitive surgery until after the puerperium.

COMPLICATIONS OF LABOUR

It is generally presumed that during labour the bladder is lifted forwards and upwards to become an abdominal organ, that the urethra subsequently becomes elongated and that the bladder neck is displaced forwards and upwards. This theory was tested as early as 1949 in a radiological study of 32 women in labour! The position of the bladder and urethra was studied by a series of cystograms (Malpas et al 1949). They found that the bladder neck is displaced forwards, but not upwards, that the urethra does not become significantly elongated, but that the bladder neck becomes more funnelled during the second stage of labour.

This dichotomy between what is presumed and what has been proven many years ago illustrates the lack of knowledge surrounding the bladder during labour and partially explains why care of the lower urinary tract is often haphazard. In labour there are three important urinary tract complications: voiding difficulties leading to urinary retention, urinary fistulae, and infection. The role of catheterization in relation to these problems also needs to be considered.

Voiding difficulties

In labour, voiding difficulties are not caused by upward displacement and elongation of the urethra, they are the result of forward displacement and compression against the symphysis pubis (Malpas et al 1949). Little has been documented on the incidence or the management of this seemingly common problem.

During labour especially under epidural analgesia the bladder is particularly prone to painless overdistension (Weil & Reis 1983), and it has been reported that this may cause long-term voiding dysfunction (Tapp & Cardozo 1989). In some centres this has led to the adoption of routine indwelling urethral catheterization in patients who have epidural analgesia in labour, particularly if they undergo forceps delivery. Our data (Barnick et al 1990) suggests that this is a safe and effective method of management, but that in/out catheterization is probably preferable, as it is less uncomfortable, does not delay early mobilization and antibiotic cover is not required.

At present the diagnosis of voiding difficulty relies on recording the frequency of micturition and clinical findings. It is made when the patient has not voided for several hours, or when the bladder is found to be palpably distended. This rather simplistic approach means that many women who are relatively dehydrated during labour are catheterized unnecessarily because they are unable to pass urine, and others who do go into urinary retention are overlooked until the bladder is very overdistended particularly if they have epidural analgesia.

A more rational approach would involve the use of an accurate fluid balance chart in labour. Theoretically this would ensure adequate hydration and allow an estimate of expected urine output to be made. However the diuresis during labour is variable and also depends on other factors such as the length of labour and the presence of oedema at the start of labour. Thus although such a regimen appears sensible it has not yet been proven to reduce the rate of unnecessary catheterization and facilitate the early diagnosis of urinary retention. As one episode of acute urinary retention can cause long-term voiding difficulties, early diagnosis and appropriate management are essential.

Urinary fistula

In Europe and the United States of America urinary fistulae are now rarely seen as a complication of pregnancy, whilst in developing countries prolonged labour continues to be a common cause of destruction of the urethra and bladder base (Shigui & Qinge 1979). This is due to changes in obstetric practice in the West, especially a marked reduction in the length of the second stage of labour and careful observation of labour progress to avoid prolonged obstructed labour. Together these two factors have almost eradicated the risk of urinary fistulae developing during delivery.

The bladder base, proximal urethra and anterior vaginal wall are particularly prone to injury by prolonged obstructed labour as the presenting part causes compression against the back of the symphysis pubis. This may lead to pressure necrosis (Malpas et al 1949, Lee et al 1988). Fistulae also occur following Caesarean section, particularly Caesarean hysterectomy and these are usually vesicovaginal.

The timing of fistula repair and the choice of approach, abdominal or vaginal, remain a matter of controversy. The general consensus of opinion is that small fistulae may be expected to close spontaneously with continuous bladder drainage and antibiotics. Large fistulae require surgical repair but should be performed once tissue oedema and infection have resolved, usually after about 3 months. Low fistulae are easier to repair vaginally whilst high or complex fistulae may require an abdominal approach (Kelly 1979, Lawson 1979, Lee et al 1988). Using such a regimen Vanderputte (1985) has reported cure rates as high as 88·7% in 89 women with different types of pregnancy related urinary fistulae in a West African population.

Currently there is growing, but as yet unsubstantiated, concern amongst gynaecologists in the West that the trend towards a longer second stage of labour particularly under epidural anaesthesia will lead to a resurgence of this devastating problem.

Catheterization

During labour and following delivery women are often catheterized using either in/out or indwelling urethral catheters. In a recent study at Kings College Hospital of 556 women in labour we showed that as many as 29% of women are catheterized at some point during labour or delivery. Of these 116 (66%) were in/out and 35 (33%) indwelling urethral catheters. Many of the catheterizations were performed in relation to forceps delivery or Caesarean section. Of the remaining women who were catheterized ($n = 74$) no good reason for catheterization was documented in over half ($n = 48$). This group consists of patients who were incorrectly thought to have developed urinary retention or were catheterized for spurious reasons such as delivery of the placenta. One possible reason behind this high rate of catheterization is the flawed theory that a full bladder may be a serious impediment to labour (Toppozada et al 1967). Read et al (1980) studied 68 women who were catheterized in labour; using a dynamic model of labour they found no significant difference in uterine activity or rate of cervical dilatation following catheterization. They concluded that the act of emptying the bladder has no effect on uterine activity, progress, or the course of labour, except possibly with very large volumes.

The present practice of early catheterization for scant indications might be expected to lead to an increased incidence of cystitis, however, we found no significant increase in urinary tract infection or urinary symptoms in patients who are catheterized during labour. It would therefore seem that catheterization during labour is safe, but it is invasive, so this should not be used as justification of the current rather unscientific practice which obviously requires review.

COMPLICATIONS OF THE PUERPERIUM

The postpartum bladder and lower urinary tract are subject to similar problems to those encountered during pregnancy and delivery. Of particular interest are voiding difficulties, urinary tract infection and urinary symptoms.

Voiding difficulties

There have been few studies to assess bladder function postpartum, and the results of these studies have been contradictory. Bennetts & Judd (1941) found that the bladder is relatively hypotonic after delivery with increased capacity and decreased sensation. These findings have not been supported by more recent studies (Kerr-Wilson & Thompson 1984), which show urodynamic parameters to be within normal limits at 48 h and 4 weeks postpartum.

Voiding difficulties, as assessed by ultrasound estimation of urinary residuals, occur in approximately 11% of women 48 h after delivery (Barnick et al 1990). These are associated with epidural analgesia, longer second stage and forceps delivery. Painless overdistension of the bladder may occur particularly when an epidural anaesthetic has been employed during the delivery. It is therefore imperative that midwifery and medical staff have a high level of awareness to this problem.

Women who have been catheterized during labour should have the catheter removed the following morning unless there is a specific contra-indication. For the next 24 h they should be kept on a strict fluid balance chart to ensure that they are not going into urinary retention although some women may have a very rapid postpartum diuresis which may cause confusion, i.e. they can pass good volumes and still have a large residual Women who are still unable to pass urine should be recatheterized using the suprapubic route. This facilitates monitoring of voiding function, reduces the rate of lower urinary tract infection and avoids repeated catheterization. The supra-pubic catheter can be safely removed once the urinary residuals fall below 50 ml on two consecutive measurements.

URINARY TRACT INFECTION

Urinary tract infection is very common in the postpartum period, occurring in approximately 12% of patients (Barnick et al 1990). The risk of pyelonephritis secondary to asymptomatic bacteriuria remains high, as the physiological changes which occur during pregnancy resolve slowly over a period of about 6 weeks. We would therefore recommend that all women should be investigated for bacteriuria in the postpartum period, using a midstream specimen of urine or dip-slide. If there is positive evidence of infection then appropriate antibiotic treatment should be instituted to prevent serious sequelae.

URINARY SYMPTOMS

Urinary symptoms are common following all types of delivery (Fig. 12.1). The symptom of stress incontinence is present in 20% of patients after spontaneous vaginal delivery, in 24% after forceps delivery and 10% following Caesarean section. Other urinary symptoms such as frequency, dysuria, straining to void and incomplete emptying occur in about 30% of women irrespective of the mode of delivery.

Patients with symptoms of stress incontinence should be taught how to perform pelvic floor exercises if they have not already performed them in the antenatal period. In general, patients can be reassured that their symptoms will usually resolve by 6 weeks postpartum, although some of these women will continue to have problems.

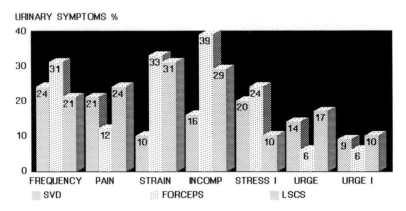

Fig. 12.1   Post partum urinary symptoms and mode of delivery.

CONCLUSION

It is interesting to note that despite the considerable anatomical and physiological changes that occur during pregnancy there are few serious urinary tract sequelae apart from urinary tract infection, which can be safely managed by routine screening and prompt, appropriate antibiotic therapy. Symptoms of stress incontinence remain a problem, although there is now scientific evidence which shows that antenatal and postnatal pelvic floor exercises maintain the strength of the pelvic floor through the latter part of pregnancy and into the puerperium.

Urological emergencies such as urinary calculi and ureteric obstruction should be managed as conservatively as possible, although it is possible to treat these by conventional means without jeopardizing the pregnancy.

During labour and the puerperium a more rational approach towards bladder care is required. Awareness amongst doctors and midwives to the problem of urinary retention and its potential long-term sequelae should be increased. Catheterization should only be performed if there is thought to be a good indication from the data recorded on frequency volume charts, clinical examination and patient symptoms, if serious sequelae such as long-term voiding difficulties are to be avoided without performing large numbers of unnecessary catheterizations. The choice of route of catheterization is important. This should initially be urethral, if when this is removed voiding difficulties persist then a suprapubic catheter should be inserted. Reluctance amongst doctors to use this route increases the risk of multiple urethral catheterizations and urinary tract infection, as the catheter has to be removed in order for voiding function to be assessed.

REFERENCES

Barnick C G W, Benness C J, Cardozo L D 1990 Post-partum voiding dysfunction. In press
Bennetts F A, Judd G E 1941 Studies of the post-partum bladder. Am J Obstet Gynecol 41: 419–427
Chow A W, Jewesson P J 1985 Pharmacokinetics and the safety of antimicrobial agents during pregnancy. Rev Infect Dis 7: 287–313
Cumming D C, Taylor P J 1979 Urologic and obstetric significance of urinary calculi in pregnancy 53(4): 505–508
Duff P 1984 Pyelonephritis in pregnancy. Clin Obstet Gynecol 27(1): 17–31
Fainstat T 1963 Ureteral dilatation in pregnancy: a review. Obstet Gynecol Surv 18: 845–849
Fayad M M, Youssef A F, Zahran M C, Kamel M, Badir M 1973 The ureterocalycael system in normal pregnancy. Acta Obstet Gynecol Scand 52: 69–73
Francis W J 1960a Disturbances of bladder function in relation to pregnancy. J Obstet Gynaecol Br Emp 67: 353–366
Francis W J 1960b The onset of stress incontinence. J Obstet Gynaecol Brit Emp 67: 899–903
Gilstrap L C, Leveno K J, Cunningham F G et al 1981 Renal infection and pregnancy outcome. Am J Obstet Gynecol 141: 709
Harris R E, Dunnihoo D R 1967 The incidence and significance of urinary calculi in pregnancy. Am J Obstet Gynecol 99(2): 237–241
Harris R E, Gilstrap L C, Pretty A 1982 Single dose antimicrobial therapy for asymptomatic bacteriuria during pregnancy. Obstet Gynecol 59: 546–548
Jakobi P, Neiger R, Merzbach D, Paldi E 1987 Single-dose antimicrobial therapy in the treatment of asymptomatic bacteriuria in pregnancy. Am J Obstet Gynecol 156(5): 1148–1152
Kelly J 1979 Vesicovaginal fistulae. Br J Urol 51: 208–210

Kerr-Wilson R, Thompson S W 1984 Effects of labor on the postpartum bladder. Obstet Gynecol 64: 115–118

Lawson J B 1979 Injuries of the urinary tract. Obstetrics and gynaecology in the tropics and developing countries. Arnold, London, pp 481–522

Lee R A, Symmonds R E, Williams T J 1988 Current status of genitourinary fistula. Obstet Gynecol 72(3) Part I: 313–319

Lenke R R, Van Dorsten J P 1981 The efficacy of the nitrite test and microscopic urinalysis in predicting urine culture results. Am J Obstet Gynecol 140: 427

Lenke R R, Van Dorsten J P, Schifrin B S 1983 Pyelonephritis in pregnancy: a prospective randomized trial to prevent recurrent disease evaluating suppressive therapy with nitrofurantoin and close surveillance. Am J Obstet Gynecol 146: 953–955

Little P J 1966 The incidence of urinary tract infection in 5000 pregnant women. Lancet i: 925–928

McNeely S G Jr 1988 Treatment of urinary tract infection during pregnancy. Clin Obstet Gynecol 31(2): 480–487

McNeely S G Jr, Baselski V S, Ryan G M 1987 An evaluation of two rapid bacteruria screening procedures. Obstet Gynecol 69: 550–552

Malpas P, Jeffcoate T N A, Lister U M 1949 The displacement of the bladder and urethra during labour. J Obstet Gynaecol Br Emp 56(6): 949–960

Marquette G P, Dillard T, Betta S et al 1985 The validity of the leucocyte esterase reagent strip in detecting significant leukocyturia. Am J Obstet Gynecol 153: 888

Neaye R L 1979 Causes of the excessive rates of perinatal mortality and prematurity in pregnancies complicated by maternal urinary tract infections. N Engl J Med 300(15): 819–823

Nielsen C A, Sigsgaard I, Olsen M, Tolstrup M, Danneskiold-Samsoee B, Bock J E 1988 Trainability of the pelvic floor. Acta Obstet Gynecol Scand 67: 437–440

Parboosingh J, Doig A 1973 Studies of nocturia in normal pregnancy. J Obstet Gynaecol Br Commonwth 80: 889–895

Phillips M H, Kwart A M 1983 Urinary tract disease in pregnancy. Clin Obstet Gynecol 26(4): 890–901

Read J A, Miller F C, Yeh S, Platt L D 1980 Urinary bladder distension: effect on labour and uterine activity. Obstet Gynecol 56(5): 565–570

Robertson A W, Duff P 1988 The nitrate and leukocyte esterase tests for the evaluation of asymptomatic bacteriuria in obstetric patients. Obstet Gynecol 71(6) part I: 878–881

Shigui F, Qinge S 1979 Operative treatment of female urinary fistulas. Chin Med J 92(4): 263–268

Snooks S J, Swash M, Henry M M, Setchell M 1986 Risk factors in childbirth causing damage to the pelvic floor innervation. Int J Colorect Dis 1: 20–24

Stanton S L, Kerr-Wilson R, Grant-Harris V 1980 The incidence of urological symptoms in normal pregnancy. Br J Obstet Gynaecol 87: 897–900

Tapp A J S, Meire H, Cardozo L D 1987 The effect of epidural analgesia in post partum voiding. Neurol Urodynamics 6(3): 235–237

Toppozada H K, Gaafar A A, El-Sahwi S 1967 The urinary bladder and uterine activity. Am J Obstet Gynecol 98: 904–907

Vanderputte S R 1985 Obstetric vesicovaginal fistulae: experience with 89 cases. Ann Soc Belg Med Trop 64: 303–309

Van Dorsten J P, Bannister E R 1986 Office diagnosis of asymptomatic bacteriuria in pregnant women. Am J Obstet Gynecol 155(4): 777–780

Williams J D 1986 Bacteruria in pregnancy. In: Asscher A W, Brumfitt W (eds) Microbial disease in nephrology. Wiley, Chichester, pp 159–181

PART THREE

Gynaecology

13. The premature menopause

R. Baber   H. Abdalla   J. Studd

A premature menopause should, ideally, be defined as ovarian failure occurring two standard deviations in years before the mean menopausal age of the study population. As the epidemiological studies necessary to make such a definition meaningful are rarely, if ever, available it is not surprising that a number of arbitrary age-related definitions of premature menopause have arisen. These range from onset before 35 years (Kinch et al 1965, Jones & Rheusen 1967) to onset before 45 years (Jacobs & Murray 1976). The most commonly accepted definition is premature ovarian failure before the age of 40 (Furuhjelm 1960, Netter & Sebaoun 1966, Moraes & Jones 1967, Van der Merwe 1981, Aiman & Smentek 1985, Jewelewicz & Schwartz 1986).

INCIDENCE

Premature ovarian failure (POF) affects approximately 1% of all women under the age of 40. It is associated with between 10% and 28% of primary amenorrhoea and 4–18% of secondary amenorrhoea (Mashchak et al 1981, Kinch et al 1965, Russell et al 1982, Starup et al 1973). The condition is thus not rare, affecting over 110 000 women in the United Kingdom alone.

AETIOLOGY

In most cases a definite aetiology cannot be established. Among the identifiable causes genetic disorders predominate in those cases which present early, and autoimmune disorders are more common in the later-onset presentations (Alper & Garner 1985). Table 13.1 summarizes the causes of premature ovarian failure.

The major genetic cause of premature ovarian failure is ovarian dysgenesis of which sex-chromosome anomalies predominate. Dewald & Spurbeck (1983) reported a 23% incidence of structural sex chromosome abnormalities and an 8% incidence of mosaicism in a group of patients with premature gonadal failure, whilst McDonough et al (1977) found sex

Table 13.1 Causes of premature ovarian failure

Genetic
—Chromosomal
—Familial
—Metabolic
—Immunological
Autoimmune diseases
Infections
Environmental
Iatrogenic
—Surgical
—Chemotherapy
—Irradiation
Idiopathic

---

chromosome abnormalities in 63% of patients in one series, all of whom were less than 63 inches tall. The commonest abnormality in both series was 45XO (Turner's syndrome).

Patients with gonadal dysgenesis may have a normal or abnormal chromosome complement. Those with a normal complement may be either 46XX or 46XY. 46XY gonadal dysgenesis is an X-linked recessive disorder and is rarer than the 46XX variety which is associated with consanguinity and is autosomal recessive in its transmission. Gonadal dysgenesis patients with a normal chromosome complement usually attain normal stature and account for up to one-third of the genetic causes of premature ovarian failure.

Ovarian determinants exist on both the long and short arms of the X chromosome (Simpson 1980). Duplication of one arm does not compensate for the loss of the other, but those with distal breaks do not show ovarian dysgenesis. Deletion of the short arm always results in short stature whilst the relationship of the long arm to stature is not known.

Rarely, autosomal anomalies, mainly Trisomy-13 and -18 are associated

Table 13.2 Genetic causes of premature ovarian failure

Chromosomal
—Turners syndrome
—Pure gonadal dysgenesis
—Familial
—Trisomy-18 and Trisomy-13
Metabolic
—17-alpha-hydroxylase deficiency
—Galactosaemia
—Myotonic dystrophy
Immunological
—Di George Syndrome
—Ataxia telangiectasia
—Mucocutaneous fungal infections

---

with ovarian dysgenesis (Kennedy et al 1977). The clinical significance of this is negligible as these disorders are incompatible with life but their occurrence indicates that ovarian determinants are found on autosomes as well as sex chromosomes.

A rare association of blepharophimosis (congenital dysplasia of the eyelids with small palpebral fissures, ptosis and sometimes dysmorphogenic features), resistant ovary syndrome and premature menopause has also been reported (Fraser et al 1988). The explanation for this association is unknown but may be related to the microdeletion of genetic material containing geographically related but independent genes. When this syndrome is transmitted in an autosomal dominant fashion women exhibiting at least type I blepharophimosis should be counselled regarding their risk of infertility and an early menopause.

The rarest of the metabolic disorders is 17-alpha-hydroxylase deficiency giving rise to patients with primary amenorrhoea, lack of secondary sexual characteristics, increased gonadotrophin levels and hypertension.

Patients with galactosaemia usually need a galactose-free diet to avoid mental retardation. This diet results in a high incidence of ovarian failure (Kaufman et al 1979) which may arise from a metabolic derangement in the ovary or a change in the bioactivity of the gonadotrophin molecule which itself contains both galactose and galactosamine. It may thus be appropriate for mothers suffering from this disorder to follow a galactose-free diet during pregnancy in order to avoid potential damage to the fetal ovaries.

Myotonic dystrophy is a myopathy involving the distal musculature and is associated with cataracts and osseous lesions. Gonadal failure is common in affected males, and 15–20% of affected females suffer from oligo-menorrhoea and increased gonadotrophin levels although hypothalamic-pituitary function is normal (Sagal et al 1975).

Ovarian failure has been reported in patients with various immune deficiency disorders such as ataxia telangiectasia, Di George syndrome and T-cell anomalies. The relationship between premature ovarian failure and human immunovirus infection (AIDS) is not yet known.

Autoimmune diseases are amongst the more commonly known causes of premature ovarian failure particularly in those cases of late onset. Alper & Garner (1985) reported a 39% incidence of autoimmune disease amongst chromosomally competent sufferers of POF, 18% of whom had a positive family history. The majority suffered from autoimmune thyroid disease in contrast to other series which reported a high incidence of Addisons disease (DeMoraes Ruehsen et al 1972, Irvine et al 1968). In these latter instances the ovarian failure appeared to precede the adrenal failure by several years. Rebar et al (1982) have suggested routine testing of adrenal reserve in all patients with POF. However recent work by Kirsop et al (1990) has cast doubt on the reliability of commercially available kits for detection of antiovarian antibodies and, indeed, on the clinical relevance of such investigations.

Mumps is the commonest infection associated with POF. Its effect is maximal during the fetal and pubertal periods when even subclinical infection can result in ovarian failure (Morrison et al 1975). Pelvic tuberculosis may cause ovarian failure in up to 3% of cases (Nogales-Ortiz et al 1979) but it should be remembered that the major cause of amenorrhoea in women suffering from this infection is intrauterine synechiae with endometrial destruction and not ovarian failure.

Jick et al (1977) showed a dose-related effect of smoking on the age of menopause. This effect is believed to be mitigated through polycyclic hydrocarbons found in cigarette smoke which have been shown to destroy oocytes in mice (Gulyas & Mattison 1979). Mahadevan et al (1982) have also reported that an early menopause is associated with poor nutrition, poor health and increased parity.

Successful treatment, with megavoltage irradiation, of women suffering from lymphoreticular disorders is often associated with ovarian failure. Patients receiving pelvic node irradiation for Hodgkins disease commonly receive 4500–5000 rads. Thomas et al (1976) found that radiation doses above 500 rads were commonly associated with ovarian failure and frequently occurred with an inverted Y field. Baker et al (1972) reported a 60% incidence of ovarian failure in patients receiving up to 500 rads and 100% when 800 rads were used. Because of the high cure rate elective oophoropexy and ovarian shielding seem worthwhile, provided the disease is one in which ovarian metastasis is uncommon. These manoeuvres have been shown to reduce the ovarian dosage to between 350 and 400 rads thus preserving ovarian function in some patients. No congenital abnormalities have been reported in the offspring of subsequent pregnancies (Floch 1976). There is no evidence that low-dose irradiation, diagnostic or therapeutic doses of radionuclides, ultraviolet light or domestic microwave appliances cause significant loss of ovarian function (Verp 1983).

Numerous chemotherapeutic agents have been implicated in the aetiology of premature ovarian failure including methotrexate, 6 mercaptopurine, actinomycin and adriamycin. Low-dose cyclophosphamide when used for non-neoplastic conditions is unlikely to cause ovarian failure but high-dose, long-term therapy for neoplasia usually will. The histological appearance of affected ovaries is similar to that seen in the resistant ovary syndrome with numerous primordial follicles (Stillman 1982). These gradually disappear although in rare cases ovarian function is resumed.

Surgery, to the uterus or adnexa, may result in early ovarian failure. Numerous authors have examined early ovarian failure after hysterectomy, reporting incidences ranging from 15–57% (Grogan & Duncan 1955, Kretzchmar & Gardiner 1935). Siddle et al (1987) found 44% of women post-hysterectomy developed ovarian failure by age 45.4 compared with only 13% of their controls. The cause of this remains obscure but may be related to an impairment of ovarian vascular supply or to the loss of some important endocrine contribution by the uterus to the ovary.

Ten percent of patients treated at the Lister Fertility and Endocrinology Clinic, London for a premature menopause developed ovarian failure following adnexal surgery, usually for benign conditions such as endometriosis and simple cysts. This incidence is similar to that reported by others (Jewelewicz & Schwartz 1986) and one can only stress that surgery to the ovaries should be a last resort rather than a first-line treatment. Needle aspiration of cysts either per laparoscope or using transvaginal ultrasound guidance is simple, quick, safe and results in an accurate histological diagnosis in over 90% of cases. Moreover, ovarian suppression using agents such as LHRH analogue will often result in the subsidence of cysts and remission of symptoms without recourse to any surgical procedure at all. Should surgery be necessary, every effort must be made to preserve all normal ovarian tissue and prevent damage to the ovarian blood supply.

PATHOPHYSIOLOGY

In most patients with premature ovarian failure, particularly in the early stages, ovarian biopsy discloses a reduced number of pre-antral follicles (Nakano et al 1978). Beyond this developmental stage gonadotrophins and gonadotrophin receptors are necessary for further development (Jewelewicz & Schwartz 1986) and it is thus possible that a lack of these receptors is the underlying cause of the disorder. The resistant ovary syndrome, first described by Jones & DeMoraes Ruehsen (1979) is similar to and may represent an early stage of premature ovarian failure. In this disorder, it is thought that there is a lack of sensitivity of the gonadotrophin receptors to gonadotrophins or a defect in the adenylate cyclase system leading to a syndrome characterized by amenorrhoea, normal secondary sexual characteristics, apparently normal follicular apparatus and increased gonadotrophin levels. It may occur in association with primary or secondary amenorrhoea (Dewhurst et al 1975) and ovarian biopsy usually discloses a normal number of follicles arrested at the antral stage of development. Pregnancies have been reported in patients with the resistant ovary syndrome, usually after a period of oestrogen administration (Shapiro & Rubin 1977), but occasionally spontaneously (Jewelewicz & Schwartz 1986) suggesting that receptor resistance to gonadotrophins is sometimes reversible.

DIAGNOSTIC CRITERIA

There are no unique clinical features that unequivocally establish the diagnosis of premature ovarian failure. In general the diagnosis is based on a triad of amenorrhoea, elevated gonadotrophin levels and signs and symptoms of oestrogen deficiency. Hot flushes and genital atrophy are present in approximately 50% of patients (Russell et al 1982, Rebar et al

1982, Board et al 1979, Aiman & Smentek 1985, Whitehead & Cust 1987) which is a similar frequency to that seen in 50-year-old women.

Whereas evidence of oestrogen deficiency is usually sought in amenorrhoeic women in order to demonstrate ovarian failure, not all women with ovarian failure will be amenorrhoeic and may ovulate and menstruate sporadically (Rebar et al 1982, Wright & Jacobs 1979). Evidence of autoimmune disease or cytotoxic drug use and stigmata of gonadal dysgenesis such as short stature and sexual immaturity should be sought.

Ultimately, concentrations of gonadotrophins in the menopausal range are necessary to establish a diagnosis of ovarian failure but because of the intermittent nature of the disease, particularly in its early stages, repeated assays may be required at intervals of 2–4 weeks and after any hormone-replacement therapy has been ceased. Serum FSH levels greater than 15 miu/ml are certainly in the perimenopausal range but may be associated with persistence of primordial follicles on biopsy and episodes of ovarian activity. Goldenberg et al (1973) demonstrated that individuals with FSH levels above 40 m i.u./ml without exception had no viable ovarian follicles on biopsy and such patients may be safely regarded as having undergone permanent ovarian failure.

Ovarian biopsy has been advocated by several authors (Maxson & Wentz 1983, Coulam 1983) in order to differentiate between the resistant ovary syndrome and premature ovarian failure since the former can only be diagnosed with certainty by the presence of a normal number of primordial follicles on biopsy. It has also been advocated as a means of diagnosing an autoimmune aetiology but the presence of a perifollicular lymphocytic infiltrate is only associative (and presumptive) evidence of autoimmune disease which is better demonstrated by the presence of humoral anti-ovarian antibody (Leer et al 1980). Biopsy is an invasive procedure. Laparoscopic biopsy specimens are rarely adequate and biopsy at laparotomy is frequently associated with adhesion formation which may result in chronic pain and render the fallopian tubes unsuitable for future donor gamete or zygote transfer. Biopsy is probably only justified in the oligoamenorrhoeic group of patients where at least intermittent ovarian function is suggested and in whom subsequent oestrogen and gonadotrophin therapy may offer some hope of response. In all other cases patients will require hormone replacement therapy and/or infertility counselling irrespective of their diagnosis.

Sex chromosomal analysis should be performed on all patients who present with primary amenorrhoea or with early-onset ovarian failure. Buccal smears are best avoided as X- and Y-chromatin tests are often unreliable for diagnosing sex chromosome abnormalities. Patients who present with later onset ovarian failure should have their adrenal reserve checked and be screened for high titres of anti-andrenal and antithyroid antibodies to preclude incipient autoimmune adrenal or thyroid failure which may follow ovarian failure by a year or more.

THE CONSEQUENCES OF PREMATURE OVARIAN FAILURE

As with a natural menopause around the age of 50, the consequences of early menopause can be divided into short- and long-term. Short-term consequences include vasomotor symptoms such as hot flushes, night sweats, palpitations and headaches, vaginal dryness and dyspareunia, urgency and stress incontinence plus psychological problems including irritability, forgetfulness, poor concentration and insomnia.

To determine the level of symptomatology in our own patients and to assess the psychological implications of a premature menopause, 65 prematurely menopausal women attending the fertility and endocrinology clinics at The Lister Hospital, London and The Royal North Shore Hospital, Sydney were sent a purpose-designed questionnaire subdivided to provide information on the frequency of oestrogen deficiency symptoms, anxieties about sterility, femininity and loss of menses, sexual problems and attitudes of partners. 46 patients replied and the results are shown in Table 13.3. Seventy-six percent of all patients reported some experience of vasomotor symptoms, which is slightly more than that reported in other series. Despite the fact that nearly 40% of women in our series had children prior to the onset of the menopause, some 54% reported that loss of fertility was the most distressing aspect of the menopause, with feeling older and loss of femininity the next most common. Approximately one-third of our patients reported a loss of interest in and enjoyment of sex,

Table 13.3 Attitudes of women suffering a premature menopause

	Yes	No	%
Did you experience hot flushes?	35	11	76
Have you ever had children?	18	28	39
Has your sexual activity			
(a) increased	3		7
(b) decreased	18		39
(c) unchanged	25		54
Has your enjoyment of sex			
(a) increased	3		7
(b) decreased	15		32
(c) unchanged	28		61
What distressed you most when your periods stopped?			
(a) loss of periods	2		5
(b) loss of femininity	6		13
(c) loss of fertility	25		54
(d) feeling older	13		28
When POF was diagnosed was your partner's attitude			
(a) supportive	30		65
(b) unchanged	13		28
(c) unhelpful	3		7

further highlighting the problems of oestrogen deficiency. The majority found that their partners were supportive but only 30% felt that the explanation of their condition by their doctor was in any way adequate.

Long term consequences of a premature menopause include infertility, osteoporosis and an increased risk of cardiovascular disease and stroke.

Infertility

Pregnancy is possible in women with follicular forms of ovarian failure, the resistant-ovary syndrome and, theoretically, in those with autoimmune ovarian failure. Exogenous oestrogens prescribed for these women may stimulate the development of ovarian FSH receptors thus allowing expression of FSH actions including follicular maturation and ovulation although pregnancy may occur coincidentally in some cases due to the intermittent nature of this disease. Check & Case (1984) reported induction of ovulation in hypergonadotrophic women with premature ovarian failure using a sequential combination of oral oestrogen and progestogen therapy followed by a course of human menopausal gonado-trophins (HMG). They postulated that chronically high levels of FSH led to a down-regulation of ovarian FSH receptors and that oestradiol therapy resulted in a temporary suppression of serum FSH and a consequent redevelopment of receptors.

Although no pregnancies have been reported, ovulation has been restored by plasmaphoresis in a patient with myasthenia gravis (Bateman et al 1983) and by glucocorticoid therapy in a patient with a perifollicular lymphocytic infiltrate (Coulam et al 1981). Nevertheless, although numerous authors have reported pregnancies in patients with premature ovarian failure (Alper et al 1986, Shangold et al 1977, Netter et al 1977, Polansky & de Papp 1976, Dewhurst et al 1975, Wright & Jacobs 1979, Tanaka et al 1982) the reality is that the probability of pregnancy in a woman with premature ovarian failure is very low indeed. Forty-three million women in the United States are of reproductive age. If 3% of these suffer primary or secondary amenorrhoea then 10% of this number (129 000) will have premature ovarian failure. Between 1964 and 1986 pregnancy has been reported in less than 20 women in the USA with this disorder and the probability of pregnancy must thus be worse than 1 in 6000. To offer these women treatment based on oestrogens and gonadotrophins is to offer them very little at all.

Oocyte donation

In 1884 Pancoast reported the first pregnancy following the use of donated sperm (Finegold 1976) but it was not until 1983 that the first pregnancy following the use of a donated oocyte was reported by Trounson et al. In 1984 Lutjen et al reported a successful pregnancy using in vitro fertilization of a donated embryo in a patient with primary ovarian failure. They used a sequential form of hormone replacement therapy, employing oral oestradiol valerate and progesterone pessaries, to produce plasma hormone levels similar to those found in a normal ovulatory cycle, performed intra-uterine embryo transfer of a two-cell embryo and then maintained the ensuing pregnancy with oral oestradiol for 12 weeks and intramuscular progesterone for 19 weeks. The obvious difficulties experienced with this protocol were synchronization of cycles between donor and recipient, its relative complexity and the narrow window of transfer. In 1987 Serhal & Craft reported a simplified protocol allowing greater flexibility. This regimen consisted of oral oestradiol valerate (6 or 8 mg) daily for 2–4 weeks whilst waiting for a donor to be stimulated augmented with progesterone 100 mg i.m. or 300 mg orally starting on the day prior to recovery of donated oocytes. This concept of a prolonged proliferative phase correctly assumed that incremental changes in oestrogen and progesterone were less important than the development of adequate secretory change in a fully developed proliferative endometrium. The Lister Fertility Clinic protocol (shown in Fig. 13.1) requires all patients with POF to take cyclical oestradiol valerate 2 mg and norgestrel 0.5 mg (Cycloprogynova 2 mg, Schering UK) and to phone the clinic each month prior to commencing their progestogens. If no eggs are likely to be available soon, they are instructed to take the progestogens and induce their regular withdrawal bleed. If eggs are available they are continued on oestradiol valerate 2 mg until 6 days before embryo transfer when the dose is increased to 4 mg for 4 days then 6 mg plus 100 mg i.m. progesterone. This protocol ensures that all patients are available to receive eggs and provides patients with balanced hormone replacement therapy whilst waiting for treatment.

Tubal transfer of donated zygotes was first reported in 1987 by Yovich et al and in 1988 Asch et al reported pregnancies following gamete intra fallopian transfer (GIFT) of donated oocytes. Pregnancy following transfer

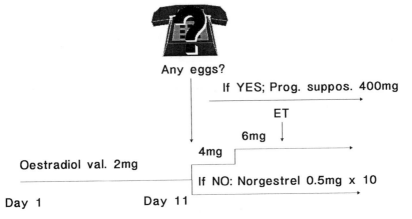

Fig. 13.1 Lister Hospital ovum donation protocol.

Table 13.4 Pregnancy rates following transfer of cryopreserved zygotes in an ovum donation programme (Lister Fertility Clinic 1988)

	Embryo transfer all cases (n = 20)	Zygote intrafallopian transfer (n = 16)	Embryo transfer 3/4 embryos (n = 10)
Age	35.65	37.40	36.40
No. frozen	3.80	4.10	4.00
No. transferred	2.70	3.50	3.40
Pregnancies	4	6	3
Pregnancies (%)	20%	37%	30%

of a frozen thawed embryo was first reported by De Vroey in 1986, and in 1988 Abdalla & Leonard reported the first successful birth following zygote intrafallopian transfer (ZIFT) of a cryopreserved zygote derived from a donated oocyte.

The attraction of cryopreservation is that it simplifies treatment protocols for recipients and ensures anonymity of donor and recipient as recommended in the United Kingdom in the Second Report of the Voluntary Licensing Authority for Human in vitro Fertilization and Embryology (1987). The effectiveness of this technique has been demonstrated in a recent study (Baber et al 1989) of patients at The Lister Hospital. In a series of 36 transfers of cryopreserved zygotes to patients on an ovum donation programme an overall pregnancy rate of 28% per transfer was reported. This rose to 35% when three or more zygotes were transferred and showed a slight but not significant advantage for tubal transfer (Table 13.4). Salat-Baroux et al (1988) reported similar results following hormonal stimulation with transdermal oestrogens and vaginal progesterone.

Oocyte donors may be recruited from patients receiving IVF treatment who wish to donate extra oocytes, or from volunteer donors motivated for altruistic reasons. In each group ovarian stimulation should be effected using clomiphene citrate and human menopausal gonadotrophins (HMG) or preferably LHRH analogue and HMG. Follicular development is then monitored using serial ultrasound scans. Oocyte collection for volunteer donors is best performed using transvaginal ultrasound-guided needle aspiration as this technique is associated with less morbidity than the laparoscopic method, may be performed under light sedation or local anaesthetic, and is at least as effective in harvesting mature oocytes (Baber et al 1988).

Oocyte donation has now become a widely used and successful treatment of infertility due to ovarian failure and initial results suggest pregnancy rates may be higher than those seen in women on IVF and GIFT programmes. Various factors may underlie this finding: there may be a less favourable intrauterine environment associated with stimulated cycles, or the age-related changes in endometrial histology (Gosden 1985) may be

Table 13.5 Possible reasons for high pregnancy rates in ovum donation programmes

—Lack of endometrial hyperstimulation
—No hyper oestrogenism
—No underlying infertility
—No premature luteinization
—Better control of the window of receptivity

lessened by the use of an artificial hormone replacement cycle (Goswamy et al 1988). Artificial cycles are free from the risks of hyperoestrogenism and premature luteinization and the oocytes obtained from fertile donors may yet prove to be 'better' than those obtained from older or infertile women (Table 13.5).

Critical factors in assessing pregnancy outcome include age, cause of infertility, the number of oocytes or embryos transferred, and the rate of embryonic cleavage. In general, patients with POF have no underlying infertility, the age of the oocytes is fixed by donor selection, and the number of zygotes transferred, by unit policy, generally at two to four. These factors may well contribute to the excellent pregnancy rates being reported.

Problems do remain, in particular the inability of supply to meet demand, a situation which is unlikely to improve now that embryo (and oocyte) freezing is available unless more volunteer donors are found and until the legal minefield which surrounds the whole issue of donated zygotes, particularly in the UK, is resolved.

Cardiovascular consequences

It is now 30 years since Oliver & Boyd (1959) first reported that castration increases the risk of coronary heart disease, a finding supported by subsequent studies (Sznajderman & Oliver 1963, Johansson et al 1975). More recently, Bengtsson & Lindquist (1978) carried out cohort- and case-control studies and demonstrated that women with myocardial infarction or angina pectoris had on average undergone the menopause earlier than other women of similar age. Gordon et al (1978) examined a cohort of 2873 women most of whom were re-examined at 2-yearly intervals during the 24-year period of follow up. They found an increase in the incidence and severity of coronary heart disease after the menopause. Within the age groups 40–44, 45–49 and 50–54 the incidence of coronary heart disease was more than twice as high in post-menopausal women as in pre-menopausal women irrespective of whether the menopause was natural or induced. These and other data provide strong evidence that a premature menopause is associated with an elevated risk of ischaemic heart disease and that the risk increases with an earlier age of ovarian failure. Although on average, smokers have an earlier menopause than non-smokers this will at best only explain a small part of the effect of age at menopause on ischaemic heart disease (Vessey & Hunt 1988).

The association between exogenous oestrogen use and cardiovascular disease has been controversial. Vessey (1980) reported an increased incidence of venous thromboembolism, stroke and myocardial infarction with the use of combined oral contraceptives and there have also been reports of increased venous thromboembolism following the use of high dose oestrogens to suppress lactation and increased cardiovascular morbidity and mortality in men being treated for prostatic cancer with large doses of oestrogens. However, numerous studies have now been conducted into the relationship between hormone replacement therapy (HRT) and cardiovascular disease. Of the recent case control studies, only one, containing 17 cases (Jick et al 1978) has shown any adverse effect from HRT. The results presented by Ross et al (1981) are, on the other hand, particularly impressive because they suggest a protective effect of oral-conjugated oestrogens against ischaemic heart disease in a study of a large group of women where relative risks were based on good evidence and corrected for a variety of confounding variables. The recent cohort studies are listed in Table 13.6. Only one of these was unable to demonstrate cardiovascular protection from oestrogen replacement therapy. Further prospective studies by Bush et al (1987) and Paganini-Hill et al (1988) showed that after adjustment for age, systolic blood pressure and smoking, oestrogen use was significantly associated with reduced mortality from cardiovascular disease or stroke.

It is clear that the vast bulk of evidence shows that oestrogen therapy after a premature menopause will help to reduce both the morbidity and mortality of cardiovascular and cerebrovascular disease. Progestogens may reduce the beneficial effects of oestrogens by elevating serum levels of low-density lipoproteins thus lowering the HDL/LDL ratio and their use should therefore be confined to women with an intact uterus and to the minimum safe dose.

Table 13.6 Cohort studies of the relationship between hormone replacement therapy and cardiovascular disease

Author	Country	Type of disease studied	Case no.	Rel. risk
Bush et al (1983)	USA	Death (all causes)	72	0.4
		Death (excl. Ca ov/uterus/breast)	55	0.4
Stampfer et al (1985)	USA	Myocardial infarction and death from ischaemic heart disease	90	0.3
Henderson et al (1985)	USA	Death from myocardial infarction	84	0.5
Wilson et al (1985)	USA	Ischaemic heart disease	116	1.9
		Stroke	45	2.3
		Death from ischaemic heart disease	48	1.9
Hunt et al (1987)	UK	Death from stroke	14	0.7
		Death from ischaemic heart disease	20	0.5

Osteoporosis

Post-menopausal osteoporosis is a common cause of major disability. Both ageing and oestrogen deficiency have been implicated in its aetiology leading to some confusion as to its significance in the prematurely menopausal woman. Peak bone mass is achieved in the fourth decade of life after which there is an age-related bone loss in both sexes (Savvas et al 1987). This is much more rapid in women and they will lose at least 2–3% of bone mass annually for the first 7–10 years following the menopause.

Richelson et al (1984) recently demonstrated that bone loss in women who had undergone oophorectomy in young adulthood was almost as great as that occurring in a group of women who had undergone a natural menopause, thus suggesting a primary role for oestrogen deficiency in the aetiology of this disorder. Cann et al (1984) demonstrated a significant decrease of 20.9% in spinal trabecular bone density in women with premature ovarian failure compared with controls but could not relate this to the period of amenorrhoea. Jones et al (1985) did however find an inverse correlation between peripheral bone density and duration of amenorrhoea in women with a premature menopause. Osteoporosis has also been described in patients with gonadal dysgenesis and has been attributed to oestrogen deficiency (Greenblatt et al 1967) but other factors presumably contribute as it has also been described before puberty in children with gonadal dysgenesis. The normal pubertal exponential increase in bone mineral density fails to occur in gonadal dysgenesis despite a normal adrenarche and women with gonadal dysgenesis have significantly less bone mineral content at age 20 than age-matched controls. Nevertheless, this group of patients will demonstrate an increase in bone density with oestrogen therapy (Garn 1970).

It seems clear that those undergoing premature ovarian failure will be equally at risk of developing osteoporosis as those who sustain a natural menopause at the normal age. They will, however, be more likely to suffer the consequences of this condition because of their greater life expectancy after its onset and it is therefore appropriate to initiate prophylactic therapy as soon as possible. Although many therapies including exercise, diet, fluoride, calcium, calcitonin and vitamin D have been advocated the most effective treatment is oestrogen-replacement therapy (Studd & Baber 1988).

Albright et al (1941) were the first to demonstrate a clear relationship between oestrogen deficiency, the menopause and an increased incidence of fractures in women. Several studies supporting these findings and demonstrating the beneficial effect of oestrogen replacement therapy followed (Lindsay et al 1976, Nachtigall et al 1979, Christiansen et al 1981). At the Dulwich Menopause Clinic and the Lister Fertility and Endocrinology Centre recent studies (Savvas et al 1988, Baber et al 1989) have demonstrated that bone loss occurs before the cessation of menses and that this loss can be prevented by hormone replacement therapy and may be at least partially corrected by the use of subcutaneous implants of oestrogen and testosterone. The method by which bone mass is replaced may be found in studies by Brincat et al (1989) who demonstrated that skin thickness and skin collagen content declined by some 30% in the first 10 years after the menopause, an amount comparable to bone loss over the same period. This collagen loss can be restored within 6 months of initiating hormone-replacement therapy and it seems likely that bone mass may be restored by a similar mechanism.

A wide range of oestrogen preparations are currently available, including tablets for oral use, creams for percutaneous or vaginal use, vaginal rings, transdermal patches and subcutaneous implants. Oral oestrogens remain the most popular but not always the best form of treatment. The major difference between oral and parenteral oestrogens is the avoidance of the 'first pass' liver metabolism of the latter, thus avoiding the induction of clotting factors and renin substrate. Parenteral oestrogens also maintain the premenopausal oestradiol to oestrone ratio, unlike tablets, and allow a more stable serum-hormone level without the troughs and peaks experienced with the intermittent use of tablets or creams. For the long term prevention of osteoporosis in patients suffering the premature menopause, transdermal patches or subcutaneous implants thus appear ideal.

Hormone implants provide a safe simple delivery system for hormone replacement therapy (Studd & Magos 1987). Their use ensures no adverse effect on clotting factors, blood pressure or glucose tolerance (Studd et al 1978) and if used in conjunction with cyclical progestogens when appropriate are not associated with any increased risk of gynaecological or breast malignancy (Baber & Studd 1989). Prematurely menopausal women do not, however, enjoy any special protection from malignancy, and regular cervical smears and breast examinations should be performed as should endometrial biopsy in the event of abnormal menstrual loss.

CONCLUSION

Premature ovarian failure, a condition of which little was known until quite recently, is a relatively common occurrence, affecting approximately 1% of women under the age of 40 years. If iatrogenic causes are included the number of women thus affected will exceed 250 000 in the USA and the UK alone. The diagnosis should always be considered in any woman presenting with a history of primary or secondary amenorrhoea or oligoamenorrhoea, vasomotor disturbances or other signs of oestrogen deficiency and may be confirmed by the detection of an elevated serum level of FSH. Although an aetiology cannot always be found chromosomal causes predominate amongst the early onset cases and autoimmune disease amongst the later presentations. Ovarian biopsy is not usually necessary as the findings will not affect future management. Women suffering a premature menopause will be at least as likely as those who undergo menopause at a normal age to suffer from an increased risk of cardiovascular disease cerebrovascular disease and osteoporosis and should be offered balanced hormone replacement therapy as soon as a diagnosis is made.

Women seeking a family may now be treated with ovum donation using either fresh or frozen transfer of zygotes to the fallopian tubes or uterus. Simplified protocols and improved techniques have resulted in excellent success rates with pregnancies being maintained by exogenous hormone replacement until the placental contribution is sufficient.

REFERENCES

Abdalla H, Leonard T 1988 Cryopreserved zygote intrafallopian transfer for anonymous oocyte donation. Lancet i: 835

Aiman J, Smentek C 1985 Premature ovarian failure. Obstet Gynecol 66: 9–14

Albright F, Smith P, Richardson A M 1941 Postmenopausal osteoporosis: its clinical features. JAMA 116: 2465–2474

Alper M M, Garner P R 1985 Premature ovarian failure: its relationship to autoimmune disease. Obstet Gynecol 66: 27–30

Alper M M, Jolly E E, Garner P R 1986 Pregnancies after premature ovarian failure. Obstet Gynecol 67(s): 595–625

Asch R, Balmaceda J, Ord T et al 1988 Oocyte donation and gamete intrafallopian transfer in premature ovarian failure. Fertil Steril 49: 263–267

Baber R, Studd J W W 1989 Hormone replacement therapy and cancer. Br J Hosp Med 41: 142–149

Baber R, Porter R, Picker R, Robertson R, Dawson E, Saunders D 1988 Transvaginal ultrasound directed oocyte collection in an IVF programme: successes and complications. J Ultrasound Med 7: 377–379

Baber R, Studd J W W, Savvas M, Fogelman I, Watson N R, Garnett T 1989 The prevention of bone loss in perimenopausal women with oestrogen and testosterone implants. Br J Obstet Gynaecol 41: 142–149

Baber R, Kirkland A, Leonard T, Studd J W W, Abdalla H 1989 High pregnancy rates following transfer of cryopreserved zygotes in an ovum donation programme. Proceedings of 6th World Congress of IVF and Assisted Conception, Jerusalem, April 1989

Baker W J, Morgan R L, Pickham M J, Smithers D W 1972 Preservation of ovarian function in patients requiring radiotherapy for paraottic and pelvic Hodgkins disease. Lancet ii: 1307

Bateman B G, Nunley W C, Kitchin D D III 1983 Reversal of apparent premature ovarian failure in a patient with myasthenia gravis. Fertil Steril 39: 108–113

Bengtsson C, Lindhurst O 1978 Coronary heart disease during the menopause. In: Oliver M F (ed) Coronary heart disease in young women. Churchill Livingstone, Edinburgh, pp 234–239

Board J A, Redwine F O, Moncure C W et al 1979 Identification of differing etiologies of clinically diagnosed premature menopause. Am J Obstet Gynecol 134: 936

Brincat M, Kabalan S, Studd J W W et al 1987 A study of the relationship of skin collagen content, skin thickness and bone mass in the post-menopausal woman. Obstet Gynecol 70: 840–845

Bush T L, Cowan L D, Barrett-Connor E 1983 Estrogen use and all cause mortality. Preliminary results from the lipid research clinic program. JAMA 249: 903–906

Bush T L, Barrett-Connor E, Cowan L 1987 Cardiovascular mortality and non-contraceptive use of estrogen in women. Circulation 75: 1102–1109

Cann C E, Martin M, Genant H, Jaffe R 1984 Decreased spinal mineral content in amenorrhoeic women. JAMA 251: 626–629

Check J H, Case J S 1984 Ovulation induction in hypergonadotropic amenorrhoea with estrogen and human menopausal gonadotrophin therapy. Fertil Steril 42: 919–922

Christiansen C, Christiansen M, Transbol I 1981 Bone mass in post-menopausal women after withdrawal of oestrogen/gestogen replacement therapy. Lancet i: 459–461

Coulam C B 1983 Autoimmune ovarian failure. Semin Reprod Endocrinol 1(2): 161–168
Coulam C, Kempers R D, Randall R V 1981 Premature ovarian failure: evidence for the autoimmune mechanism. Fertil Steril 36: 238–246
DeMoraes Ruehsen M, Blizzard R M, Garcia Bunuch R, Seegar-Jones G 1972 Autoimmunity and ovarian failure. Am J Obstet Gynecol 112: 693–696
Dewald G W, Spurbeck J L 1983 Sex chromosome anomalies associated with premature ovarian failure. Semin Reprod Endocrinol 1: 79–92
Dewhurst C J, DeKoos E B, Ferreira H P 1975 The resistant ovary syndrome. Br J Obstet Gynaecol 82: 341–345
De Vroey P, Braeckmans P, Camus M et al 1986 Pregnancies after replacement of fresh and frozen thawed embryos in a donation programme. In: Feichtinger W, Kemeter P (eds) Future aspects in human in vitro fertilization. Springer-Verlag, Berlin, pp 133–143
Finegold W J 1976 Artificial insemination with husband sperm. C. Thomas, Springfield, Illinois
Floch O L, Donaldson S S, Kaplan H S 1976 Pregnancy following oophorectomy and total radiation in women with Hodgkins disease. Cancer 38: 2263
Fraser I S, Shearman R P, Smith A, Russell P 1988 An association among blepharophimosis resistant ovary syndrome and true premature menopause. Fertil Steril 50: 747–751
Furuhjelm M 1960 Classification and treatment of oligomenorrhoea and amenorrhoea. Acta Obstet Gynecol Scand 39: 593–595
Garn S M 1970 The earlier gain and later loss of cortical bone. C C Thomas, Springfield, Illinois
Goldenberg R L, Grodin J M, Rodbard D, Ross G T 1973 Gonadotropins in women with amenorrhoea. Am J Obstet Gynecol 116: 1003
Gordon T, Kannel W, Hjortland M, McNamara P 1978 Menopause and coronary heart disease. The Framingham Study. Ann Intern Med 89: 157–161
Gosden R G 1985 Maternal age a major factor affecting the prospects and outcome of pregnancy. Ann NY Acad Sci 442: 45–57
Goswamy R, Williams G, Steptoe P 1988 Decreased uterine perfusion—a cause of infertility. Hum Reprod 3: 955–959
Greenblatt R, Rogers-Byrd J, McDonough P, Mahesh V 1967 The spectrum of gonadal dysgenesis. Am J Obstet Gynecol 98: 151–172
Grogan R H, Duncan C J 1955 Ovarian salvage in routine abdominal hysterectomy. Am J Obstet Gynecol 70: 1277–1279
Gulyas B J, Mattison D R 1979 Degeneration of mouse oocytes in response to polycystic aromatic hydrocarbons. Anat Rec 193: 863–864
Henderson B E, Ross R K, Paganini-Hill A 1985 Estrogen use and cardiovascular disease. J Reprod Med 30 (suppl) 814–820
Hunt K, Vessey M, McPherson K, Coleman M 1987 Long-term surveillance of mortality and cancer incidence in women receiving hormone replacement therapy. Br J Obstet Gynaecol 94: 620–635
Irvine W J, Cahn M M W, Scanth L et al 1968 Immunological aspects of premature ovarian failure associated with Addison's disease. Lancet ii: 883
Jacobs H S, Murray M A F 1976 The premature menopause. In: Campbell S (ed) The management of the menopause and post-menopausal years pp 359–367
Jewelwicz R, Schwartz M 1986 Premature ovarian failure. Bull NY Acad Med 62: 219–236
Jick A, Porter J, Morrison A S 1977 The relation between smoking and age of natural menopause. Lancet ii: 1354
Jick A, Dinan B, Rothman K 1978 New contraceptive estrogens and new fatal myocardial infarction. JAMA 239: 1407–1408
Johanssohn B, Kaij L, Kullander S, Lenner H C, Svanberg L, Astedt B 1975 On some late effects of bilateral oophorectomy in the age range 15–30 years. Acta Obstet Gynecol Scand 54: 449–461
Jones G S, DeMoraes Ruehsen M 1979 A new syndrome of amenorrhoea in association with hypergonadotropism and apparently normal ovarian follicular apparatus. Am J Obstet Gynecol 104: 597
Jones G S, Reuhsen M D M 1967 A new syndrome of amenorrhoea in association with hypogonadotropism and apparently normal follicular apparatus. Fertil Steril 18: 440
Jones K, Ravnikar V, Tulchinsky D, Schiff I 1985 Comparison of bone density in

amenorrheic women due to athletics, weight loss and premature menopause. Obstet Gynecol 66: 5–8

Kaufaman F, Kogut M D, Donnel G H, Kock R 1979 Ovarian failure in galactosaemia. Lancet *ii*: 737

Kennedy J F, Freedman M C, Benirschke K 1977 Ovarian dysgenesis and chromosomal abnormalities. Obstet Gynecol 50: 13

Kinch R A, Plunkett E R, Sment M S et al 1965 Primary ovarian failure. A clinico-pathological and cystogenetic study. Am J Obstet Gynecol 91: 630

Kirsop R, Brock T, Robinson B, Baber R 1990 The detection of antiovarian antibodies by indirect immunofluorescence. Reprod, Fertil, Dev (submitted for publication)

Kretzschmar N, Gardiner S 1935 A consideration of the surgical menopause after hysterectomy and the occurrence of cancer in the stump following sub-total hysterectomy. Am J Obstet Gynecol 29: 168–174

Leer J, Patel B, Innes M, Cameron D P 1980 Secondary amenorrhoea due to autoimmune ovarian failure. Aust N Z J Obstet Gynaecol 20(3): 177–179

Lindsay R, Aitken J, Anderson J, Hart D, MacDonald E, Clarke A C 1976 Long-term prevention of post-menopausal osteoporosis by oestrogen. Lancet *i*: 1038–1041

Lutjen P, Trounson A, Leeton J, Findlav J, Wood C, Rhenou P 1984 The establishment and maintenance of pregnancy using in vitro fertilisation and embryo donation in a patient with primary ovarian failure. Nature 307: 104–105

McDonough P G, Gynd R J, Thi Tho P, Mahesh V B 1977 Phenotypic cystogenic findings in 82 patients with ovarian failure—changing trends. Fertil Steril 28: 638–641

Mahadevan K, Murthy M, Reddy P, Bhaskaran S 1982 Early menopause and its determinants. J Biosoc Sci 14: 473–476

Mashchak C A, Keltzky O A, Davajan V et al 1981 Clinical and laboratory evaluation of patients with primary amenorrhoea. Obstet Gynecol 57: 715–721

Maxson W S, Wentz A C 1983 The gonadotropin resistant ovary syndrome. Semin Reprod Endocrinol 1(2): 147–160

Morrison J C, Gimes J R, Wiser L W, Fish S A 1975 Mumps oophoritis: a cause of premature menopause. Fertil Steril 26: 655–659

Nachtigall I, Nachtigall R H, Nachtigall R D, Beckman E 1979 Estrogen replacement therapy: a ten-year prospective study in the relationship to osteoporosis. Obstet Gynecol 53: 277–281

Nakano R, Hashiba N, Washio M, Tojo S 1978 Ovarian follicular apparatus and hormonal parameters in patients with primary amenorrhoea. Acta Obstet Gynecol Scand 57: 293–300

Netter A, Sebaoun M 1966 Menopause precose. Gynecol Obstet 66: 249

Netter A, Cahen G, Rozenbaum H 1977 Le syndrome des ovaires resistant aux gonadotropines. Actual Gynecol 8: 29–38

Nogales-Ortiz F, Tarncon I, Nogales F F 1979 The pathology of female genital tuberculosis. Obstet Gynecol 53: 422–428

Oliver M F, Boyd G S 1959 Effects of bilateral ovariectomy on coronary artery disease and serum lipid levels. Lancet *ii*: 690–694

Paganini-Hill A, Ross R, Henderson B 1988 Post-menopausal oestrogen treatment and stroke: a prospective study. Br Med J 297: 519–522

Polansky S, de Papp E W 1976 Pregnancy associated with hypergonadotropic hypogonadism. Obstet Gynecol 47: 475–515

Rebar R W, Erickson G F, Yen S C 1982 Idiopathic premature ovarian failure: clinical and endocrine characteristics. Fertil Steril 37: 35–41

Richelson L, Wahner H, Melton L, Riggs B 1984 Relative contributions of aging and oestrogen deficiency to post-menopausal bone loss. N Engl J Med 311: 1273–1275

Ross R K, Paganini-Hill A, Mack T, Arthur M, Henderson B 1981 Menopausal oestrogen therapy and protection from death from ischaemic heart disease. Lancet *i*: 858–860

Russell P, Bannatyne P, Shearman R P, Fraser I, Corbett P 1982 Premature hypergonadotropic ovarian failure. Clinico-pathological study of 19 cases. Int J Gynecol Pathol 1: 185–201

Sagal J, Distiller L A, Morley J E, Isaacs H, 1975 Myotonia dystrophica: Studies on gonadal function using LHRH. J Clin Endocrinol Metab 40: 1110–1111

Salat-Baroux J, Cornet D, Alvarez S et al 1988 Pregnancies after replacement of frozen thawed embryos in a donation programme. Fertil Steril 49: 817–821

Savvas M, Brincat M, Studd J W W 1987 Postmenopausal osteoporosis. Br J Hosp Med 38: 16–24

Savvas M, Studd J W W, Fogelman I, Dooley M, Montgomery J, Murby B 1988 Skeletal effects of oral oestrogen compared with subcutaneous oestrogen and testosterone in post-menopausal women. Br Med J 297: 331–333

Second Report of the Voluntary Licensing Authority for Human In Vitro Fertilization and Embryology 1987 Sumfield and Day, East Sussex

Serhal P, Craft I 1987 Simplified treatment for ovum donation. Lancet i: 687–688

Shangold M M, Turksoy R N, Bashford R A, Hammond C B 1977 Pregnancy following the insensitive ovary syndrome. Fertil Steril 28: 926–931

Shapiro A G, Rubin A 1977 Spontaneous pregnancy in association with hypergonadotropic ovarian failure. Fertil Steril 28: 500–501

Siddle N, Sarrel P, Whitehead M 1987 The effect of hysterectomy on the age at ovarian failure: identification of a subgroup of women with premature loss of ovarian function and literature review. Fertil Steril 47: 94–100

Simpson J L 1980 Genes chromosomes and reproductive failure. Fertil Steril 33: 107–116

Stampfer M J, Willett W, Colditz G, Rosner B, Speizer F, Hennekens C 1985 A prospective study of post-menopausal estrogen therapy and coronary heart disease. N Engl J Med 313: 1044–1049

Starup J, Sele V 1973 Premature ovarian failure. Acta Obstet Gynecol Scand 52: 259

Stillman R J, Shiff I, Schinfield J 1982 Reproductive and gonadal function in the female after therapy for childhood malignancy. Obstet Gynecol Surv 37: 385–393

Studd J W W, Baber R J 1988 Calcitonin for post-menopausal bone loss. Lancet i: 1277–1278

Studd J W W, Magos A 1987 Hormone pellet implantation for the menopause and premenstrual tension. Obstet Gynecol Clin N Am 14: 229–249

Studd J W W, Dubiel M, Kakkar V, Thom M, White P 1978 The effect of hormone replacement therapy on glucose tolerance, clotting factors, fibrinolysis and platelet behaviour in post-menopausal women. In: Cooke I D (ed) The role of oestrogen/progestogen in the management of the menopause. M.T.P. Press, Lancaster, pp 41–59

Sznajderman M T, Oliver M F 1963 Spontaneous premature menopause, ischaemic heart disease and serum lipids. Lancet i: 962–965

Tanaka T, Sakaguri N, Fujimoto S 1982 HMG-HCG therapy in patients with hypergonadotropic ovarian anovulation. Int J Fertil 27: 100–104

Thomas P R M, Winstanley D, Peckham M J, Austin D E, Murray M A F, Jacobs H S 1976 Reproductive and endocrine function in patients with Hodgkins disease: effects of oophoropexy and irradiation. Br J Cancer 33: 226–231

Trounson A, Leeton N, Besanko M, Wood C, Conti A 1983 Pregnancy established in an infertile patient after transfer of a donated embryo fertilised in vitro. Br Med J 286: 835–838

Van der Merwe J 1981 Premature gonadal failure. S Afr Med J 59: 104–108

Verp M S 1983 Environmental causes of ovarian failure. Semin Reprod Endocrinol 1: 101–111

Vessey M P 1980 Female hormones and vascular disease—an epidemiological overview. Br J Family Planning (suppl) 6: 1–12

Vessey M, Hunt K 1988 The menopause, hormone replacement therapy and cardiovascular disease. In: Studd J W W, Whitehead M I (eds) The menopause. Blackwell Scientific, London, pp 190–196

Whitehead M I, Cust M 1987 Consequences and treatment of early loss of ovarian function. In: Zichilla L, Whitehead M I, Van Keep P A (eds) The climacteric and beyond. Parthenon, Carnforth, Lancashire, pp 63–81

Wilson P W F, Gamson R J, Castelli W P 1985 Post-menopausal estrogen use cigarette smoking and cardiovascular morbidity in women over 50. The Framingham Study. N Engl J Med 313: 1038–1043

Wright C S W, Jacobs H S 1979 Spontaneous pregnancy in a patient with hypergonadotrophic ovarian failure. Br J Obstet Gynaecol 86: 389–392

Yovich J, Blackledge D, Richardson P, Matson P, Turner S, Draper R 1987 Pregnancies following pronuclear stage tubal transfer. Fertil Steril 48: 851–857

14. Fertilization by micro-insemination

S.-C. Ng   T. A. Bongso   A. H. Sathananthan
S. S. Ratnam

The severely oligozoospermic patient usually has a combination of multiple spermatozoal defects (WHO 1987), with poor chances of spontaneous conception. In vitro fertilization (IVF) has not contributed to significant improvement for patients with severe oligozoospermia (Yovich & Stanger 1987). Fertilization rate decreases when inseminating concentrations are reduced (Diamond et al 1985, Wolf et al 1984). Motility also has an important influence on fertilization rates (Bongso et al 1989a, Mahadevan et al 1985).

There is a significant reduction in fertilization in triple sperm defects (35·1%, 61 men in 116 cycles), when compared to single sperm defects (61·3%, 121 men in 206 cycles) and double sperm defects (48·9%, 98 men in 177 cycles) (Yates et al 1989). Low sperm density ($< 5 \cdot 0 \times 10^6$/ml) is usually combined with low motility and high abnormal forms (WHO 1987), except when due to obstructive causes. Such a combination is to be expected when there is seminiferous tubular failure, usually of an idiopathic nature.

Oehninger et al (1988) reported that 5% of 1067 IVF attempts resulted in failed fertilization. Sperm anomalies were thought to be the cause in 61·5% of cases, while 13·4% had a combination of sperm and oocyte anomalies.

Tubal embryo transfer (Wong et al 1988), otherwise known as pronuclear stage transfer (PROST) and tubal embryo stage transfer (TEST) (Yovich et al 1988), does not offer increased hope for patients with severe sperm problems as the spouses' oocytes still need to be fertilized before transfer into the Fallopian tubes.

The introduction of spermatozoa directly into the oocyte by micro-manipulation will be very useful since very minimal spermatozoa will be required.

Before defining assisted fertilization, we need to define what are assisted reproductive techniques (ART): ART is any procedure where the oocyte is manipulated, i.e. removed from the body before returning either as an oocyte or an embryo (Ng et al 1990a). The procedures can be independent of sperm handling, e.g. in oocyte donation or freezing. However, sperm manipulation per se is not ART, e.g. hysteroscopic or ultrasonic-guided insemination into Fallopian tubes. We would like to introduce some new terms: assisted fertilization, micro-insemination, sperm transfer, and micro-injection. 'Assisted fertilization' is when fertilization is assisted by micro-manipulation techniques. The term 'micro-insemination' has been proposed (Yanagimachi 1988), in contrast to 'macro-insemination' which refers to vaginal and dish insemination. The term 'micro-fertilization' was first used by Alan Trounson (1987) to describe introduction of spermatozoa into the oocyte. However, we believe 'micro-insemination' is more appropriate because insemination is the process of adding sperm, while fertilization is the result of sperm union with oocyte (Yanagimachi 1988). In micro-insemination, spermatozoa are introduced either singly or in multiples into the perivitelline space (pvs) under the zona ('sperm transfer') or directly into the cytoplasm ('sperm micro-injection'). We propose the following acronyms: MIST for micro-insemination sperm transfer, and MIMIC for micro-insemination micro-injection into cytoplasm (Ng et al 1990b).

INDICATIONS

The indications for human micro-insemination are (see Ng et al 1990b):

1. Severe oligozoospermia

When the sperm count is less than 5 million/ml, there is a reduced chance of fertilization by normal IVF procedures (see above). While TET (Devroey et al 1986) improves the pregnancy rate following fertilization, the fertilization process still requires the initial semen sample to be more than 5 million/ml (Hamori et al 1988).

2. Severe multiple sperm factors (oligoasthenoteratozoospermia)

Severe forms of oligoasthenoteratozoospermia have very poor prognosis in terms of treatment and realization of pregnancy. Such patients have previously relied on artificial insemination with donor sperm. Now, micro-insemination offers some hope. In borderline situations, it should be demonstrated that there is repeated failed fertilization in vitro.

3. Immotile sperm (total asthenozoospermia)

Immotile spermatozoa may be caused by environmental or congenital factors, e.g. ciliary dyskinesis (Rossman et al 1981), with its three major variants (see Zamboni 1987). Environmental problems, e.g. drug therapy, usually result in decreased motility, and this can be improved by removal of the drug or introduction of additives into the sperm washing procedures (see Bongso et al 1988). Congenital problems are more difficult to treat and there is the ethical issue of whether propagation of such genes is desirable.

The immotile cilia syndrome (ciliary dyskinesis) is an autosomal recessive condition (Palmblad et al 1984), which is one such problem and is compatible with normal life span if preventive therapy is instituted for the respiratory complications. Hence, for this genetic disease we feel that micro-insemination is justified.

4. Inability to penetrate egg vestments

While this has not been described conclusively in the literature, there are many instances where there is failed fertilization in spite of oocytes being mature and spermatozoa of good motility (Chia et al 1984). Oehninger et al (1988) stressed that in spite of critical reappraisal of the causes of failed fertilization in 52 patients, 6 (11·5%) were unexplained. The zona-penetration test (Overstreet 1983) may shed more light on this defect. The 'hemi-zona' assay will also help in the understanding of sperm penetration through the zona (Burkman et al 1988). 'Spontaneous' hardening of the zona pellucida has been described in mouse oocytes cultured in vitro (De Felici & Siracusa 1982), after increasing resistance to solubilization by chymotrypsin. The authors suggested that follicular fluid contains glyco-saminoglycans that prevent such hardening (De Felici et al 1985). Alterations of the surface structure of the zona have been linked to sperm-binding capacity of the zona (Familiari et al 1988). For micro-insemination to be justified in this condition, there must be failed fertilization on repeated IVF attempts of all oocytes. Specific sperm abnormalities that do not allow attachment of sperm to oolemma, e.g. acrosomeless sperm (Lalonde et al 1988), might also justify sperm injection. Lanzendorf et al (1988a) have recently reported that MIMIC into hamster oocytes with such sperm can result in sperm head decondensation.

CONTRAINDICATIONS

The absolute contraindication is a genetic abnormality in the male. In male patients attending a subfertility clinic, Chandley et al (1975) reported that 2% of them were chromosomally abnormal. This frequency increased to 6% among men with a mean sperm count of less than 20 million per ml, and was 15% among azoospermic men. Kjessler (1972) also demonstrated that the majority of chromosomally abnormal infertile men were oligo-zoospermic and azoospermic. In a study on 1000 human male pronuclear chromosomes complements from 33 normal donors, Martin et al (1983) reported an abnormality rate of 8·5% (5·2% aneuploidy and 3·3% structural abnormalities). The incidence of sperm chromosome aberrations from proven donors varies between 6·6% and 14·3% (Templado et al 1988). However, testicular karyotypes of subfertile men with normal peripheral karyotypes do not show any difference from the controls (Skakkebek et al (1973). There have been no reported studies on the sperm chromosomes of oligozoospermic men. It is unlikely to have an increased abnormality in sperm haploid chromosomes when the peripheral karyotype is normal (see Ng et al 1990c). This is supported by the report of De Boer et al (1976) where tertiary trisomic male mice carry the small translocation chromosome from the T(1;13)7OH reciprocal translocation as an extra chromosome. These mice are oligozoospermic with euploid and aneuploid spermatozoa in equal numbers and there is no relationship between sperm morphology and karyotype. For our clinical program, a peripheral karyotype of the male is needed. If this was abnormal he would be excluded from micro-insemination.

Other contraindications are as for the Assisted Reproductive Technology program, and would include medical or surgical contraindications to pregnancy.

LIMITATIONS

There are limitations to the widespread application of micro-insemination. It requires expensive equipment and training, is time-consuming, and, currently yields low fertilization rates (see below). It is still a research procedure and optimal conditions for its successful application are still not determined.

Recently, Martin et al (1988) reported a high incidence of abnormal sperm complements following sonication and direct micro-injection (MIMIC) into hamster oocytes (Martin et al 1988). The karyotype yield was very poor (3·4 human karyotypes per 100 micro-injected oocytes), though 90% of the oocytes looked healthy after the micro-injection. These workers obtained 10 of 11 abnormal spreads after sonication; the majority were multiple breaks and rearrangements. Abnormal spreads were seen in only 14 of 33 spreads (42·4%) after TEST-yolk buffer exposure. The authors suggested that the sonication resulted in the markedly increased abnormalities in the sperm karyotypes. It must be noted that sonication is not used in the sperm transfer (MIST) technique; it is used only in MIMIC when the spermatozoal head (not the whole spermatozoon) is micro-injected into the ooplasm. They also suggested that the micro-injection technique resulted in the high abnormality rate with TEST-yolk buffered sperm.

ZONAL PROCEDURES

The zona pellucida is thought to be the main block to spermatozoal penetration of mammalian oocytes (Jaffe & Gould 1985). Hence in situations of reduced ability of spermatozoa to penetrate the zona, such as oligozoospermia, zonal procedures to assist the spermatozoa to pass through the zona may be of assistance. Complete removal of the zona will result in polyspermy (Yanagimachi 1984) and reduced developmental ability because the preimplantation embryo is protected by this vestment during early development. Zonal procedures to assist fertilization include zona-drilling, zona-cutting, zona-cracking/splitting, and partial zona-dissection. These procedures are macro-insemination procedures (see above) as the manipulated oocytes are then introduced into an insemination dish. There are other zonal procedures which can be used in ART, e.g. assisted hatching, where a cleaved embryo has a slit made in the zona before embryo replacement (Cohen 1989).

Zona 'drilling' was first reported by Gordon & Talansky (1986) in which the mouse zona was 'punctured' with acid Tyrode's solution delivered through a fine micropipette. The zona can also be punctured with enzymes, e.g. trypsin (Gordon et al 1988) or pronase. As the zona is an acellular glycoprotein layer, it does not 'heal' (see Walton et al 1987) but probably may 'seal' off with time. The breach in the zona after acid-drilling is 5–10 times wider than after mechanical perforation (Sathananthan et al 1989). As this breach is larger, there is a possibility that sperm that enter in may also find their way out (Sathananthan et al 1989). Zona-drilling was also recently reported to be useful in the rat (Vanderhyden et al 1989).

Recently, Gordon et al (1988) reported their results of zona drilling of 47 human oocytes, with acid Tyrode's, chymotrypsin and mechanical perforation after zona softening with chymotrypsin. Thirty-one of the 47 oocytes (66%) survived the procedure, and of these, 10 were fertilized (5 monospermic and 5 polyspermic). Three patients had embryos replaced, with no resulting pregnancies. Acid PBS for zona-'drilling' may result in arrest of the second meiotic division of the oocyte, possibly at anaphase II (Ng et al 1989a). It has also been shown by Cummins et al (1989) that there was reduced microvillar height on the underlying oocyte surface.

Similar problems to zona-drilling may also be encountered with zona 'cutting', though absence of acid with this technique should reduce arrest in meiosis. Zona-cutting was originally described in fertilized eggs to improve nuclear manipulations (Tsunoda et al 1986). A comparative study of these two methods was reported by Depypere et al (1988) using murine gametes.

In zona 'cracking', the zona is 'cracked' with 2 fine glass hooks controlled by a micromanipulator (Odawara & Lopata 1987). Odawara & Lopata (1989) described an expanded series of 425 mouse oocytes with their zona cracked after exposure to sucrose solution. At inseminating concentrations of 1×10^4/ml there was a significant improvement in fertilization for zona-cracked oocytes over controls (63·2% vs 37·5%). There was no significant difference in fertilization rates at 1×10^3/ml. Similar observations were noted for blastocyst development and polyspermy rates were not significantly increased.

Cohen et al (1988) 'partially opened the zona using mechanical force only' similar to that described by Tsunoda et al (1986) and termed it 'partial zona dissection' (PZD). Cohen et al (1988) achieved monospermic fertilization in 10/16 (63%) PZD oocytes and 4/17 (24%) control oocytes. They reported 2 pregnancies (both twins) in 4 replacements, and both had 2 PZD and 1 control embryo replaced. They also reported an enlarged series (Malter & Cohen 1989a) of 34 oocytes from 11 patients with male infertility. Macro-insemination was possible with $5-20 \times 10^6$/ml motile spermatozoa and fertilization was achieved in 27/34 (79%), (4 were polyspermic) as compared to controls with a 53% fertilization rate (16/30), (6 polyspermic). Of the 11 patients, 2 had all their PZD embryos frozen, while another 2 had no oocytes fertilized. Seven had embryos replaced, but 5 of them had a combination of PZD and normally-inseminated embryos. Three pregnancies were obtained.

In a recent series, Cohen et al (1989) reported 5 pregnancies following replacement of 23 micro-manipulated embryos and 8 control embryos in 23 patients with male factor problems. Polyspermy in couples with abnormal semen analyses was relatively low ($<20\%$), and the authors thought this was due to partial oocyte activation by sucrose. However, polyspermy was high (57%) in normospermic patients with either immunological infertility, or failure of fertilization in previous IVF cycles.

Interestingly, in the mouse, immunological block to zona-binding can be overcome by zona-drilling. Conover & Gwatkin (1988) reported that zona-drilling with acid Tyrode's solution resulted in fertilization in vitro with development to blastocyst, when sperm penetration through the zona was prevented by a monoclonal antibody to ZP3.

Many of the zonal procedures require exposure to sucrose to shrink the oocyte before manipulation. Malter et al (1989) reported that this may result in activation and reduce the risk of polyspermic fertilization.

However, zonal procedures may result in the embryo being squeezed out of the zona as it traverses down the oviduct, at least in the mouse (Nichols & Gardner 1989). The rate of development to mid-gestation of operated zygotes and 2-cell embryos transferred directly to the oviduct was significantly lower than controls. Though hatching may be easier when the zona has been breached, the hatching process is abnormal (Malter & Cohen 1989b).

MICRO-INSEMINATION SPERMATOZOA TRANSFER (MIST)

Single sperm transfer in the human was first done by Metka et al (1985); the sperm transferred were treated as in routine IVF. Of 9 oocytes manipulated, one pronuclear oocyte cleaved to 4-cells. After embryo replacement there was no pregnancy. To improve the fertilization rates for such single sperm transfer, the acrosome reaction has to be improved above the 10–30% seen after 6 hours in capacitating medium (Lee et al 1987, Byrd & Wolf 1986). Hence, procedures to improve or synchronize acrosome reaction are therefore required for single sperm transfer in the human. This was achieved by Laws-King et al (1987), where they used a calcium-depleted strontium-based medium (Mortimer et al 1986) to incubate the sperm overnight. Of 7 human oocytes cultured 6–9 hours after collection which had single sperm transfers, 5 fertilized. Two out of 3 that were cultured underwent normal cleavage whilst the rest were examined by TEM or were karyotyped (Laws-King et al 1987). Another 12 human oocytes were cultured for 23–28 hours before single sperm transfer; of these, 3 were fertilized and 3 were parthenogenetically activated. TEM confirmed fertilization in both categories. There have been worries about polyspermy if multiple sperm were transferred into the peri-vitelline space. However, there is now some evidence for an oolemma block as in the rabbit; this may be related to sperm receptors on the oolemma.

Sperm receptors on oolemma membrane

Earlier studies with zona-free oocytes suggested that there is some form of block to excessive polyspermy (Pavlok & McLaren 1972, Toyoda & Chang 1968, Niwa & Chang 1975). Recently, 97% of human sperm nuclei from donors with poor penetration of zona-free hamster oocytes ($<10\%$) underwent decondensation after direct cytoplasmic injection into hamster oocytes (Lanzendorf et al 1987).

The first direct evidence for sperm receptors on the oolemma came from a study with murine gametes by Ng and Solter (see Ng et al 1990b). We transferred between 3–5 motile spermatozoa into oocytes before and after ethanol activation (Cuthbertson 1983) of the oocytes. Of 101 oocytes, with no ethanol activation, 32 (31·7%) developed 2 pronuclei and a second polar body at 8 hours. Only 2 oocytes had 3 pronuclei, and none with more than 3 pronuclei, at 8 hours. The fertilization (monospermy and polyspermy) of oocytes was not signficantly different from oocytes exposed to ethanol 1–2 hours after multiple sperm transfer. However, when the oocytes were exposed to ethanol $\frac{1}{2}$ to 1 hour before sperm transfer, only 8 of 60 oocytes were fertilized. The data support the hypothesis that sperm receptors or sperm blocks were present on the oolemma of zona-intact oocytes because the polyspermy rates were low in spite of transfer of 3–5 spermatozoa. Ethanol activation prior to sperm transfer probably resulted in removal or inactivation of sperm receptors because of the low fertilization rate. It is possible that the sperm receptors on the oolemma may be inactivated by the lysozomal contents following cortical granule reaction (see Ng et al 1990d). The presence of sperm receptors on the oolemma may explain the low fertilization rates of inter-species fertilization in zona-free oocytes, with the possible exception of golden hamster oocytes (Yanagimachi 1984). Interestingly, it was reported recently that heteroantibodies found in human sera reacted against the hamster oolemma, although these oolemma antigens were distinct from antigens present on the surface of human spermatozoa (Bronson & Cooper 1988).

It must be noted that human oocytes manipulated with zonal procedures followed by macro-insemination have high polyspermy rates. This was

20% (4/20) after acid Tyrodes' drilling, 25% (1/4) after mechanical drilling, and 0% (0/7) after chymotrypsin drilling (Gordon et al 1988). In the other zonal technique where human oocytes were involved, Cohen et al (1989) also reported high polyspermy rates: 22·2% (2/9) for previous failure of fertilization, 100% (3/3) for sperm antibodies in the female, 42·9% (3/7) for sperm antibodies in the male, and 12% (6/50) for abnormal semen problems. This may be related to the constant exposure of acrosomally-reacted sperm which come into continuous contact with the oolemma because of the macro-insemination. When the sperm receptors regenerate with time following their initial removal after the first sperm-oocyte union at the oolemma membrane, there is still more acrosomally-reacted sperm to bind with them. Moreover, the cortical granules would have been discharged initially, and there are no further cortical granule reactions. Hence polyspermy rates are higher in such situations.

Multiple sperm transfer

Lassalle et al (1987) first reported multiple sperm transfer into human oocytes; 3–5 sperm were transferred into 7 oocytes and 3 fertilized, all monospermic. When the number of sperm transferred was increased to 10–12 sperm per oocyte, 2 of 3 oocytes fertilized but they were polyspermic. It is possible that with high sperm numbers, more than one sperm could attach onto their receptors on the oolemma before the receptors are inactivated, possibly by cortical granule release.

We embarked on a clinical trial in late 1987 (Ng et al 1990e). This was to evaluate the usefulness of the MIST procedure for patients with severe oligoasthenoteratozoospermia who would otherwise have to resort to artificial insemination with donor spermatozoa. Patients were included when their husbands' final sperm concentration was very poor ($<1·0 \times 10^6$/ml) or poor concentration and motility ($<2·5 \times 10^6$/ml with sluggish or no forward motility). These patients were separated into 2 groups: (1) initial semen analysis with severe oligozoospermia ($<5·0 \times 10^6$/ml); (2) initial semen analysis revealed oligozoospermia though not severe enough to consider sperm transfer, but very poor sperm parameters as described above after swim-up on the day of the oocyte recovery necessitated their inclusion. The males had original semen analyses with motile sperm densities of between 0·07 and 2·01 $\times 10^6$/ml (for group 1) and between 1·20 and 21·0 $\times 10^6$/ml (for group 2); and total sperm densities of between 0·5 and 5·3 $\times 10^6$/ml (for group 1) and between 12·9 and 76·0 $\times 10^6$/ml (for group 2). Viable and normal forms were also low. Semen collected on the day of sperm transfer yielded very low motile sperm densities (Table 14.1). For MIST, the entire semen sample was used and sperm were prepared by the Ficoll entrapment procedure.

Twenty-nine patients were on 3 stimulation regimes: (1) clomiphene + hMG; (2) FSH + hMG; (3) GnRH agonist + FSH + hMG. Four to 5 hours

Table 14.1 Micro-insemination sperm transfer: sperm parameters. (From Ng et al 1990e with permission.)

	Severe oligozoospermia	Final oligozoospermia
No. of cases	15	14
Average age	31·5	34·0
Previous SA:		
Density ($\times 10^6$/ml)	$2·64 \pm 1·31$	$37·76 \pm 55·84$
Motility (%)	$23·00 \pm 18·12$	$30·44 \pm 16·45$
Fresh SA:		
Motile density ($\times 10^6$/ml)	$2·28 \pm 3·79$	$3·84 \pm 3·03$
Total density ($\times 10^6$/ml)	$6·13 \pm 8·88$	$15·90 \pm 18·71$
Post-washing:		
Motile density ($\times 10^6$/ml)	$0·34 \pm 0·29$	$0·50 \pm 0·65$
Post-microcentrifugation:		
Motile density ($\times 10^6$/ml)	$1·18 \pm 0·99$	$1·69 \pm 1·98$

after oocyte collection, the cumulus-corona complex was removed with 0·1% hyaluronidase in T6 medium. There were 195 oocytes at metaphase II, 20 at metaphase I and 10 at prophase I; the rest were subjected to IVF. Only metaphase II oocytes were manipulated, within 1 hour (Ng et al 1990e).

Following MIST, 16 (8·2%) were damaged (Table 14.2). Eight oocytes had 2 pronuclei (9·4%) in group 1, while 33 of 110 oocytes had 2 pronuclei in group 2 (30·0%). IVF was used as controls only, when the sperm concen-

Table 14.2 Micro-insemination sperm transfer: fertilization. (From Ng et al 1990e with permission.)

	Severe oligozoospermia	Final oligozoospermia
Metaphase II eggs	85	110
Sperm transferred	$6·00 \pm 3·33$	$6·81 \pm 2·81$
Accidental MIMIC	16	23
1PN	2 (2·4%)	6 (5·5%)
2PN	8 (9·4)	33 (30·0)
3PN or more	2 (2·4)	0
Unfertilized	65 (75·6)	63 (57·3)
Damaged	8 (9·4)	8 (7·3)
Concomitant IVF		
No. of eggs	7	26
Fertilized	0	5 (19·2)
MIST embryos transferred		
No. of embryos	15	29
No. of patients	9	12
Pregnancies (pts)	2 (22·2)	1 (8·3)

tration and motility were thought to be adequate for fertilization; for group 1, none fertilized (7 oocytes, 2 patients), and for group 2, five of 26 fertilized (5 patients, 19·2%). Though fertilization following MIST was better (30·0% versus 19·2%), this was not significant. In spite of multiple sperm transfer, polyspermy was seen only in 2 oocytes in group 1 (2·3%). Parthenogenetic activation was seen in 2 (2·3%) and 6 (5·5%) in groups 1 and 2 respectively. In group 1, a total of 15 embryos and zygotes were replaced in 9 patients, with 2 pregnancies; the numbers are more than the 8 fertilized because 7 embryos were looking healthy the next day. In group 2, 29 zygotes/embryos were replaced in 12 patients, with 1 resulting pregnancy (Ng et al 1990e).

The first pregnancy after MIST has been reported (Ng et al 1988). She has since delivered a healthy baby boy weighing 3·356 kg on 20th April 1989 by LSCS. This is the first such delivery by micro-insemination. In the second pregnancy 2 monospermic zygotes and 1 dispermic zygote were obtained after MIST. The monospermic zygotes were transferred into the left Fallopian tube at pronuclear stage. Unfortunately, she developed a left tubal ectopic pregnancy and an intra-uterine pregnancy which aborted. The third pregnancy was from group 2. She was a 41-year-old female, with the husband 48 years old and with oligoasthenoteratozoospermia. Four zygotes with 2 pronuclei were obtained, and 1 other had 1 pronucleus following MIST. The 4 normo-spermic aygotes were replaced by TET. She became pregnant but the ultrasound at 8 weeks ammenorrhoea revealed a gestational sac without a fetal heart. Karyotyping of the chorionic villi revealed normal karyotype (46,XX).

Efficiency of sperm transfer

Single spermatozoal transfer in the mouse was recently reported by Mann (1988) in which 25% (55/221) of mouse oocytes 'injected' with a single spermatozoon into the pvs had 2 pronuclei and a second polar body at 8 hours after the sperm transfer. About half of those that were fertilized developed to live fetuses or young after transfer into pseudopregnant recipients (54%, or 26/48). The fertilization efficiency of the sperm transfer was lower than that for in vitro fertilization under similar conditions (78%). Lacham et al (1989) induced acrosome reaction by incubation in T6 medium for 30 minutes, 2 hours and 6 hours, and in 12 mM dibutryl guanosine 3,5-cyclic monophosphate (dbcGMP) with 10 mM imidazole for 30 minutes, and acrosomal status was $54 \pm 7·9\%$, $58 \pm 5·6\%$, $73 \pm 9·1\%$, and $81 \pm 15·1\%$ respectively. However, fertilization after sperm transfer was much lower than the acrosome-reacted rates of the spermatozoa—36%, 34%, 29% and 43% respectively. Blastocyst rates were high, at 73%, 96%, 92% and 96% respectively. TEM of the unfertilized oocytes revealed that the majority of the spermatozoa under the zona were not acrosomally-reacted, though some were reacted or reacting. Yamada et al (1988) transferred single motile mouse spermatozoa into mouse oocytes after exposing the spermatozoa to dbcGMP and imidazole. They reported 19·6% (41/209) fertilization rate with treated sperm, compared to only 5·3% (8/150) fertilization rate with untreated sperm. Again the fertilization efficiency was low, compared to 79·3% (680/858) fertilization in IVF with untreated spermatozoa, but surprisingly only 1·6% (6/368) with treated sperm. In the data from Ng and Solter (unpublished) only 31 of 101 oocytes (30·7%) that had multiple sperm transfer without ethanol ezposure developed to 2 cells. This was significantly lower than the 120, 2-cell embryos that developed from 134 oocytes (89·6%; $P<0.001$) fertilized in vitro within 2 hours of ovulation.

We also studied incorporation of multiple transferred human spermatozoa into hamster oocytes (Ng et al 1990f). Of 49 hamster oocytes, 43 (87·8%) had spermatozoa incorporation (decondensed spermatozoal heads) following MIST, compared to 88 of 121 (72·7%) control zona-free hamster oocytes ($P<0.05$). When the human spermatozoa were micro-centrifuged at 6500 rpm before introduction to the hamster oocytes, there was reduced sperm incorporation—12 of 41 (77·4%) after MIST and 79 of 130 (60·8%) for control zona-free hamster oocytes ($P<0.05$). Hence, in both groups, MIST resulted in significantly better sperm incorporation. However, when results were compared between micro-centrifuged spermatozoa and spermatozoa that were not, sperm incorporation into hamster oocytes was better when spermatozoa were not micro-centrifuged.

Sperm transfer into zona-intact hamster oocytes was also reported by Lassalle et al (1987). They transferred spermatozoa from 3 normal donors with a penetrated oocyte rate of $>20\%$ in the zona-free hamster assay. When 1–4 spermatozoa were transferred, penetration of 0 to 9% of hamster oocytes was obtained, while 36–37% penetration was obtained when 5–12 spermatozoa were transferred. However, when more than 12 spermatozoa were transferred, penetration decreased (0 to 6·6%). No polyspermy was obtained when 1–4 spermatozoa were transferred but there was 55% polyspermy (10/18) when 5–12 sperm were transferred and 100% (2/2) when >12 sperm were transferred. Their sperm incorporation rates were much lower than our experiment, but it could be due to fixation of the hamster oocytes at 3 hours after sperm transfer by Lassalle et al, and 5–6 hours in our experiment. The difference could also be due to exposure to cytochalasin D during the sperm transfer in our experiments.

In a later study, Lassalle & Testart (1988) reported on sperm pretreated with calcium ionophore (A23187) and freeze-thaw before micro-insemination into hamster oocytes. The penetration rates were better with A23187-treated (average 28·2%) and freeze-thawed (average 50·0%) sperm compared with control sperm (7·7%). The optimal penetration rates were obtained when 5 sperm were transferred (57·1% for A23187, and 71·4% for freeze-thaw). However, polyspermy rates were also higher when more spermatozoa were transferred. It must be realized that polyspermy block at

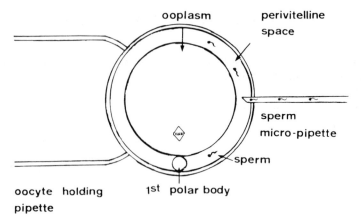

Fig. 14.1 Diagrammatic representation of Micro-Insemination Sperm Transfer (MIST). The sperm micro-pipette punctures through the zona pellucida, and sperm (multiple in this case) deposited into the peri-vitelline space. (Reproduced with permission from Ng et al 1990d.)

the hamster oolemma is not species-specific, and therefore may not prevent multiple spermatozoa from fusing with the oocyte.

Technique of MIST (Fig. 14.1)

Because the semen quality is very poor, the entire semen sample is used and spermatozoa are collected by the Ficoll entrapment procedure (Cummins & Breen 1984). This procedure improves sperm samples from WHO motility grade 1 to 2 with concomitant improvement in fertilization (Bongso et al 1989b). After the motile spermatozoa are collected from the supernatant, they are concentrated in a micro-centrifuge (MSE, Landsborough, UK) at 6500 rpm ($3352 \times g$) for 10 minutes, and the supernatant is removed. Such micro-centrifugation does reduce the fertilizability of such sperm after MIST (see above). Ficoll solution (5% in PBS, 0·1 ml) is added and the suspension is kept at 4°C until use.

The rest of the technique was as described in Ng et al (1988).

Karyotype results

For a comprehensive review of chromosomal anomalies in gametes, see Ng et al (1990c). It must be realized that there is no evidence of increased chromosomal abnormality following MIST. Kola et al (1990) karyotyped 18 fertilized human oocytes after transfer of single sperm from patients with severe male factors. Two (11%) were monosomic and 2 (11%) were trisomic; these rates were not significantly different from 30 oocytes fertilized by conventional IVF.

Transmission electron microscopy (TEM) of human oocytes after MIST

We have studied the ultrastructural features of spermatozoa-oocyte incorporation after spermatozoa transfer (Sathananthan et al 1989). It is noteworthy that the acrosome reaction could occur at the surface of the egg after multiple sperm transfer into the pvs (Sathananthan et al 1989), though Kawamura et al (1989) reported that there is inhibition of acrosome reaction within the pvs. Transfer of multiple spermatozoa has a theoretical advantage in that selection of spermatozoa may occur at the level of the oolemma where a membrane block could occur (Ng et al 1990e, Wolf 1978). This is especially relevant to human male subfertility where there may be a higher percentage of structurally or genetically abnormal spermatozoa and sperm selection is not possible. Of 100 spermatozoa examined by TEM in the pvs of 16 oocytes after transfer of 5–10 spermatozoa from oligozoospermic men, 76% had intact acrosomes and 33% of intact spermatozoa were morphologically abnormal (Sathananthan et al 1989). Nuclear, acrosomal, midpiece and tail defects were encountered in these abnormal sperm forms.

We have also studied the possibility of spermatozoa undergoing spermhead decondensation and formation of a pronucleus within blastomeres (Ng et al 1990g). Between 10–30 sperm were transferred into 11 donated human embryos between pronuclear and 16-cell stages. After culture for 6–24 hours in vitro, the embryos were fixed TEM. Both acrosome-intact and acrosome-reacted sperm were located in the pvs and between blastomeres. Sperm-blastomere membrane fusion was not observed. Sperm heads incorporated into blastomeres were often located in membrane-bound vesicles (both acrosome-intact and acrosome-reacted). Acrosome-reacted sperm heads were lying passively in vacuoles or were undergoing degenerative changes at their surfaces. Sperm chromatin decondensation was not observed in any of the sperm heads that were detected in the blastomeres. The results clearly show that sperm heads are incapable of expanding their chromatin to form typical male pronuclei following MIST into early human embryos.

MICRO-INSEMINATION MICRO-INJECTION INTO CYTOPLASM (MIMIC)

MIMIC is the direct injection of spermatozoon into the ooplasm of the oocyte (Fig. 14.2). It is indicated in situations where the spermatozoal count is so low that MIST is not possible, and possibly when there is a structural abnormality preventing gamete fusion, e.g. round-headed acrosomeless spermatozoa (Lalonde et al 1988). Oocyte mortality is high due to injury (Markert 1983). In spite of using very fine micropipettes (4–6 μm diameter) and under ideal conditions, only about 30% of micro-injected rat

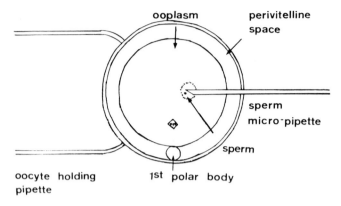

Fig. 14.2   Diagrammatic representation of Micro-Insemination Micro-Injection into Cytoplasm (MIMIC). The sperm micro-pipette punctures through the zona pellucida into the ooplasm, and 1 sperm is deposited into the ooplasm. (Reproduced with permission from Ng et al 1990d.)

eggs survive the procedure (Thadani 1981). TEM studies by our group show that a spermatozoon could be injected with minimal injury to the ooplasm and possible sperm-oocyte membrane fusion could occur in the ooplasm (Sathananthan et al 1989). However, many of the oocytes micro-injected with multiple spermatozoa showed evidence of degeneration and the spermatozoa heads, whether unreacted, reacting or fully reacted, remained unexpanded even 24 hours after the injection. Morphologically abnormal spermatozoa were seen frequently among these unexpanded sperm.

There was only one reported study of MIMIC involving both human spermatozoa and human oocytes, by Lanzendorf et al (1988b). Twenty oocytes from 11 patients were micro-injected, and 5 (possibly 8) oocytes became degenerated. Seven oocytes from 5 patients developed pronuclei; all the oocytes were fixed for TEM at 13 hours. It is interesting that the patients who had micro-injected oocytes showing pronuclei formation also became pregnant after transfer of embryos obtained from routine IVF.

However, as discussed above, there is a report of increased chromosomal abnormalities in the decondensed sperm head after micro-injection into hamster oocytes following sonication (Martin et al 1988).

CONCLUSIONS

In conclusion, micro-insemination, especially MIST, is a viable technique for patients with severe oligoasthenoteratozoospermia. These patients would previously have no choice other than to opt for donor spermatozoa. However, the techniques need much more work and research before it can be widely applied. Only a few specialized centres should embark on its use, in order to have sufficient patients to acquire the skills needed to make this technique a success. There are still some worries that need to be addressed scientifically, especially the risk of chromosomal abnormalities associated with this procedure. However, we are sure that time will show that we have a useful technique which can help many such patients.

ACKNOWLEDGEMENTS

We are particularly grateful to our colleagues involved in the ART program, and our technicians without whom the laboratories will not run. We are also grateful to the National University of Singapore and the Singapore Science Council for financial support.

REFERENCES

Bongso A, Ng S C, Ratnam S S 1988 The state of the art in laboratory IVF technology. In: Chen C, Cheng W C, Tan S L (eds) Advances in perinatal and reproductive medicine. MacMillan, Singapore, pp 191–205

Bongso T A, Ng S C, Mok H et al 1989a Effect of sperm motility on human in-vitro fertilization. Arch Androl 22: 185–190

Bongso T A, Ng S C, Mok H et al 1989b Improved sperm density, motility and fertilization rates following Ficoll treatment of sperm in a human in vitro fertilization program. Fertil Steril 51: 850–854

Bronson R A, Cooper G W 1988 Detection in human sera of antibodies directed against the hamster egg oolemma. Fertil Steril 49: 493–496

Burkman L J, Coddington C C, Franken D R et al 1988 The hemizona assay (HZA): development of a diagnostic test for the binding of human spermatozoa to the human zona pellucida to predict fertilization potential. Fertil Steril 49: 688–697

Byrd W, Wolf D P 1986 Acrosomal status in fresh and capacitated human ejaculated sperm. Biol Reprod 34: 859–869

Chandley A C, Edmond P, Christie S et al 1975 Cytogenetics and infertility in man. Pt 1. Karyotype and seminal analysis. Ann Hum Genet 39: 231–254

Chia C M, Sathananthan H, Ng S C et al 1984 Ultrastructural investigation of failed in vitro fertilisation in idiopathic subfertility. 18th Singapore–Malaysia Congress of Medicine, Singapore. Abstract p 52

Cohen J 1989 The zona pellucida. In: Proceedings of the NATO advanced research workshop on mechanisms of fertilization: from plants to animals. Springer Verlag, Berlin, NATO ASI series, Vol H45: 377–388

Cohen J, Malter H, Fehilly C et al 1988 Implantation of embryos after partial opening of oocyte zona pellucida to facilitate sperm penetration. Lancet ii: 162

Cohen J, Malter H, Wright G et al 1989 Partial zona dissection of human oocytes when failure of zona pellucida penetration is anticipated. Hum Reprod 4: 435–442

Conover J C, Gwatkin R B L 1988 Fertilization of zona-drilled mouse oocytes treated with a monoclonal antibody to the zona glycoprotein, ZP3. J Exp Zool 247: 113–118

Cummins J M, Breen T M 1984 Separation of progressively motile spermatozoa from human semen by 'sperm-rise' through a density gradient. Aust J Lab Sci 5: 15–20

Cummins J M, Edirisinghe W R, Odawara Y et al 1989 Ultrastructural observations on gamete interactions using micromanipulated mouse oocytes. Gamete Res 24: 461–470

Cuthbertson K S R 1983 Parthenogenetic activation of mouse oocytes in vitro with ethanol and benzyl alcohol. J Exp Zool 226: 311–314

De Boer P, van der Hoeven F A, Chardon J A 1976 The production, morphology, karyotypes and transport of spermatozoa from tertiary trisomic mice and the consequences for egg fertilization. J Reprod Fertil 48: 249–256

De Felici M, Siracusa G 1982 'Spontaneous' hardening of the zona pellucida of mouse oocytes during in vitro culture. Gamete Res 6: 107–113

De Felici M, Salustri A, Siracusa G 1985 'Spontaneous' hardening of the zona pellucida of mouse oocytes during in vitro culture. II. The effect of follicular fluid and glycosamino-glycans. Gamete Res 12: 227–235

Depypere H, McLaughlin J, Seamark R F et al 1988 Comparison of zona cutting and zona drilling as techniques for assisted fertilization in the mouse. J Reprod Fertil 84: 205–211

Devroey P, Braeckmans P, Smitz J et al 1986 Pregnancy after translaparoscopic zygote intra-fallopian transfer in a patient with sperm antibodies. Lancet i: 1329

Diamond M P, Rogers B J, Vaughn W K, Wentz A C 1985 Effect of the number of inseminating sperm and the follicular stimulation protocol on in vitro fertilization of human oocytes in male factor and non-factor couples. Fertil Steril 44: 499–503

Familiari G, Nottola S A, Micara G et al 1988 Is the sperm-binding capacity of the zona pellucida linked to its surface structure? A scanning electron microscopic study of human in vitro fertilization. J In Vitro Fertil Embryo Transfer 5: 134–143

Gordon J W, Talansky B E 1986 Assisted fertilization by zona-drilling: a mouse model for correction of oligospermy. J Exp Zool 239: 347–354

Gordon J W, Grunfeld L, Garrisi G J et al 1988 Fertilization of human oocytes by sperm from infertile males after zona pellucida drilling. Fertil Steril 50: 68–73

Hamori M, Stuckensen J A, Rumpf D et al 1988 Zygote intrafallopian transfer (ZIFT): evaluation of 42 cases. Fertil Steril 50: 519–521

Jaffe L A, Gould M 1985 Polyspermy-preventing mechanisms. In: Metz C B, Monroy A (eds) Biology of fertilization 3: 223–250

Kawamura M, Mishima M, Iwaki A, Okada A 1989 The effect of human sperm acrosome, microinjected into the hamster perivitelline space. In: Symposium on Fertilization in Mammals. Massachusetts Abstract II-12, 56

Kjessler B 1972 Facteurs genetiques dans la subfertile male humaine. In: Fecondite et Sterilite du male. Masson, Paris, pp 205–225

Kola I, Lacham O, Jansen R et al 1990 Chromosome analysis of human oocytes fertilized by micro-injection of spermatozoa into the perivitelline space. Human Reprod 5: 575–577

Lacham O, Trounson A, Holden C et al 1989 Fertilization and development of mouse eggs injected under the zona pellucida with single spermatozoa treated to induce the acrosome reaction. Gamete Res 23: 233–243

Lalonde L, Langlais J, Antaki P et al 1988 Male infertility associated with round-headed acrosomeless spermatozoa. Fertil Steril 49: 316–321

Lanzendorf S E, Mayer J F, Swanson J et al 1987 The fertilizing potential of human spermatozoa following microsurgical injection into oocytes. 5th World Congress IVF & ET, Virginia Abstract, p 103

Lanzendorf S E, Maloney M K, Ackerman S et al 1988a Fertilizing potential of acrosome-defective sperm following microsurgical injection into eggs. Gamete Res 19: 329–337

Lanzendorf S E, Maloney M K, Veeck L L et al 1988b A preclinical evaluation of pronuclear formation by microinjection of human spermatozoa into human oocytes. Fertil Steril 49: 835–842

Lassalle B, Courtot A M, Testart J 1987 In vitro fertilization of hamster and human oocytes by microinjection of human sperm. Gamete Res 16: 69–78

Lassalle B, Testart J 1988 Human sperm injection into the perivitelline space (SI-PVS) of hamster oocytes: effects of sperm pretreatment by calcium-ionophore A23187 and freezing-thawing on the penetration rate and polyspermy. Gamete Res 20: 301–311

Laws-King A, Trounson A, Sathananthan H, Kola I 1987 Fertilization of human oocytes by micro-injection of a single spermatozoon under the zona pellucida. Fertil Steril 48: 637–642

Lee M A, Trucco G S, Bechtol K B et al 1987 Capacitation and acrosome reactions in human spermatozoa monitored by a chlortetracycline fluorescence assay. Fertil Steril 48: 649–658

Mahadevan M M, Leeton J F, Trounson A O, Wood C 1985 Successful use of in vitro fertilization for patients with persisting low-quality semen. Ann NY Acad Sci 442: 293–300

Malter H, Cohen J 1989a Partial zona dissection of the human oocyte: a nontraumatic method using micromanipulation to assist zona pellucida penetration. Fertil Steril 51: 139–148

Malter H, Cohen J 1989b Blastocyst formation and hatching in vitro following zona drilling of mouse and human embryos. Gamete Res 24: 67–80

Malter H, Talansky B, Gordon J, Cohen J 1989 Monospermy and polyspermy after partial zona dissection of reinseminated human oocytes. Gamete Res 23: 377–386

Mann J R 1988 Full term development of mouse eggs fertilized by a spermatozoon microinjected under the zona pellucida. Biol Reprod 38: 1077–1083

Markert C L 1983 Fertilization of mammalian eggs by sperm injection. J Exp Zool 228: 195–201

Martin R H, Balkan W, Burns K et al 1983 The chromosome constitution of 1000 human spermatozoa. Hum Genet 63: 305–309

Martin R H, Ko E, Rademaker A 1988 Human sperm chromosome complements after microinjection of hamster eggs. J Reprod Fertil 84: 179–186

Metka M, Haromy T, Huber J, Schurz B 1985 Artificial insemination using a micromanipulator. Fertilitat 1: 41–44

Mortimer D, Curtis E F, Dravland J E 1986 The use of strontium-substituted media for capacitating human spermatozoa: an improved sperm preparation method for the zona-free hamster egg penetration test. Fertil Steril 46: 97–103

Ng S C, Bongso T A, Ratnam S S et al 1988 Pregnancy after transfer of multiple sperm under the zona. Lancet ii: 790

Ng S C, Bongso T A, Chang S I et al 1989a Transfer of human sperm into the peri-vitelline space of human oocytes after zona-drilling or zona-puncture. Fertil Steril 1989 52: 73–78

Ng S C, Bongso T A, Ratnam S S et al 1990a The future of Assisted Reproductive Technologies. Ann Acad Med Singapore 19: 841–844

Ng S C, Bongso T A, Sathananthan A H, Ratnam S S 1990b Micro-manipulation: its relevance to human IVF. Fertil Steril 53: 203–219

Ng S C, Bongso T A, Ratnam S S 1990c Micro-insemination: genetic aspects. Arch Androl 25: (in press)

Ng S C, Bongso T A, Sathananthan A H, Ratnam S S 1990d Micro-insemination sperm transfer (MIST) into human oocytes and embryos. In: Dale B (ed) Proceedings of the NATO Conference on Mechanism of Fertilization: Plants to Humans. Springer, Berlin, NATO ASI series, Vol H45: 351–376

Ng S C, Bongso T A, Sathananthan A H, Ratnam S S 1990e Micro-insemination of human oocytes. In: In vitro fertilization and alternate assisted reproduction (Proceedings of 6th World Congress on In Vitro Fertilization and Alternate Assisted Reproduction). Plenum Press, NY (in press)

Ng S C, Bongso T A, Sathananthan A H et al 1990f Micro-centrifugation of human spermatozoa: its effect on fertilization of hamster oocytes after micro-insemination spermatozoal transfer. Human Reprod 5: 209–211

Ng S C, Sathananthan A H, Bongso T A et al 1990g Subzonal transfer of multiple sperm into early human embryos. Molecular Rep Dev 26: 253–260

Nichols J, Gardner R L 1989 Effect of damage to the zona pellucida on development of preimplantation embryos in the mouse. Human Reprod 4: 180–187

Niwa K, Chang M C 1975 Requirement of capacitation for sperm penetration of zona-free rat eggs. J. Reprod Fertil 44: 305–308

Odawara Y, Lopata A 1987 Zona cracking: a new technique for assisted fertilization. Proceedings Austr Fertil Society, Sydney Abstract 073

Odawara Y, Lopata A 1989 A zona opening procedure for improving in vitro fertilization at low sperm concentrations: a mouse model. Fertil Steril 51: 699–704

Oehninger S, Acosta A A, Kruger T et al 1988 Failure of fertilization in in vitro fertilization: the 'occult' male factor. J In Vitro Fertil Embryo Transfer 5: 181–187

Overstreet J W 1983 The use of the human zona pellucida in diagnostic tests of sperm fertilizing capacity. In: Crosignani P G, Rubin B L (eds) In vitro fertilization and embryo transfer. Academic Press, London, pp 145–166

Palmblad J, Mossberg B, Afzelius B A 1984 Ultrastructural, cellular, and clinical features of the immotile-cilia syndrome. Ann Rev Med 35: 481–492

Pavlok A, McLaren A 1972 The role of cumulus cells and the zona pellucida in fertilization of mouse eggs in vitro. J Reprod Fertil 29: 91–97

Rossman C M, Forrest J B, Less R et al 1981 The dyskinetic cilia syndrome: abnormal ciliary motility in association with abnormal ciliary ultrastructure. Chest 80: 860–865

Sathananthan A H, Ng S C, Trounson A O et al 1989 Human micro-insemination by injection of single or multiple sperm: ultrastructure. Human Reprod 4: 574–583

Skakkebek N E, Bryant J I, Philip J 1973 Studies on the meiotic chromosomes in infertile men and controls with normal karyotypes. J Reprod Fertil 35: 23–36

Templado C, Benet J, Genesca A et al 1988 Human sperm chromosomes. Human Reprod 3: 133–138

Thadani V M 1981 A study of oocyte interactions using in vitro fertilization and sperm micro-injection. Yale Univ. PhD thesis

Toyoda Y, Chang M C 1968 Sperm penetration of rat eggs in vitro after dissolution of zona pellucida by chymotrypsin. Nature 220: 589–591

Trounson A 1987 Micro-fertilization. Plenary lecture 56, 5th World Congress In Vitro Fertilization, Virginia

Tsunoda Y, Yasui T, Nakamura K 1986 Effect of cutting the zona pellucida on the pronuclear transplantation in the mouse. J Exp Zool 240: 119–125

Vanderhyden B C, McLaughlin K J, Rutledge J M, Armstrong D T 1989 Zona-drilling increases the penetrability of rat oocytes matured in vitro. Biol Reprod 40: 953–960

Walton J R, Murray J D, Marshall J T, Nancarrow C D 1987 Zygote viability in gene transfer experiments. Biol Reprod 37: 957–967

WHO 1987 World Health Organization Task Force on the diagnosis and treatment of infertility. Towards more objectivity in diagnosis and management of male infertility. Int J Androl Suppl 7: 1–53

Wolf D P 1978 The block to sperm penetration in zona-free mouse eggs. Dev Biol 64: 1–10

Wolf D P, Byrd W, Dandekar P, Quigley M M 1984 Sperm concentration and the fertilization of human eggs in vitro. Biol Reprod 31: 837–848

Wong P C, Bongso T A, Ng S C et al 1988 Pregnancies after human tubal embryo transfer (TET): a new method of infertility treatment. Singapore J Obstet Gynecol 19: 41–43

Yamada K, Stevenson A F G, Mettler L 1988 Fertilization through spermatozoal microinjection: significance of acrosome reaction. Human Reprod 3: 657–661

Yanagimachi R 1984 Zona-free hamster eggs; their use in assessing fertilizing capacity and examining chromosomes of human spermatozoa. Gamete Res 10: 187–232

Yanagimachi R 1988 Personal communication

Yates C A, Trounson A O, de Kretser D M 1989 Male factor infertility and in vitro fertilization. 4th International Congress in Andrology, Florence Abstract, p 263

Yovich J L, Stanger J D 1987 The limitations of in vitro fertilization from males with severe oligospermia and abnormal sperm morphology. J In-Vitro Fertil Embryo Transfer 1: 172–179

Yovich J L, Yovich J M, Edirisinghe W R 1988 The relative chance of pregnancy following tubal or uterine transfer procedures. Fertil Steril 49: 858–864

Zamboni L 1987 The ultrastructural pathology of the spermatozoon as a cause of infertility: the role of electron microscopy in the evaluation of semen quality. Fertil Steril 48: 711–734

15. Chronic pelvic pain

J. Frappell   S. L. Stanton

During 1984 the British Journal of Hospital Medicine ran a series of articles under the heading 'Symptoms that depress the doctor'. One of these was entitled 'Too much pain' (Merskey 1984). The problem of women complaining of chronic pelvic pain is one that is met by most gynaecologists with dismay and apprehension. Why is this so?

Firstly, the prospect of a condition which is likely to be protracted and difficult to cure requires adjustment in the mind of both doctor and patient. How much easier it is to provide the instant answer, rather like a magician pulling a rabbit from a hat.

Secondly, the patient may well have higher expectations than those of the doctor and thereby make unacceptable demands on the latter's resources of time and patience. Many studies have confirmed that people complaining of chronic pain are more likely to have a neurotic type of personality (Gomez & Dally 1977) and may therefore come to be labelled as 'difficult patients'. Pain has often been found to be a sign of psychological illness (Merskey 1980) and there is no doubt that most patients with chronic pain who present to hospital show evidence of psychological disturbance. How far this is a cause rather than an effect of the pain has not been fully elucidated.

Thirdly, where pain is caused by a condition which has proved resistant to attempts at a cure, the doctor's concern may be increased by feelings of failure and inadequacy. Such is the case with advanced malignant disease where the response to pain by both doctor and patient is complicated by the prospect of impending death.

Chronic pelvic pain is a common complaint amongst women in their reproductive years and may account for as many as one third of outpatient referrals, of whom only a small proportion will have a significant abnormality (Morris & O'Neill 1958). In addition investigation of pelvic pain was the commonest indication for laparoscopy (52% of cases) in the Royal College of Obstetricians and Gynaecologists Survey (Chamberlain & Brown 1978).

Pelvic pain therefore represents a heavy part of the workload of most gynaecologists. Severe pain is not necessarily caused by organic disease, whilst conversely less troublesome pain may be the harbinger of serious pathology. Pain may of course be related to a non-gynaecological problem

Table 15.1   Gynaecological causes of chronic pelvic pain

1. Cyclical pain: Dysmenorrhoea
                    Mittelschmerz
2. Chronic pelvic inflammatory disease
3. Endometriosis
4. Neoplasia: Benign—fibroids
                       —ovarian cyst
                Malignant disease of the genital tract
5. Pelvic venous congestion/pelvic pain syndrome (PPS)
6. Polycystic ovarian syndrome
7. Residual ovary syndrome
8. Uterovaginal prolapse

Table 15.2   Non-gynaecological causes of chronic pelvic pain

Intestine	Diverticulitis
	Inflammatory bowel disease
	Irritable bowel syndrome
	Malignancy
	Subacute intestinal obstruction
Urinary tract	Calculus
	Chronic retention
	Infection
	Malignancy
Musculo-skeletal	Lumbo-sacral osteoarthritis
	Prolapsed intervertebral disc
	Spondylolisthesis

which reminds us of the need to keep an open mind in all cases. In the majority however no obvious pathological cause for the pain will be found (Gillibrand 1981) but this does not mean that the woman does not deserve a positive approach to further investigation and management. Left unresolved, pain may cast a blight over her entire life and that of her family and friends. It is clear therefore that the patient complaining of pain requires prompt and thorough investigation leading to a firm diagnosis which results in the correct treatment.

INNERVATION

Gynaecological pain may be somatic, from the vulva, perineum and lower vagina, and transmitted via the pudendal nerves (S2, 3 and 4), or visceral from the uterus, fallopian tubes, ovaries and visceral peritoneum supplied by the autonomic nervous system (T10–L1). Visceral and somatic pain perceptions are different. The viscera are insensitive to thermal and tactile sensations, and poorly localized in the cerebral cortex. Referred pain results from irritation of the overlying peritoneum, and is perceived in dermatomes supplied by the same nerve root.

Stimuli that produce pain include the following:

1. Distension and contraction of a hollow organ
2. Rapid stretching of the capsule of a solid organ
3. Chemical irritation of the parietal peritoneum
4. Tissue ischaemia
5. 'Neuritis' secondary to inflammatory, neoplastic or fibrotic processes in adjacent organs.

CLASSIFICATION

Classification by site of pathology is of little practical use other than to remind the clinician of the large variety of conditions that may present in this way. Possible conditions that should be considered can be divided into gynaecological and non-gynaecological (Tables 15.1 and 15.2).

HISTORY

The importance of good history taking in assessing the patient with chronic pelvic pain cannot be overemphasized. This should not be hurried and the doctor should watch the patient as she talks, as a sympathetic listener will pick up many valuable clues from the patient's 'body language'. She may also be able to talk about difficult areas such as sexual difficulties or revelations about unhappy memories that have been 'bottled up' for years.

In addition to this relatively unstructured approach the following specific points should be covered.

1. Characteristics of the pain:
   Mode of onset
   Duration
   Site
   Radiation
   Relationship to menstrual cycle and previous pregnancy.
   Intensity: this can be best assessed by instructing the patient in the use of a visual analogue scale, as this can be used later as an objective measure of the patient's symptoms. Huskisson (1974) makes the point that for assessing response to treatment a pain relief scale has advantages over a pain scale, and that 'pain cannot be said to have been relieved unless pain or pain relief has been directly measured'.
2. Full gynaecological, contraceptive and obstetric history, including any sexual problems.
3. Full history relating to bowel and urinary function.

4. Past medical history, including psychiatric illness.
5. Family history with particular reference to cancer amongst female relatives.
6. Social history including childhood memories and bereavements.

EXAMINATION

Observation of the patient should begin from the moment she enters the consulting room and is continued throughout the interview, as her demeanour may tell much about the true nature of the problem. She may be defensive and resent questions about sensitive areas, or on the other hand be openly hostile. A flattened effect may suggest a depressive illness with pain as the presenting symptom.

The formal examination should cover the following points:

1. General examination, specifically looking for signs of malignancy such as lymphadenopathy, anaemia and swelling of the lower limbs.
2. Abdominal palpation for masses, ascites and tenderness.

   Tenderness over the ovarian point (at the junction of middle and inner thirds of a line between the anterior superior iliac spine and the umbilicus) is said to be characteristic of women with pelvic venous congestion. It is thought to be due to compression of the ovarian vein as it crosses the transverse processes of the lumbar vertebrae (Beard et al 1984). Tenderness over a palpable caecum and sigmoid colon may be due to gaseous distension relating to the irritable bowel syndrome (IBS).
3. Vaginal examination:

   Speculum examination—vaginal discharge

   —cervical pathology

   Bimanual palpation   —uterine enlargement

   —adnexal masses

   —tenderness of uterus, tubes or ovaries

   —full bladder
4. Rectal examination, particularly to exclude malignant disease and to assess any masses in the pouch of Douglas.
5. Examination of lumbo-sacral spine and hip joints.

CLINICAL PRESENTATION

Although it may be impossible to make a firm diagnosis on history and examination alone, it is usually possible to make a differential diagnosis which points the way to the most appropriate further investigation. The conditions listed in Tables 15.1 and 15.2 will often have a specific clinical picture, although there may well be a considerable overlap of symptomatology and physical signs.

Gynaecological conditions

Cyclical pain

Dysmenorrhoea is a common complaint, although only in 5% of women is it severe. In the majority of cases there is no underlying pathology although so called congestive dysmenorrhoea is said to be associated with such conditions as endometriosis or adenomyosis.

Ovulation pain (Mittelschmerz). This occurs mid cycle, is of acute onset and is a sharp lower abdominal pain followed by several hours of dull aching in the pelvis. Although it is usually thought to be caused by rupture of the ovarian follicle at ovulation, it has been shown that the onset of pain most frequently corresponds to the peak LH levels 24 hours prior to ovulation, suggesting that the pain is caused by increased contractility of ovarian perifollicular smooth muscle mediated through prostaglandin f_2 (O'Herlihy et al 1980).

Pelvic inflammatory disease (PID)

Patients with PID are usually young (less than 25 years old) sexually active and have had more than one sexual partner. Clinical signs and symptoms are frequently misleading however. In women who have a combination of lower abdominal pain, vaginal discharge and pelvic tenderness only 60% will be found to have pelvic infection at laparoscopy (Westrom & Mardl 1984). Acute PID is most commonly caused by *Chlamydia trachomatis* or *Neisseria gonorrhoea*, and particularly if inadequately treated may progress to the chronic condition where recurrent or persistent infection is more likely to be due to coliform or anaerobic organisms. The long term sequelae of chronic PID are persistent lower abdominal and pelvic pain, deep dyspareunia, altered menstruation and infertility.

Endometriosis

The pain of endometriosis is very variable in presentation and there is a poor correlation with the laparoscopic findings. Severe pain may be associated with minimal disease, whilst the reverse is also true. The commonest symptoms are dysmenorrhoea, dyspareunia and a persistent dull ache in the pelvis, although severe acute pain may be caused by the rupture of an endometriotic cyst.

Neoplasia of the genital tract

Benign. Large fibroids may cause a persistent dull aching pain in the pelvis, whilst an ovarian cyst may produce recurrent episodes of sharp pain secondary to torsion of the ovarian pedicle.

Malignant. Although pain is not a leading feature of malignant disease of the cervix and body of the uterus, lower abdominal and pelvic pain is the commonest presenting symptom in advanced ovarian cancer. Such cases comprise 70% of the total at initial diagnosis, and on examination one would expect to find ascites in association with a mass arising from the pelvis.

Pelvic pain syndrome (PPS)

In many women with chronic pelvic pain no clearly defined pathological cause will be found. Such 'unexplained' pain may well be associated with pelvic venous congestion which produces a clinical picture that has become known as the pelvic pain syndrome. Although the idea that such pelvic pain could be caused by venous congestion still generates scorn amongst sceptical gynaecologists, there is an ever increasing body of evidence that supports this view (Beard et al 1984, Hughes & Curtis 1962, Kaupilla 1970). The concept of pelvic venous congestion however is by no means new. In 1831 Robert Googe in his treatise on 'Diseases Peculiar to Women' gave a very good description of a syndrome which he ascribed to 'a morbid state of pelvic blood vessels indicated by their fullness'.

This condition is restricted to women in their reproductive years (Steege 1983) and is characterized by a dull aching pain with occasional severe acute attacks, more commonly present in the right iliac fossa, but sometimes moving from one side to the other. The pain responds to postural change, in that lying flat eases the pain whereas standing, walking and bending all make the pain worse. Congestive dysmenorrhoea, deep dyspareunia and typically post-coital ache are also common findings (Beard et al 1988) and not surprisingly these symptoms are related to a high incidence of sexual problems.

Polycystic ovarian syndrome (PCOS)

It has been suggested that this condition is closely related to PPS as in one study of women with PPS 56% also have PCOS (Adams et al 1986). Indeed recent histological studies have shown the ovaries removed from women suffering from PPS to be identical to those seen in PCOS. It has been postulated that the excess oestrogen seen in PCOS causes dilatation of the pelvic veins (Reginald et al 1989), as oestrogen has been shown to inhibit the contraction of smooth muscle in the walls of human veins (Barwin & McCalden 1972).

Residual ovary syndrome

This is the name given to the symptoms from ovaries left at the time of hysterectomy. Chronic pelvic pain and dyspareunia are the presenting symptoms in approximately 75% of cases, whilst a minority will present with an asymptomatic pelvic mass which is frequently associated with a benign, but sometimes malignant ovarian neoplasm (Christ & Lotze 1975).

Uterovaginal prolapse

The patient usually complains of a dull aching or dragging sensation in the pelvis in association with a 'lump' in the vagina.

Non-gynaecological conditions

Gastrointestinal

Bowel pathology typically is associated with change in bowel habit and the passage of blood and mucus per rectum, and it is therefore unusual to see such cases in a gynaecology clinic. Diverticular disease is common in people over the age of 60 years and approximately half the patients have chronic or intermittent lower abdominal pain. Constipation, or alternating diarrhoea and constipation with the passage of pebbly stools may accompany the pain or occur independently. Abdominal pain is one of the commonest presenting symptoms of colorectal malignancy, particularly in the sigmoid colon where the pain is often associated with an obstructing lesion.

The irritable bowel syndrome (IBS) is a common complaint of women presenting with pelvic pain to a gynaecology clinic (Hogston 1987), although in some women the pain said to be due to IBS is probably caused by pelvic venous congestion (Farquhar et al 1987). IBS is twice as common in women as in men and usually presents in the third or fourth decade. The most frequent site of pain is in the left lower abdomen. Pain can vary from a dull ache to one of such severity that strong analgesia is required. It may last from a few minutes to many hours and may be precipitated by food or relieved by defaecation or the passage of flatus. Bowel habit tends to swing between diarrhoea and constipation, and patients complain of feeling 'full of wind'. Other symptoms such as nausea, vomiting, frequency, dysuria, dysmenorrhoea and dyspareunia may also occur, but weight loss and evidence of systemic illness are absent. Although the diagnosis is made primarily by exclusion, use of Manning's Questionnaire may aid positive diagnosis (Manning et al 1978).

Renal tract

The two main causes of pain arising from the urinary tract are infection and the presence of calculi. Although the peak symptomatic period is during the late teens and twenties, infection increases in frequency with age. Infection in the elderly may be asymptomatic or have minimal symptoms such as lower abdominal pain and frequency. Chronic infection can result in persistent pelvic pain, whilst chronic interstitial cystitis usually occurs in middle-aged women and causes severe supra-pubic pain.

Ureteric and bladder calculi may cause recurrent episodes of lower abdominal and pelvic pain. They are particularly likely to occur in women with predisposing conditions such as diabetes mellitus, multiple sclerosis and other causes of a neurogenic bladder.

Skeletal causes

Women with chronic pelvic pain are often polysymptomatic and may well complain of back-ache (Renaer et al 1980). Low back-ache of musculo-skeletal origin radiates most commonly to the lower limbs and not to the abdomen or pelvis. Hip pain may sometimes be mistaken for pain arising in the lower back and characteristically is most severe in the groins but may also be felt in the buttocks (Klenerman 1981).

INVESTIGATIONS

Laparoscopy

Of the few investigations which are genuinely helpful, laparoscopy is by far the most informative and is an essential part of the investigation in all cases of chronic pelvic pain. Although a diagnosis may often be made on history and examination alone it is impossible to exclude endometriosis completely. Conversely, many women have been said to have chronic PID and treated with multiple courses of antibiotics, when laparoscopy reveals a healthy pelvis. Other conditions that may be diagnosed at laparoscopy are polycystic ovarian syndrome (PCOS), and the dilated veins associated with pelvic pain syndrome (PPS).

The finding of a completely normal pelvis is also important as this knowledge will reassure many women whose pain is brought on by anxiety or fear of cancer (Beard et al 1977).

Imaging

Ultrasound is a very informative investigation which has the added advantage of being non-invasive. As well as detecting pelvic masses the characteristic features of the ovaries in PCOS are easily seen. The dimensions of uterus and ovaries tend to be larger than normal in cases of PPS (Adams et al 1986) whilst the diameter of pelvic veins can be measured using the Doppler mode.

X-rays:

1. Plain x-ray of lumbo-sacral spine and hip joints ⎫
2. Intravenous urogram   ⎬ where indicated
3. Barium enema   ⎭
4. Transuterine pelvic venography

This is a simple outpatient technique similar to a hysterosalpingogram. It is a reliable means of demonstrating dilatation and congestion of pelvic veins (Beard et al 1984).

Computerized tomography and magnetic resonance imaging

Although these techniques have no place in assessing the majority of women with chronic pelvic pain they are invaluable in assessing the spread of malignant disease.

Other investigations

Examination of mid-stream urine specimen. This is mandatory. Urinary infection is common in women and may present, particularly in older age groups, with pelvic pain without any obvious symptoms such as dysuria and frequency. Specimens which contain $> 10^5$ bacteria per ml indicate infection in 80% of cases. If two successive specimens show $> 10^5$ organisms per ml this is diagnostic of infection in 95% of cases. In the remainder unless there are white blood cells present the growth may be due to contamination of the specimen at the time of collection or to delay in culturing which may give a few contaminant bacteria time to multiply. If it is impossible to obtain a 'clean catch' specimen, then suprapubic aspiration or a urethral catheter specimen is indicated.

Full blood count. This may reveal an iron deficiency which although commonly caused by menorrhagia, may alert to the possibility of a colonic malignancy.

TREATMENT

In a minority of women complaining of chronic pelvic pain a specific pathology can be identified as the cause, and the appropriate treatment undertaken. Malignant disease and utero-vaginal prolapse are good examples of conditions where a specific treatment is indicated. Pain caused by endometriosis has been well reviewed elsewhere by Nezhat who advocates laser ablation of endometriosis using video laseroscopy techniques (Nezhat 1989). In his study of 190 patients with endometriosis who complained of pelvic pain, 82% had complete relief of symptoms when reviewed 12 months after treatment. In inexperienced hands this is a potentially hazardous technique, and one which should only be considered if prior medical treatment with hormonal therapy has failed.

Chronic PID can cause recurrent episodes of pain which may be related to recrudescence of infection which is amenable to antibiotic therapy. The long-term complications of infection such as menorrhagia and dysmenorrhoea are best managed using non-steroidal anti-inflammatory drugs

(NSAID), but surgery will be necessary in cases of abscess formation. Certainly in advanced cases of endometriosis or chronic infection where the pelvic organs are stuck down by dense adhesions—the 'frozen pelvis'—the resulting pain can be severe and intractable, and again surgery is the best answer. This means a complete clearance of uterus, tubes and ovaries, with indefinite hormone replacement therapy (HRT) thereafter. Now that such effective methods of HRT are available, there is absolutely nothing to be gained by trying to leave a small volume of functioning ovary, as it is the ovaries which are the source of most of the pain—the so-called ovarian entrapment or residual ovary syndrome (Christ & Lotz 1975). Subsequent attempts at oophorectomy following hysterectomy can be very difficult as the ovaries are usually stuck down to the pelvic side walls, and there is a real risk of damage to the ureters and great vessels.

Whether surgery is justified where adhesions are thought to be causing pain is open to debate. Adhesions can of course produce a painful band obstruction of the small or large bowel but whether they cause pain otherwise is a vexed question and one which may be no more than 'a poorly substantiated myth' (Alexander-Williams 1987). Rapkin (1986) questioned the role of pelvic adhesions as a cause of chronic pelvic pain when she reported on a retrospective analysis of 100 consecutive laparoscopies for pelvic pain, and compared the findings with 88 consecutive laparoscopies in women with primary infertility. Twenty-six per cent of the women with chronic pelvic pain had pelvic adhesions compared with 39% in the infertile group. In addition only 4 out of 34 patients in the latter group complained of pain, yet there was no difference in the density or localization of adhesions between the two groups. In a similar study however, Kresh et al (1984) found pelvic adhesions in 38% of women with chronic pelvic pain as against only 12% in a control group undergoing laparoscopy for tubal ligation. Chan & Wood (1985) claimed that pelvic adhesiolysis was effective in relieving chronic pelvic pain in a retrospective questionnaire study. However, in the vast majority of their cases the indication for surgery was infertility caused by tubal adhesions rather than chronic pelvic pain, which tends to invalidate their conclusions. A problem which bedevils proper analysis of pain relief by adhesiolysis is that the adhesions are frequently associated with chronic PID and endometriosis, both of which are common causes of pelvic pain. Furthermore, attempts to divide adhesions at laparotomy are often doomed to failure because standard surgical technique leads to formation of yet more adhesions. The new technique of laser laparoscopic adhesiolysis circumvents these problems and very promising results have been achieved following division of adhesions in a group of women without evidence of PID or endometriosis but in whom adhesions had been caused by previous pelvic or abdominal surgery (Sutton 1989).

Although this study is open to criticism as it was retrospective and uncontrolled, the use of the laser in these circumstances is certainly worthy of further investigation.

The problem remains however of the woman who complains of persistent pelvic pain but in whom, usually after a succession of investigations culminating in a negative laparoscopy, no pathological cause can be found. Many doctors label the woman as 'hysterical' and vow never to see her again. This is often achieved by referring her to another specialist for his opinion and hoping that she is not sent back again when he cannot find anything wrong either. Others, feeling forced into a corner, may resort to surgery. The results are often disappointing however and the woman is left with her pain despite having lost her entire reproductive tract, sometimes during the course of repeated operations. This only reinforces her feelings of inadequacy as she grieves for the loss of her womanhood and her ability to bear children. Taylor (1957) wrote that 'premature resort to surgery is the characteristic error in the present day treatment of these patients with pelvic pain'.

Following a negative laparoscopy in a woman in the reproductive age range the next step should be to perform pelvic venography and pelvic ultrasound if this has not already been done. Increased uterine area on ultrasound scan correlates well with the finding of pelvic venous congestion, whilst direct measurement of venous diameters can be made with the Doppler mode. Using these techniques, the demonstration that these women commonly have pelvic venous congestion will often produce a marked improvement in their response to the pain, because they feel that at last an explanation for the symptoms has been found and they are not 'just imagining things'. Pelvic venography has also led on to the development of specific therapy, and allows an objective assessment of the effects of treatment. Treatment of PPS can be either with surgery, drugs or psychotherapy.

Surgical treatment

Although surgery clearly has a limited role in a disorder confined exclusively to the child bearing years, there have been advocates of this approach. Resection of dilated ovarian veins has been successful in some cases (Railo 1968, Rundquist et al 1984) as has hysterectomy (Mills 1978). In the older woman who has no wish for further pregnancies, total abdominal hysterectomy together with bilateral salpingo-oophorectomy, followed by hormone replacement therapy, will definitely have a place. Previous comments about avoiding the problems of the residual ovary syndrome by performing a pelvic clearance followed by HRT again hold true. Beard has recently reported on 15 women, with an average age of 30 years, suffering from PPS who were thus treated. At 9 month follow-up they all had a dramatic improvement in their pain, with a concomitant increase in frequency of sexual activity and overall improvement in their quality of life (Beard 1989).

Drug treatment

Continuous high dose progestogen

The rationale behind this treatment is to reduce oestrogen levels by supressing ovulation. Using medroxyprogesterone acetate (MPA) (Provera-Upjohn) 300 mg/day, Reginald et al (1989) have achieved promising results. In a group of 22 women with PPS they achieved significant improvement in 17 with minimal side effects. Pain relief correlated with a reduced diameter of the pelvic veins on venography together with a decrease in uterine size and endometrial thickness. A subsequent placebo-controlled study (Farquhar et al 1989) using MPA 50 mg daily for 4 months has shown a significantly better response to MPA than placebo after initial treatment. However, there was no difference after treatment had been stopped at 9 months follow-up unless the drug treatment had been combined with psychotherapy. This would suggest therefore that although MPA is effective whilst it is being taken by the patient, it has no long lasting benefit thereafter. There are anecdotal reports of patients being maintained on high dose MPA for up to 18 months, but many women find the side effects of weight gain, bloating and menstrual irregularity intolerable in the long term.

Dihydroergotamine (DHE)

The use of ergot alkaloids is not a new idea. Over 100 years ago Lawson Tait used ergot to relieve the pain of congestive dysmenorrhoea (Tait 1883). DHE is a selective venoconstricting agent which increases venous tone and mobilizes blood which is present in capacitance vessels. Following intravenous injection of DHE in 12 women with PPS in a single blind cross over trial, Reginald et al showed a significant reduction in the diameter of the pelvic veins. This correlated well with pain relief which lasted up to 48 hours after the injection (Reginald et al 1987). This obviously merits further investigation and it would be interesting to see whether oral administration might have similar effects.

Psychotherapy

Many authors have confirmed that women who complain of pelvic pain but have no pathological cause for it are, as a group, psychologically different from women without pain. They tend to be more neurotic, to have abnormal attitudes to their own and their partner's sexuality, and to form less rewarding relationships. This does not mean that these women should be referred directly to a psychiatric department, a suggestion which would give grave offence to most of them. Many of these women are helped by a sympathetic doctor who is prepared to take their complaint seriously. This in itself is a simple form of psychotherapy as is the knowledge that her complaint does have some physical basis i.e. pelvic venous congestion. The best approach therefore is to work closely with an interested colleague, either psychologist, psychotherapist or psychiatrist, with whom one can share such cases, thereby gaining the trust and confidence of the patient. A recent study comparing two behavioural methods of treatment—stress analysis and pain analysis—with a minimal intervention control group showed a significant improvement in the two treatment groups over the latter (Reginald et al 1989). Such treatment has also been shown to have long term benefits in the irritable bowel syndrome (Suedlund et al 1983), a problem which frequently presents with pain to gynaecologists, and which may have a psychosomatic background similar to PPS.

REFERENCES

Adams J, Beard R W, Franks S, Pearce S, Reginald P W 1986 Pelvic ultrasound findings in women with chronic pelvic pain: correlation with laparoscopy and venography. Abstracts of the 24th British Congress of Obstetrics & Gynaecology. Cardiff April 1986. RCOG, London, p 80
Alexander-Williams J 1987 Do adhesions cause pain? Br Med J 294: 659–660
Barwin B N, McCalden T A 1972 The inhibitory action of oestradiol -17b and progesterone on human venous smooth muscle. Proceedings of the Physiological Society, p 41
Beard R W 1989 British Congress of Obstetrics and Gynaecology
Beard R W, Belsy E N, Lieberman M B, Wilkinson J C M 1977 Pelvic pain in women. Am J Obstet Gynecol 128: 566–570
Beard R W, Highman J H, Pearce S, Reginald P W 1984 Diagnosis of pelvic varicosities in women with chronic pelvic pain. Lancet ii: 946–949
Beard R W, Reginald P W, Wadsworth J 1988 Clinical features of women with chronic lower abdominal pain and pelvic congestion. Br J Obstet Gynaecol 95: 153–161
Chamberlain G V P, Brown J C (eds) 1978 Report of the Working Party of the Confidential Enquiry into Gynaecological Laparoscopy. Royal College of Obstetricians and Gynaecologists, London
Chan C L, Wood C 1985 Pelvic adhesiolysis—the assessment of symptom relief by 100 patients. Aust NZ J Obstet Gynaecol 25: 295–298
Christ J E, Lotze E C 1975 The residual ovary syndrome. Obstet Gynecol 46: 55
Farquhar C M, Reginald P W, Beard R W 1987 Irritable bowel syndrome as a cause of chronic pain in women attending a gynaecological clinic (letter). Br Med J 294: 1228
Farquhar C M, Rogers V, Franks S, Pearce S, Wadsworth J, Beard R W 1989 A study of medroxy progesterone acetate and psychotherapy for the treatment of lower abdominal pain associated with pelvic congestion. Br J Obstet Gynaecol (in press)
Gillibrand P N 1981 The investigation of pelvic pain. Communication on the scientific meeting on chronic pelvic pain: a gynaecological headache. RCOG, London
Gomez J, Dally P 1977 Psychologically mediated abdominal pain in surgical and medical outpatient clinics. Br Med J i: 1451–1453
Hogston P 1987 Irritable bowel syndrome as a cause of chronic pain in women attending a gynaecology clinic. Br Med J 294: 934
Hughes R R, Curtis D D 1962 Uterine phlebography. Am J Obstet Gynecol 83: 154–156
Huskisson E C 1974 Measurement of pain. Lancet ii: 1127–1131
Kaupilla A 1970 Uterine phlebography with venous compression. A clinical and roentological study. Acta Obstet Gynecol Scand 49: 33–34
Klenerman L 1981 Lower abdominal pain—the orthopaedic viewpoint. In: Fisher A M, Gordon H (eds) Clinics in Obstetrics & Gynaecology vol 8. (ii) p 27
Kresch A J, Seifer D B, Sachs L B, Barresse I 1984 Laparoscopy in 100 women with chronic pelvic pain. Obstet Gynecol 64: 672–674

Manning P, Thompson W G, Heaton K W, Morris A F 1978 Towards positive diagnosis of the irritable bowel. Br Med J 2: 653–654

Merskey H 1980 In: Bonica J J (ed) Pain: Association for research in nervous and mental disease vol 58. Raven Press, New York, pp 249–250

Merskey H 1984 Too much pain. Br J Hosp Med 31: 63–66

Mills W G 1978 The enigma of pelvic pain. J R Soc Med 71: 257–260

Morris N, O'Neill D 1958 Outpatient gynaecology. Br Med J i: 1038–1039

Nezhat C 1989 Videolaseroscopy for the treatment of endometriosis. In: Studd J (ed) Progress in Obstetrics & Gynaecology vol. 7. Churchill Livingstone, Edinburgh, pp 293–303

O'Herlihy C, Robinson H P, de Crespigny L J Ch 1980 Mittelschmerz is a preovulatory symptom. Br Med J 280: 986

Railo J E 1968 The pain syndrome in ovarian varicocele. Acta Chir Scand 134: 157–159

Rapkin A 1986 Adhesions and pelvic pain: a retrospective study. Obstet Gynecol 68: 13–15

Reginald P W, Beard R W, Kooner J S et al 1987 Intravenous dihydroergotamine to relieve pelvic congestion with pain in young women. Lancet ii: 351–353

Reginald P W, Pearce S, Beard R W 1989 Pelvic pain due to venous congestion. In: Studd J (ed) Progress in Obstetrics and Gynaecology, vol 7. Churchill Livingstone, London, pp 275–292

Renaer M, Nij P, Van Assche A, Vertommen H 1980 Chronic pelvic pain without obvious pathology in women. Personal observation and a review of the problem. Eur J Obstet Gynaecol Reprod Biol 10: 415–463

Rundquist E, Sandholm L E, Larsson G 1984 Treatment of pelvic varicosities causing lower abdominal pain with extra peritoneal resection of the left ovarian vein. Ann Chirurgie et Gynaecologiae 73: 339–341

Steege J F 1983 Chronic pelvic pain: clinical perspectives. In: Dinnerstein, Burrows (eds) Handbook of psychosomatic obstetrics and gynaecology. Elsevier Biomedical Press, Amsterdam, pp 401–412

Suedlund J, Ottoson J O, Sjodin I, Doterwall E 1983 Controlled study of psychotherapy in irritable bowel syndrome. Lancet ii: 589–592

Sutton C J G 1989 Personal communication

Tait L 1883 The pathology and treatment of the diseases of the ovaries. William Wood, New York

Taylor H C 1957 The problem of pelvic pain. In: Meigs J V, Samers H S (eds) Progress in gynecology vol III. Grunne and Stratton, New York, pp 191–208

Westrom L, Mardl P A 1984 Salpingitis. In: Holmes K (ed) Sexually transmitted diseases. McGraw-Hill, New York

Wilkes E 1974 Some problems in cancer management. Proc R Soc Med 67: 1001–1005

16. Pelvic inflammatory disease

C. M. Stacey   S. E. Barton   A. Singer

Most gynaecologists are familiar with the expression '?PID', which is often to be found written in both GP referral letters and the hospital notes of women admitted to gynaecology wards via casualty. Usually it is used as shorthand to indicate that an upper genital tract infection is being considered as a differential diagnosis, often because there are no specific symptoms or signs of another condition. The majority of women who are given a diagnosis of '?PID' have not had sufficient investigations performed to confirm or refute the diagnosis, but are managed by a trial of antibiotic therapy with further investigations following only if the clinical condition does not improve.

The sequelae of pelvic inflammatory disease (PID) now cause a significant morbidity in women of childbearing age (Westrom 1988), and attempts must be made to reduce both the prevalence and complications of this condition.

It is becoming increasingly clear that there is a group of women who acquire the infection asymptomatically, who are not diagnosed in the acute stage but only present later with complications. Appropriate strategies to detect and treat these women need to be considered urgently.

This chapter will review the pathogenesis and microbiology of this condition, as well as discussing diagnostic techniques, therapy and outcome.

DEFINITION

The term pelvic inflammatory disease is used to describe an upper genital tract infection, giving no indication of the site or severity. This term should not be used to describe the lower genital tract infections (vulvitis, vaginitis and cervicitis).

It is more specific to use terms that describe the anatomical sites of the infection such as endometritis, parametritis, salpingitis, salpingo-oophritis, pelvic peritonitis and pelvic abscess. This is not possible when a clinical diagnosis is made as the exact location of the upper genital tract infection is usually unknown, however if the diagnosis is made by laparoscopy, laparotomy or endometrial biopsy then the more accurate terms should be used.

PATHOGENESIS AND MICROBIOLOGY

PID may be caused by a variety of organisms which can be present in the genital tract in different combinations during the course of the disease. Thus the aetiology of the condition has been described as polymicrobial (Eschenbach et al 1975).

The natural course of the disease is incompletely understood, but it has been suggested (Westrom 1987) that there is an initial infection with a sexually transmitted agent, which often causes only clinically mild disease. However, if this does not resolve spontaneously, a polymicrobial stage may follow, eventually resulting in pelvic peritonitis and abscess formation.

Pathogenesis

It is assumed, even in cases where no sexually transmitted agent is found, that the organisms causing the disease have originated in the lower genital tract. These organisms may be present for a variable length of time, with or without causing symptoms. In some cases the organism may be introduced into the endometrium by gynaecological procedures such as insertion of intra-uterine contraceptive device, dilatation and curettage, laparoscopy and dye testing and termination of pregnancy (Westrom & Mardh 1989).

The mechanism by which organisms ascend from the cervix into the upper genital tract is not known. Both motile spermatozoa and trichomonads have been postulated as carriers (Keith et al 1986). In particular, spermatozoa have been shown to attach to pathogenic organisms and facilitate their migration through cervical mucus in vitro (Toth et al 1982). Passive transport of particles from the lower to the upper genital tract has also been demonstrated (Egli & Newton 1971), but the exact mechanism and its importance is unknown.

Lymphatic spread via the parametrium, avoiding the endometrium has been demonstrated in animal studies using *Mycoplasma hominis* (Mh) in grivet monkeys (Mardh et al 1983), but again its clinical importance remains uncertain.

The development of PID is often associated with menstruation (Sweet et al 1986), suggesting that organisms already present in the cervix may ascend at this time. This may be due to either cervical factors or retrograde menstruation.

Contraceptive method seems to be important in the epidemiology of PID as women wearing an intra-uterine contraceptive device have a 1·5 to 7·3 times increased risk of developing PID when compared to non-contraceptors. Women using the combined oral contraceptive pill have a reduced rate of 0·2 to 0·4 (Westrom 1987). These observations suggest that whereas an intra-uterine contraceptive device may encourage organisms present in the cervix to ascend to the upper genital tract, hormonal methods of contraception appear to discourage this process, possibly due to changes in cervical mucus.

Sexual activity is another epidemiological factor affecting the prevalence of PID, and although increased sexual activity is likely to result in an increased exposure to pathogenic organisms, it is also possible that sexual activity itself affects the course of the disease (Keith et al 1986).

Once the infectious agent has gained access to the upper genital tract, the initial lesion caused is an endometritis (Wolner-Hanssen et al 1982). This may produce the symptom of irregular vaginal bleeding reported in a proportion of cases of PID. Although endometritis is associated with laparoscopic evidence of PID (Paavonen et al 1985), the association is not invariable, and women with an intra-uterine contraceptive device in situ are known to have a low grade endometrial infection with no apparent ill effects (Mishell et al 1966).

The infection can then ascend into the endosalpinx, causing a mucosal inflammation followed by oedema of the tubal wall and the production of an exudate which leaks through the fimbrial end of the fallopian tube. This exudate is associated with inflammation of other pelvic structures, which results in the formation of sticky adhesions between the inflamed tissues. At the fimbrial end of the fallopian tube these adhesions may lead to the tube becoming sealed. It is important to note that adhesion formation occurs concurrently with the acute infection. This can result in permanent damage to the tubes and tubo-ovarian mass formation. Further spread along the paracolic gutter or lymphatics may cause the infection to reach the liver, causing Fitz-Hugh Curtis syndrome (Fitz-Hugh 1934).

From these observations it is possible to postulate that there is a stage, before tubal damage has taken place, when prompt treatment of the infection could prevent the formation of adhesions. It may even be possible to prevent the passage of the infection to the Fallopian tubes by treatment at the stage of endometrial infection.

Microbiology

Tuberculous disease is now not properly defined as PID, as this term implies an ascending infection.

Table 16.1   Isolation of sexually transmitted agents from the lower genital tract of women with laparoscopically confirmed PID

Study	Location	No. of women	Ct %	Ng %	Mh %
Kristensen et al (1985)	Sweden	85	13	24	
Wolner-Hanssen et al (1985)	Sweden	544	38	19·5	
Magnusson et al (1986)	Iceland	225	18·9	38·5	
Brihmer et al (1987)	Sweden	187	26·7	11·2	21·9
Brunham et al (1988)	USA	50	10	36	

The causative organisms have been studied by taking specimens from the lower and upper genital tracts in women with laparoscopic evidence of disease. The proportion of cases due to each organism depends on the population studied. The rates of isolation of *Chlamydia trachomatis* (Ct) and *Neisseria gonorrhoeae* (Ng) from the lower genital tracts of women in recent studies are shown in Table 16.1.

Using tubal cultures and/or serological evidence the estimated proportions of PID caused by the various agents are as follows: Ct 40–60%, Ng 15–18%, *Mycoplasma hominis* 10–15%, anaerobes 3–5% and unknown 15–20% (Westrom & Mardh 1989).

In a recent Swedish study of 187 women with PID and 136 with a normal pelvis at laparoscopy (Brihmer et al 1987), Ng was found in the cervix of 21% of the women with PID and 3% of those without. This organism was isolated from the Fallopian tube in 2% of the PID cases. In the same study *Chlamydia trachomatis* was detected in the cervix of 50% of the women with PID and 16% of those without. The rate of isolation from the Fallopian tube of Ct was 5%. Cervical cultures detected either Ct or Ng in 71% of the PID cases. In the same study, Bacteriodes species were found in the Fallopian tubes of 5%, *Actinomyces israelii* in 2%, *Gardnerella vaginalis* in 1%, *Ureaplasma urealyticum* in 1% and *Mycoplasma hominis* in no cases.

The proposed natural history accounts for the paucity of sexually transmitted agents isolated from the tubes suggesting that the initiating organism causes an acute and short-lived inflammation, and the continuance of the disease only occurs if superinfection with other, perhaps less pathogenic agents occurs.

Isolation of any pathogen from the Fallopian tubes presents considerable difficulty unless there is free pus present, because adequate microbiological specimens are difficult to obtain without the risk of adding to tubal damage.

There have been reports of the isolation of Ct from the upper genital tract in cases where it was not found in the lower genital tract (Moller et al 1986), however this is an infrequent finding. Although specimens from the upper genital tract are mandatory for research purposes, in the clinical situation, testing of the lower genital tract is more likely to yield a microbiological diagnosis.

Anaerobes such as Bacteriodes and Peptococcus species are frequently found in the lower genital tract of asymptomatic sexually active women, and the numer of organisms depends on the menstrual cycle. However in the upper genital tract these organisms are usually secondary invaders, either in the chronic phase of an initial episode of PID, or in recurrent disease. Aerobic bacteria normally found in the endogenous flora of the lower genital tract can become pathogenic if they ascend to the upper genital tract. Isolation of non-sexually transmitted organisms from the upper genital tract is more common in patients who are seriously ill or who have pelvic abscesses (Mardh 1980).

Mycoplasma hominis has been shown to be a pathogen in animal studies and has been isolated from the upper genital tract of infected women (Mardh 1980). Its mode of spread is different from Ct and Ng, as it causes parametritis rather than endometritis. Its importance as an aetiological agent has yet to be determined (Lind et al 1985).

Different clinical syndromes have been associated with specific infectious agents (Westrom & Mardh 1989). Although there is considerable overlap certain patterns of disease do suggest particular causative organisms.

Gonococcal disease usually presents with a short history and a pyrexial illness with a severe clinical picture, but resolution of symptoms within 72 hours after starting appropriate antibiotic therapy is the rule.

Chlamydial disease is characterized by a longer history and a more benign clinical picture. The infection may be asymptomatic.

As anaerobic infections are associated with abscesses the disease is often severe, with palpable adnexal masses and evidence of pelvic peritonitis.

In cases where no organisms are isolated, the clinical picture and tubal damage both tend to be milder.

Serology

Serological methods have been used to complement culture techniques in the evaluation of the cause of PID (Paavonen & Makela 1985). However there are several problems with serological data. Firstly, due to the natural history of PID, the patient may present long after the initiating infection. Secondly the presence of antibodies is not always indicative of PID as an antibody response may occur with asymptomatic colonization. Thirdly, as the disease is often of polymicrobial aetiology, antibody responses to many different organisms may occur. Thus serology does not currently play a major part in the acute diagnosis of the condition although serological findings may be more useful in detecting a past infection, for example in infertile women, for use in epidemiological surveys.

CLASSIFICATION

Westrom & Mardh (1989) classified ascending pelvic infection into two groups: exogenous infections (usually sexually transmitted) and endogenous infections. A more detailed classification has been suggested by Hare (1988):

Primary pelvic inflammatory disease (first attack, no precipitating cause)

1. Due to exogenous sexually transmitted agents (common, especially in younger women).
2. Due to endogenous organisms (rare, usually in the older age group; beware of missed underlying cause).

Secondary pelvic inflammatory disease

1. Leading on from primary, where endogenous organisms replace exogenous organisms in an ongoing infection.
2. Secondary to a significant event such as the insertion of an intra-uterine contraceptive device, pregnancy termination etc.
3. Secondary to the wearing of an intra-uterine contraceptive device, usually endogenous infection.
4. Secondary to a focus of infection elsewhere in the body. This may be intra-abdominal e.g. appendix, or remote e.g. tuberculous infection.

Recurrent pelvic inflammatory disease

1. Recurrence related to a further exposure to an exogenous source of sexually transmitted disease.
2. Recurrence involving endogenous organisms, due to reduced host defences to infection after the primary attack.

DIAGNOSIS OF PID

PID has a wide spectrum of clinical features, ranging from no symptoms at all to life threatening disease. It is probable that up to one third of cases are undiagnosed at the time of the acute infection. Laparoscopy has come to be used as the gold standard of diagnosis, although clinical diagnosis becomes more accurate with more severe disease.

Clinical diagnosis

Although many studies have been published (see Table 16.1), the criteria for the clinical diagnosis of PID have not been standardized, which limits the comparisons that can be made between different findings.

The percentage of women with suspected PID whose diagnosis was confirmed at laparoscopy ranges from 49 to 74% (Odendaal 1990). The first study of this type was performed in 1969, and involved 814 cases (Jacobson & Westrom 1969). The women studied presented with acute low abdominal pain and two or more of the following signs and symptoms: abnormal vaginal discharge, fever, vomiting, menstrual irregularities, urinary symptoms, proctitis symptoms, pelvic tenderness, adnexal mass, and $ESR > 15$ mm per hour. Acute salpingitis was visually confirmed in 65% of women during laparoscopy.

In a later study of 738 women (Wolner-Hanssen et al 1985), the minimum criteria for performing laparoscopy were acute lower abdominal pain, abnormal adnexal tenderness and purulent vaginal discharge or irregular uterine bleeding. Laparoscopic signs of acute salpingitis were found in 73·7% of women.

The correlation between non-laparoscopic and laparoscopic diagnosis increases as the number of clinical and laboratory criteria used to confirm the diagnosis of PID are increased.

Multivariate analysis has been used in an attempt to predict the women with PID, or the women with sufficient doubt in the diagnosis to necessitate diagnostic laparoscopy (Hadgu et al 1986). In this study 628 women underwent laparoscopy, and 414 were confirmed as having PID. Using seven features that are associated with PID, namely: purulent vaginal discharge, $ESR > 15$, gonorrhoea culture result, adnexal swelling, rectal temperature > 38, age < 25 and marital status, the regression model accurately predicted 87% of women who had PID but only 52·5% of those who did not. If a woman exhibits all seven variables, then the estimated probability of her having acute PID is 97%. If the only criterion that she lacks is a vaginal discharge the probability is 86%. If all the predictor variables are negative in a woman complaining of acute abdominal pain, the probability of PID is only 7%.

If laparoscopic findings were taken into account in women with a low probability of PID then all cases of PID would have been diagnosed, making the sensitivity of the model 100%. This would involve laparoscoping only 212 of the 628 women studied. The overall correct classification in this circumstance is 89·1%, as some of the women not laparoscoped would be incorrectly diagnosed as having PID, making the specificity 67·2%.

The authors comment that the clinical parameters used may need to be adjusted, for instance the addition of the results of isolation tests for Ct, but the theory that the decision whether to laparoscope can be made by taking a set of clinical criteria is an attractive one.

Several attempts have been made to assess the economic considerations of the inaccuracy of the diagnosis of PID. There is no doubt that unnecessary hospital stays, especially if intravenous antibiotics are used, are expensive. Furthermore, there is considerable morbidity resulting from the delay in diagnosing other conditions which have been missed after the provisional diagnosis of PID has been made. Method et al (1987) found that the routine use of laparoscopy to diagnose PID in hospitalized patients would not greatly increase the expense. However this does not take into account women with disease that is judged too mild for hospital admission, and for whom the clinical diagnosis is likely to be even less accurate.

Clinicians differ in their criteria for subjecting a woman with '?PID' to laparoscopy, although for research purposes this is considered mandatory. In current clinical practice, women are generally deemed to require a laparoscopy if a pelvic mass is present, if there is any suspicion of ectopic pregnancy or if there is failure of response to treatment.

Laparoscopic diagnosis

The laparoscopic appearances of PID were originally described by

Jacobson & Westrom in 1969. Three signs were described: pronounced hyperaemia of the tubal surface, oedema of the tube and a sticky exudate on the tubal surface. All need to be present for a diagnosis to be made.

These criteria were further modified by Hager et al (1983), and a grading system was introduced. Mild disease was characterized by tubal erythema and oedema, with the presence of an exudate assessed after the tube was manipulated. In moderate disease gross purulent material was evident and the tubes were not mobile. In severe disease there was a tubo-ovarian mass, pyosalpinx or a pelvic abscess.

The chronicity of the infection can also be estimated from the appearance at laparoscopy. Henry-Suchet (1985) describes five classifications:

1. Acute disease with normal fimbriae and no adhesions.
2. Acute disease with purulent discharge coming from the fimbrial ends.
3. Subacute disease with gelatinous adhesions and with or without pyosalpinges or abscesses.
4. Pelvic peritonitis with bowel adhesions and abundant purulent exudate.
5. Chronic or recurrent disease with dense fibrous adhesions.

Laparoscopic diagnosis is not always completely unequivocal. In mild cases there may be no spontaneous exudate, and the degree of oedema and hyperaemia needs to be assessed visually.

In a case of pelvic adhesions and hydrosalpinges it is often difficult to determine whether there is an acute infection, or if the adhesions are the result of past and inactive disease. The presence of a purulent exudate under these circumstances does indicate an active infection, but if this is absent the degree of oedema and hyperaemia need to be assessed and used to decide if there is continuing infection. Thus inert adhesions may be wrongly diagnosed when there is infection within a tubo-ovarian mass.

A situation is also possible in which there is potential infection in the endometrium, parametrium, or endosalpinx, but the outside of the tube looks normal (Paavonen et al 1985). In this case early disease may be missed at laparoscopy.

SEQUELAE

The most frequent short-term complication of PID is the development of a tubo-ovarian abscess, occurring in up to 30% of hospitalized patients (Landers & Sweet 1985). Long-term complications include adhesion formation leading to infertility and ectopic pregnancy, increased susceptibility to recurrent infection, chronic infection and chronic pelvic pain.

The probability of developing infertility depends on the number of episodes of infection and their severity (Westrom 1975). The proportion of women diagnosed as having tubal occlusion after one infection was reported as 12·8%, rising to 75% after three infections. These were all diagnosed laparoscopically. The rate of ectopic pregnancy was increased sixfold in the women with a past history of pelvic infection.

The long-term complications of PID may affect reproductive capacity. Further information about the prevalence of PID can be obtained by looking at women who have such sequelae. In a study of 52 women with pelvic adhesions (Sellors et al 1988), only 31% had a history of PID. Robertson et al (1988) reported a history of PID in only 3 out of 50 women who had an ectopic pregnancy. These figures suggest that a large proportion of women are undiagnosed at the time of the initial infection, and present later with complications.

Serological studies have shown that women with tubal infertility are more likely to have serum antibodies to Ct and Ng than women with other forms of infertility (Tijam et al 1985, Kelver & Nagamani 1989).

The development of chronic pelvic pain after an attack of PID has been well described (Westrom 1975). It is important to distinguish between three different groups of women: firstly, women who develop a recurrent infection in which the inflammation subsides but then develop a new infection due to either reacquisition of a sexually transmitted agent or reinfection with endogenous organisms; secondly those who develop a chronic infection, with multiple pockets of pus in the pelvis, and who are not properly cured by their initial treatment (this condition is frequently diagnosed but rarely confirmed); thirdly, women who develop pain related to adhesion formation to other pelvic or abdominal structures.

The complaint of chronic pelvic pain is common in women of child-bearing age, and in many cases the diagnosis of post PID pain or chronic PID is made with very little evidence of an original infection. Women with chronic pelvic pain have been extensively studied, and signs of past PID such as the presence of adhesions are found in few cases (Levitan et al 1985).

Beard et al (1988) reported that 46% of women with chronic pelvic pain and a normal laparoscopy had previously been diagnosed as having PID. In this paper the clinical features of pelvic congestion were described, which included the presence of a vaginal discharge and ovarian tenderness, features that may suggest a diagnosis of PID. If a detailed history of the pain is taken, other factors suggestive of pelvic congestion such as duration of pain greater than 6 months, postcoital ache and exacerbation by a rise in intra-abdominal pressure may be elicited.

MANAGEMENT

The management of a woman with '?PID' must depend on the clinical situation. Obtaining samples for the detection of sexually transmitted pathogens in the lower genital tract and the appropriate screening of the partner is mandatory (Barton et al 1986).

Adequate specimens for culture should be taken: a high vaginal swab may miss a gonococcal infection, so samples should be taken from the endo-cervix and urethra and placed in transport media for passage to the laboratory. Immediate microscopy and plating is helpful.

Another endocervical specimen should be taken for the detection of Ct. The laboratory methods for the detection of this organism are changing, and it is to be hoped that a cheap and accurate technique will soon be available. In the past, tissue culture was necessary to detect Ct as it is an obligate intracellular parasite, but this is an expensive use of laboratory time and prone to failure. A monoclonal antibody technique of staining direct smears has been developed (Syva UK) and this, though very accurate (Thomas et al 1984) also demands expensive technician time and thus is unsuitable for mass screening. A number of ELISA kits are now available, and it is these that are in current use in most centres. The accuracy of this technique still awaits further evaluation.

Blood tests for ESR and white cell count may be helpful in monitoring the course of the disease, but normal values do not exclude an acute infection.

Whether a laparoscopy should be performed depends on the factors already discussed, and on the woman's wish to undergo such investigation. In a recent study of PID in a genitourinary medicine clinic in London, only 1 in 5 women were prepared to undergo laparoscopy (Stacey et al 1989).

Pelvic abscesses can now be diagnosed by ultrasound examination, and this may be superior to laparoscopy and safer in cases where the vision is obscured by adhesions. Ultrasound also has the advantage that it can be more easily repeated. If the abscess is large, then surgical drainage is likely to be required, but if small, medical treatment may be curative.

Women with severe symptoms, pyrexia or pelvic masses should be admitted to hospital, and intravenous antibiotic therapy commenced if immediate diagnostic laparoscopy is not possible. A usual combination is penicillin, gentamicin and metronidazole (Hare 1988). The penicillin may need to be reviewed after the Ng culture results are available. If there is satisfactory improvement within 72 hours then it can be replaced by oral metronidazole and tetracycline or erthromycin for 14 days.

In cases of moderate symptoms, hospital admission is still advisable and oral treatment with metronidazole and a tetracycline commenced, with the treatment reviewed regularly.

Admission to hospital is not mandatory in all cases of '?PID'. If the signs and symptoms are mild, then oral antibiotic treatment can be given, with repeat examination twice weekly to assess the patient's condition and review the results of microbiological tests.

Women with particular worries about their fertility are best managed by laparoscopy however mild their symptoms. Laparoscopy is important in women who do not improve on antibiotics and women with recurrent symptoms. Chronic pelvic pain should not be diagnosed as PID without laparoscopic evidence.

CONCLUSION

The spectrum of PID is wide, and the emergency gynaecologist should be aware of all the different forms of this disease.

In women who complain of abdominal pain, an assessment of the likelihood of PID can be made by using clinical and laboratory tests with the liberal use of laparoscopy. Treatment is designed to arrest the infection, but irreversible tubal damage may already have occurred. It is important to take adequate samples to detect sexually transmitted diseases, enquire about symptoms in the partner, and suggest that he is also examined for genital infections.

It is possible that a large proportion of upper genital tract infection is asymptomatic, and it is in this group of women that we may look to prevent tubal damage. Ct is thought to be the major pathogen in these women, so that screening for this organism in sexually active women (and men) at genitourinary medicine clinics, family planning clinics and gynaecological outpatients, followed by appropriate treatment, may prevent some cases of PID. Screening for Ct is thought to be economically viable, at least in high risk women (e.g. women under 25 years of age, Estany et al 1989). Studies of the risk of infection in asymptomatic women with lower genital tract Ct colonization are urgently required.

Screening for sexually transmitted diseases should be performed before gynaecological manipulations such as IUCD insertion, termination of pregnancy and laparoscopy and dye test to prevent iatrogenic disease.

PID needs to be re-established as a positive and accurate diagnosis. Further research is needed to better define the causative agents and the most useful therapies for preventing tubal damage. The questionable use of the term '?PID' is only justified if clinicians then perform appropriate tests to confirm or refute this important diagnostic question.

REFERENCES

Barton S E, Greenhouse P, Attia W et al 1986 *Chlamydia trachomatis* infection in women: a case for more action? Lancet i: 1215

Beard R W, Reginald P W, Wadsworth J 1988 Clinical features of women with chronic lower abdominal pain and pelvic congestion. Br J Obstet Gynaecol 95: 153–161

Brihmer C, Kallings I, Nord C E et al 1987 Salpingitis; aspects of diagnosis and etiology: a 4-year study from a Swedish capital hospital. Eur J Obstet Gynaecol Reprod Biol 24: 211–220

Brunham R C, Binns B, Guijon F et al 1988 Etiology and outcome of acute pelvic inflammatory disease. J Infect Dis 158: 510–517

Egli G, Newton M 1961 The transport of carbon particles in the human female reproductive tract. Fertil Steril 12: 151–155

Eschenbach D A, Buchanan T M, Pollock H M et al 1975 Polymicrobial etiology of acute pelvic inflammatory disease. N Engl J Med 293: 166–171

Estany A, Todd M, Vasque et al 1989 Early detection of genital chlamydial infection in women: an economic evaluation. Sex Transm Dis 16: 21–27

Fitz-Hugh T 1943 Acute gonococcic peritonitis of the right upper quadrant in women. JAMA 102: 2094–2096

Hadgu A, Westrom L, Brooks C A et al 1986 Predicting acute pelvic inflammatory disease: a multivariate analysis. Obstet Gynecol 155: 954–960

Hager W D, Eschenbach D A, Spence M R et al 1983 Criteria for diagnosis and grading of salpingitis. Obstet Gynecol 61: 113–114

Hare M J 1988 Pelvic inflammatory disease. In: Hare M J (ed) Genital tract infection in women. Churchill Livingstone, Edinburgh, pp 134–158

Henry-Suchet J 1985 Laparoscopic diagnosis and treatment of PID. In: Keith L G, Berger G S (eds) Infections in reproductive health, vol 1 Common infections. MTP Press, Lancaster, pp 197–208

Jacobson L, Westrom L 1969 Objectivised diagnosis of acute pelvic inflammatory disease. Am J Obstet Gynecol 105: 1088–1098

Keith L G, Berger G S, Lopez-Zeno J 1986 Pathogenesis of pelvic inflammatory disease. In: New concepts on the causation of pelvic inflammatory disease, current problems in obstetrics, gynecology and fertility. Year Book Medical, Chicago, pp 18–30

Kelver M E, Nagamani M 1989 Chlamydial serology in women with tubal infertility. Int J Fertil 34: 42–45

Kristensen G B, Bollerup A C, Lind K et al 1985 Infections with *Neisseria gonorrhoeae* and *Chlamydia trachomatis* in women with acute salpingitis. Genitourin Med 61: 179–184

Landers D V, Sweet R L 1985 Current trends in the diagnosis and treatment of tubo-ovarian abscess. Am J Obstet Gynecol 151: 1098–1110

Levitan Z, Eibschitz I, de Vries K et al 1985 The value of laparoscopy in women with chronic pelvic pain and a 'normal pelvis'. Int J Gynaecol Obstet 23: 71–74

Lind K, Kristensen G B, Bollerup P et al 1985 Importance of *Mycoplasma hominis* in acute salpingitis assessed by culture and serological tests. Genitourin Med 61: 185–189

Magnusson S S, Oskarsson T, Geirsson R T et al 1986 Lower genital tract infection with *Chlamydia trachomatis* and *Neisseria gonorrhoeae* in Icelandic women with salpingitis. Am J Obstet Gynecol 155: 602–607

Mardh P A 1980 An overview of infectious agents of salpingitis, their biology and recent advances in methods of detection. Am J Obstet Gynecol 7: 933–951

Mardh P A, Westrom L, Torvald Ripa K et al 1983 Pelvic inflammatory disease: clinical, etiologic, and pathophysiologic studies. In: Holmes K K, Mardh P A (eds) International perspectives on neglected sexually transmitted diseases: impact on venereology, infertility and maternal and infant health. McGraw, Washington DC, pp 251–268

Method M W, Urnes P, Casas E R et al 1987 Pelvic inflammatory disease, laparoscopy and the expenditure of health care dollars. Int J Fertil 32: 17–37

Mishell D R, Bell J H, Good R G et al 1966 The intrauterine device: a bacteriologic study of the endometrial cavity. Am J Obstet Gynecol 96: 119–126

Moller B R, Kaspersen P, Kristiansen F V et al 1986 *Chlamydia trachomatis* in the upper female genital tract with negative cervical culture. Lancet 2: 390

Odenaal H J 1990 The management of acute pelvic inflammatory disease. In: Bonnar J (ed) Recent advances in obstetrics and gynaecology. Churchill Livingstone, Edinburgh, pp 165–183

Paavonen J, Makela J 1985 Use of serologic methods in the diagnosis of pelvic inflammatory disease. In: Keith L G, Berger G S (eds) Infections in reproductive health, vol 1, Common infections. MTP Press, Lancaster, pp 209–236

Paavonen J, Aine R, Teisala K et al 1985 Comparison of endometrial biopsy and peritoneal cytologic testing with laparoscopy in the diagnosis of acute pelvic inflammatory disease. Am J Obstet Gynecol 151: 645–650

Robertson J N, Hogston P, Ward M E 1988 Gonococcal and chlamydial antibodies in ectopic and intrauterine pregnancy. Br J Obstet Gynaecol 95: 711–716

Sellors J W, Mahony J B, Chernesky M A et al 1988 Tubal factor infertility: an association with prior chlamydial infection and asymptomatic salpingitis. Fertil Steril 49: 451–457

Stacey C M, Munday P E, Beard R W 1989 Pelvic inflammatory disease: diagnosis and microbiology. Oral presentation. Silver Jubilee British Congress of Obstetrics and Gynaecology, London 4–7 July

Sweet R L, Blankfort-Doyle M, Robbie M O 1986 The occurrence of chlamydial and
   Gonocccoccal salpingitis during the menstrual cycle. JAMA 255: 2062–2064
Thomas B J, Evans R T, Hawkins D A et al 1984 Sensitivity of detecting *Chlamydia
   trachomatis* elementary bodies in smears by use of a fluorescein labelled monoclonal
   antibody: comparison with conventional chlamydial isolation. J Clin Pathol 37: 812–816
Tijam K H, Zeilmaker G H, Alberda A T et al 1985 Prevalence of antibodies to *Chlamydia
   trachomatis, Neisseria gonorrhoeae,* and *Mycoplasma hominis* in infertile women. Genitourin
   Med 61: 175–178
Toth A, O'Leary W M, Ledger W 1982 Evidence for microbial transfer by spermatozoa.
   Obstet Gynecol 59: 556–559
Westrom L 1975 Effect of acute pelvic inflammatory disease on fertility. Am J Obstet
   Gynecol 121: 707–713
Westrom L 1987 Pelvic inflammatory disease: bacteriology and sequelae. Contraception 36:
   111–128
Westrom L 1988 Long-term consequences of pelvic inflammatory disease. In: Hare M J (ed)
   Genital tract infection in women. Churchill Livingstone, Edinburgh, pp 350–367
Westrom L, Mardh P A 1989 Salpingitis. In: Holmes K K et al (eds) Sexually transmitted
   diseases. McGraw Hill, New York, pp 615–632
Wolner-Hanssen P, Mardh P A, Moller B et al 1982 Endometrial infection in women with
   chlamydial salpingitis. Sex Transm Dis 9: 84–88
Wolner-Hanssen P, Svensson L, Mardh P A et al 1985 Laparoscopic findings and
   contraceptive use in women with signs and symptoms suggestive of acute salpingitis.
   Obstet Gynecol 66: 233–238

17. Treatment of endometriosis

R. W. Shaw

Endometriosis is one of the commonest benign gynaecological conditions. It has been estimated to be present in between 10 and 25% of women presenting with gynaecological symptoms in Britain and the USA. This incidence is based on finding its presence in patients who have undergone laparoscopy for diagnostic indications (Jeffcoate 1975, Tyson 1974). Although it is an extremely common condition, there is much that is still not understood and the condition still arouses much interest and controversy.

Endometriosis is defined as the presence of functioning endometrial tissue outside the uterine cavity. Clinical diagnosis is usually made at laparoscopic observations of small or large haemorrhagic or fibrotic foci on the pelvic peritoneum or serosal surface of the pelvic organs. This ectopic endometrial tissue responds to ovarian hormones and undergoes cyclical changes which, whilst not exactly comparable to those seen in the endometrium, are closely similar. Cyclical bleeding from the endometriotic deposits contributes to a local inflammatory reaction, fibrous adhesion formation, and in the case of deep ovarian implants leads to the formation of endometriomas or chocolate cysts.

Endometriosis commonly affects women during their childbearing years. In the main this reflects in deleterious social, sexual and reproductive consequences as a result of the associated infertility and painful symptoms.

AETIOLOGY—FACTORS AND PATHOGENESIS

The precise aetiology of endometriosis still remains unknown. It has often been called the disease of theories because of the many postulated theories

Table 17.1 Theories of the pathogenesis of endometriosis

Implantation theory—retrograde menstruation
Genetic and immunological factors
Lymphatic and venous embolization—embolic
Metaplasia coelomic epithelium
Composite theories

encompassed to explain its pathogenesis. Table 17.1 lists some of the best known of these theories. Indeed, no single theory can explain the location of endometriotic deposits in all of the sites reported.

Menstrual regurgitation and implantation

Sampson (1927) suggested that endometriosis developed as a result of menstrual regurgitation and subsequent implantation of endometrial tissue on the peritoneal surface. In support of this theory experimental endometriosis has been induced in animals by replacement of menstrual fluid or endometrial tissue in the peritoneal cavity. In addition endometriosis has been described in young girls in association with abnormalities of the genital tract causing obstruction to the outflow of menstrual fluid (Schifrin et al 1973).

Retrograde menstruation through the fallopian tubes is however a common finding at laparoscopies performed during the perimenstrual period (Halme et al 1984), and therefore some other mechanism, which may be immunological, must account for the subsequent development of endometriosis in susceptible individuals.

Genetic and immunological factors

Dmowski et al (1981) suggested that genetic and immunological factors may alter the susceptibility of a woman to develop endometriosis, indeed they demonstrated a decreased cellular immunity to endometriotic tissue in women with endometriosis. Another group of workers (Simpson et al 1980) demonstrated an increased incidence of endometriosis in first degree relatives of patients with the disorder, compared to a control group, and racial differences also exist.

Vascular and lymphatic spread

Vascular and lymphatic embolization to distant sites has been demonstrated and explains the rare finding of endometriosis in sites outwith the peritoneal cavity, e.g. lung, kidney, joints and skin.

Transformation of coelomic epithelium

The epithelial cells lining the Mullerian duct arise from primitive cells which differentiate into peritoneal cells and the cells on the surface of the ovaries. It is proposed that these adult cells undergo de-differentiation back to their primitive origin and then transform into endometrial cells. This is an attractive theory that can explain the occurrence of endometriosis in nearly all ectopic sites due to the presence of aberrant Mullerian cells. Their transformation into endometrial cells may be due to hormonal stimuli or inflammatory irritation.

SYMPTOMATOLOGY AND DIAGNOSIS

Symptoms in patients with endometriosis are extremely variable. Symptoms vary depending upon the site of the ectopic endometrium but what is apparent is that the extent of the disease does not necessarily bear any relationship to the intensity of the symptoms. Indeed the disease may be an incidental finding during surgery or other investigations for various conditions; this is particularly true with patients presenting with infertility. Common symptoms related to the site of deposits are summarized in Table 17.2.

There exists an association between endometriosis and infertility which occurs in between 30–40% of patients suffering with endometriosis (Kistner 1975). Pathogenesis of infertility in patients with endometriosis is probably multifactoral and perhaps more readily explained in patients with the more severe degrees of endometriosis when there is obvious anatomical distortion, e.g. peri-adnexal adhesions, or destruction of ovarian tissue by endometriomas. These mechanical factors may then interfere with the release or pick up of oocytes. However, when only minimal endometriosis is found in patients complaining of infertility, the cause and effect relationship is more difficult. A number of possible mechanisms have been postulated including various endocrine disorders e.g. anovulation, uterine unruptured follicle syndrome, prostaglandin induced luteolysis, oocyte maturation defects, prostaglandin induced alteration in tubal and cilial motility, disordered coital function due to dyspareunia and phagocytosis by

Table 17.2 Symptoms of endometriosis in relationship to site of endometriotic implants

Site	Symptoms
Female reproductive tract	Dysmenorrhoea Lower abdominal and pelvic pain Dyspareunia Infertility Menstrual irregularity Rupture/torsion endometrioma Low back pain
Gastrointestinal tract	Cyclical tenesmus/rectal bleeding Diarrhoea Colonic obstruction
Urinary tract	Cyclical haematuria/pain Ureteric obstruction
Surgical scars, umbilicus	Cyclical pain and bleeding
Lungs	Cyclical haemoptysis

macrophages of spermatozoa. Currently, no simple explanation can be proposed for infertility with mild to minimal endometriosis. Some investigators still state that it is controversial as to whether such cases benefit from any form of treatment, though most clinicians would offer therapy to patients if only perhaps to prevent further progress of the disease which may in the future jeopardize fertility.

Diagnosis

Endometriosis should be a differential diagnostic consideration in any patient presenting with infertility or with worsening dysmenorrhoea, pelvic pain, dyspareunia or other cyclical associated symptoms related to bladder or bowel. The only definitive way of confirming endometriosis is to visualize deposits laparoscopically and histologically confirm the presence of endometriotic tissue by performing a biopsy of such lesions.

There have been several classification schemes devised for evaluating the disease, but the most widely used is the American Fertility Society classification which is aimed to standardize classification with relationship to sites, size of deposits and the presence of adhesions.

Ultrasound examination of the pelvis may be useful in delineating the presence of cystic ovarian structures containing blood. Such chocolate cysts in the minority of cases may be echo-free, but the walls of endometriomas are irregular as opposed to the smooth wall of a simple ovarian cyst. The commonest pattern is for the chocolate cyst to contain low level echoes, or clumps of dense high level echoes, representing blood clots. Several cysts may be present in different phases of evolution.

Barbieri et al (1985) using a monoclonal antibody CA 125 prepared to a membrane antigen, detected elevated levels in 80% of patients with epithelial ovarian cancer and in less than 2% of normal women. He also found that patients with endometriosis tended to have higher levels, with up to 49% of patients with endometriosis outside the normal range. The majority of these patients were AFS stage 3 and 4. We have confirmed the findings that a proportion of patients with endometriosis do have elevated levels and it is more common in those with more advanced stages of the disease. The levels regress during treatment and rise again following treatment, particularly in those patients in which recurrence develops (Fig. 17.1). Thus, whilst measurement of CA 125 may not be helpful in initial diagnosis of endometriosis, in patients in whom it is initially elevated, this may be a pointer for recurrence of the disease during follow-up (Acien et al 1989).

TREATMENT

Endometriosis can be a difficult disease to treat as often the long-term response to therapy lies in recognition of the disease in its earliest stages. In

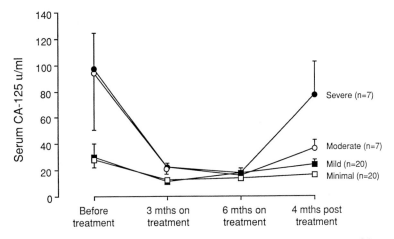

Fig. 17.1   Serum CA 125 levels before, at 3 months and 6 months on treatment and 4 months post-treatment in patients with various degrees of endometriosis as classified by the revised American Fertility Society. (Reproduced with permission from Shaw et al 1989.)

up to 60% of cases following most treatment modalities, recurrence of endometriosis will eventually occur, and thus there is therefore often no permanent cure for this disease. The final resort may well be to perform surgical oophorectomy which offers the most effective treatment. Management should be individualized, taking into account a number of aspects which include patient's age, future fertility wishes, extent of the disease and severity of the symptoms.

Treatment is essentially surgical, medical, or a combination of both approaches. Combined medical and surgical treatment might use medical therapy before, after, or both before and following surgical intervention.

In trying to assess the efficacy of any particular treatment modality it is necessary to take into account the following: (1) rate of symptomatic relief during and following therapy; (2) degree of resolution of endometriotic lesions; (3) the rate of recurrence of the disease over a specified period of follow-up; (4) in those patients where infertility was a factor, the pregnancy rate achieved.

Surgical treatment

Conservative surgery

This form of therapy may be carried out at laparoscopy or at laparotomy. The aim is to conserve as much ovarian tissue as possible as well as to return the reproductive tract to its normal anatomy to preserve and enhance reproductive potential. The procedures performed during laparoscopy may involve division of adhesions, diathermy and destruction of endometriotic deposits. More recently, the use of laser destruction of lesions in laparoscopic surgery has been advocated (Feste 1984). This has been more advantageous than diathermy destruction since the area of laser vaporization is more localized with less surrounding tissue damage, and it is claimed with less adhesion formation.

Laparotomy may be necessary for more extensive adhesiolysis or the excision of endometriomas and for access to deposits not amenable to a laparoscopic approach. Employment of microsurgical techniques and principles may well improve infertility prospects in such patients (Gomel 1980).

The pregnancy rate following conservative surgery seems directly related to the severity of the disease as shown by pregnancy rates of 40%, 56% and 73% for severe, moderate and mild degrees of endometriosis respectively (Buttram 1979). It has been reported that between 40–47% of patients undergoing conservative surgery require a second surgical procedure for recurrence at some stage (Schenken & Malinak 1982).

Radical surgery

Radical surgery is often utilized when other forms of therapy have failed and with patients who have no desire to retain fertility potential. In such cases the preferred operation is hysterectomy and bilateral salpingo-oophorectomy, and resection of other endometriotic lesions wherever possible. Since these patients are often still relatively young when these procedures are performed, it is advisable that they are given hormone replacement therapy. Such therapy should be kept at a minimum as a small proportion of patients develop a recurrence of endometriosis related to oestrogen replacement. Combined oestrogen-testosterone implants may minimize the risk of recurrence due to the beneficial effects of the androgen supplementation.

Hormonal treatment

Endometriotic tissue is classically described as being morphologically and histologically similar to the endometrium. However there are dissimilarities as evidenced both by electron-microscopic, nuclear oestrogen binding studies, and cytosolic oestrogen-progesterone receptor studies. The ectopic endometrial tissue does, however, respond to endogenous and exogenous ovarian sex steroid hormones in a fashion sufficiently similar to that of normal endometrium to suggest that a hormonal approach which suppresses oestrogen and progesterone levels preventing cyclical changes, should be beneficial in its treatment. The hypo-oestrogenic state following the menopause produces atrophy of the normal endometrium and atrophy and regression of endometriotic deposits. Administration of progesterone or exogenous progestogens oppose the effect of oestrogen on endometrial tissue by inhibiting replenishment of cytosolic oestrogen receptors. The progestogens also induce secretory activity in the endometrial glands and decidual action in endometrial stroma.

The success of various hormone therapies depends to a large extent on the localization of endometriotic lesions. The superficial peritoneal and serosal implants respond better to hormone therapy than deep ovarian, deep peritoneal or lesions within other organs (e.g. rectum, bladder).

In the last 40 years the medical treatment of endometriosis has undergone a remarkable evolution. In the past testosterone, diethylstilboestral and high dose combined oestrogen-progestogen pill preparations were used with some success. However, therapies which induce decidualization (pseudo-pregnancy regimes) or suppress ovarian function (pseudo-menopausal regimes), appear to offer the best chance of clinical remission of endometriosis.

Current medical treatments

Progestogens

Pseudo-pregnancy may effectively be induced by these progestogen preparations, which can either be derivatives of 19 Nor-Testosterone, e.g. norethisterone, Norgestrol, Norethynodral Lynoestenol; or the derivatives of progesterone such as medroxyprogesterone acetate and Didrogesterone. These agents induce a hypo-oestrogenic hyperprogestogenic state and the various preparations may be either taken orally or as injectable depot formulations for a period of 6–9 months. The results appear to be comparable to those reported with combined oral oestrogen-progestogen preparations in the past. Side effects are those commonly seen in oestrogen-progestogen agents and include breakthrough bleeding, weight gain, increased appetite, oedema, acne, bloating and reduced libido.

Danazol

Danazol is an Isoxazol derivative of 17 alpha-ethyl testosterone [17 alpha bregn-4-nen-20-Yno-(2,3-D) Isoxazol-17-OL] and has mildly androgenic and anabolic properties. Danazol is currently the most widely used medical treatment for endometriosis. Mechanism of action is complex but includes interference with pulsatile gonadotrophin secretion, inhibition of the mid-cycle gonadotrophin surge, direct inhibition of ovarian steroidogenesis by inhibiting several enzymatic processes, competitive blockage of androgen and oestrogen progesterone receptors in the ovaries and endometrium and suppression of sex hormone binding globulin (Barbieri & Ryan 1981). The multiple effects of Danazol produce a hypo-oestrogenic, hypo-progestogenic environment with induced endometrial atrophy and accompanying amenorrhoea. The degree of achievement of all these endocrine changes is dose-related.

Clinical use of Danazol for the treatment of endometriosis began in 1971 and it has to be administered in the dose range of between 200 mg and 800 mg daily in the majority of patients. In cases of mild to moderate endometriosis it has been shown to be highly effective with subjective symptomatic improvement in over 85% of cases (Low et al 1984). However, it has been reported that symptoms may recur in up to one third of patients within 1 year of ceasing a course of therapy (Dmowski & Cohen 1978).

Subjective resolution and improvement of endometriotic lesions is observed at post-treatment laparoscopic evaluation in between 70 and 95% of patients (Dmowski & Cohen 1975, Barbieri et al 1982, Matta & Shaw 1987).

Dmowski & Cohen (1978) reported a 39% recurrence rate up to 37 months after completion of a course of Danazol therapy, with annual recurrences in first, second and third years of 23%, 5% and 9% respectively.

Pregnancy rates in fertile patients are between 31–53% in mild endometriosis and between 23–50% in moderate endometriosis, reported in the review of the literature by Schmidt (1985).

Danazol therapy should be commenced in the early follicular phase of the menstrual cycle with additional barrier contraception in order to avoid the drug being administered during early pregnancy, and it should be administered every 6–8 hours as the drug's half-life is approximately 4–5 hours. The dose should be titrated to the patient's clinical response and severity of side effects, starting with a dose of 400 mg in mild disease and 600–800 mg daily in moderate to severe disease, with a recommended treatment course of 6 months.

Danazol therapy is associated with side effects related to androgenic, and anabolic properties. These side effects include weight gain, acne, oily skin, fluid retention symptoms, muscle cramp and mood changes commonly, and less commonly, hirsutism, depression, hot flushes, skin rash and deepening of voice. The incidence and severity of side effects are dose-related and a few patients will discontinue because of side effects alone.

An elevation of low density lipoproteins (LDL) and a reduction of high density lipoprotein (HDL) cholesterol concentrations has been reported whilst on Danazol therapy (Fahraeus et al 1984). These effects are quickly reversed after ceasing treatment. In addition Danazol has been known to alter liver function and serum levels of various enzymes and thus should be contra-indicated in patients with liver disease. Patients on long-term therapy should perhaps have serum liver function enzymes and serum lipoproteins assessed periodically.

Gestrinone

Gestrinone is a synthetic trienic 19 Nor steroid (13-ethyl-17 alpha ethinyl-17 hydroxy-gona-4,9,11-trien-3-one). Recent clinical trials have shown it to be effective in treatment of endometriosis. Gestrinone exhibits mild androgenic, marked anti-progesterogenic and anti-oestrogenic, as well as moderate anti-gonadotrophic properties. One effect of these actions is to induce progressive endometrial atrophy.

The endocrine effects of Gestrinone are similar to those of Danazol in that the mid-cycle gonadotrophin surge is abolished though basal gonado-trophin secretions are not significantly reduced. It inhibits ovarian steroid-ogenesis as evidenced by suppressed serum levels of progesterone and oestradiol 17β, and induces profound progressive production of serum sex binding globulin levels by up to 85% with resulting increase in free unbound testosterone index (Kaupilla et al 1985). The half-life of Gestrinone is quite prolonged and therefore it can be administered as an oral preparation in doses of 2·5–5 mg twice weekly. These doses induce endometrial atrophy and amenorrhoea in between 85–95% of patients. From early uncontrolled studies using Gestrinone it appears to compare favourably with Danazol treatment of endometriosis with regard to symptomatic relief and improved pregnancy (Coutinho et al 1984) and arrest and resolution of deposits (Thomas & Cooke 1987).

Reported side effects occur in up to 50% of patients which include seborrhoeic acne, increased weight gain, reduced breast size, hot flushes, nausea, muscle cramps, hirsutism and voice hoarseness. Side effects are reportedly moderate, dose-dependent and transient.

Gestrinone then is an effective drug which is comparable to Danazol in its effect in treating endometriosis and its side effect profile, but more randomized comparative studies are required to establish that it is more beneficial.

Luteinizing hormone-releasing hormone (LHRH) analogues

Whilst surgical castration has so far been the most effective treatment for endometriosis, the possibility to induce a reversible medical castration with the administration of luteinizing hormone-releasing hormone (LHRH) analogues is currently being investigated as an alternative medical treat-ment for endometriosis. Replacement of amino acids in positions 6 and/or 10 of the native LHRH molecule, produces a series of superactive agonistic analogues having a reduced susceptibility to degradation by enzymes and hence a prolonged therapeutic half-life. Continued administration of these analogues in humans causes pituitary gonadotrophes to become desen-sitized and pituitary down-regulation occurs which induces a state of hypogonadotrophic hypogonadism. Following initial administration of LHRH analogues, increased output of both LH and FSH occurs for a period of between 4–7 days. This increase in gonadotrophin secretion stimulates ovarian steroidogenesis, particularly oestradiol if commenced during the menstrual phase of the cycle, and both oestradiol and progesterone if commenced during the mid-luteal phase of the cycle. Once pituitary desensitization occurs serum levels of FSH begin to fall and by the

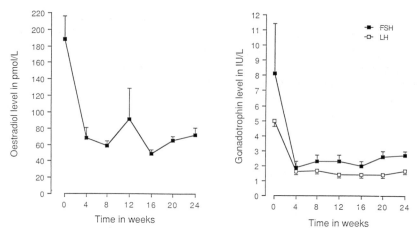

Fig. 17.2   A Circulating levels of serum oestradiol-17β in a group of 20 women with endometriosis administered Zoladex depot (3·6 mg D-Ser(tBu)⁶ Aza Gly¹⁰ LHRH) 4 weekly × 24 weeks. (mean +/− s.e.m.). **B** Suppressed levels of serum LH and FSH (mean +/− s.e.m.) maintained in patients who received Zoladex depot every 4 weeks (*n* = 20 subjects with endometriosis treated for 24 weeks).

7th day of administration are comparable to those seen in the early follicular phase of the cycle but with no discernible pulsatile pattern of release. As a result oestrogen levels fall to values in the post-menopausal range (see Fig. 17.2A). Continued administration of LHRH analogues maintains a situation of hypogonadotrophic hypo-oestrogenism (Fig. 17.2B). A number of LHRH analogues are undergoing clinical trials for the treatment of endometriosis and the results of such studies are being published. Various amino acid substitutions of the molecule compared with the native LHRH are shown in Figure 17.3.

	1	2	3	4	5	(6)	7	8	9	(10)
LHRH	— p-GLU	— HIS	— TRP	— SER	— TYR	— GLY	— LEU	— ARG	— PRO	— GLY NH₂
Buserelin						D-Ser(Buᵗ)			PRO-Net	
Nafarelin						(D-NAL)₂				
Goserelin						D-SER(Buᵗ)			AZA-GLY	
Tryptorelin						D-TRP				
Leuprolide						D-LEU			PRO-Net	
Histrelin						D-HIS (Imbzl)			PRO-Net	

Fig. 17.3   Amino-acid sequence of nature LHRH and some of the agonistic analogues.

First reports of LHRH analogues utilized for endometriosis appeared in late 1982. Meldrum et al (1982) administered D Tryp[6] PRO[9] NET LHRH in a series of 5 women for a period of one month. In this study the drug was administered subcutaneously and endocrine responses compared with a group of normal patients who had undergone surgical oophorectomy as treatment for endometriosis. After one month's treatment, oestradiol concentration reached castrate levels in 4 out of the 5 patients treated with the LHRH analogue. One of the earliest definitive reports of attempts to treat patients with endometriosis using the LHRH analogue, Buserelin, D-Ser (But[6]) PRO[9] LHRH administered intranasally came from our own group (Shaw et al 1983). This initial study used a low dose of 200 µg t.d.s. intranasally administered to 5 of the subjects and 400 µg once daily in the remaining subjects. A good clinical response and laparoscopic evidence of resolution of endometrial deposits was achieved in patients receiving the 200 µg t.d.s., intranasally. However, the patient receiving the lower dose at 400 µg once per day failed to show adequate response.

A number of open non-randomized studies using LHRH analogues have now been reported confirming the value of these agents in the treatment of endometriosis. These include those using Buserelin by intranasal route (Lemay et al 1984, Shaw & Matta 1986), intranasal Nafarelin D(Nal$_2$)[6] LHRH (Schriock et al 1985) and (Imbzl—DHis[6] PRO[9] LHRH) sub-cutaneous injection (Steingold et al 1987).

Randomized comparative controlled trials comparing LHRH analogue with Danazol have recently been performed and the results have been published. The results which we reported (Matta & Shaw 1987) were part of a large multicentre study and compared Buserelin 400 µg t.d.s. intra-nasally versus Danazol 200 mg t.d.s. orally. Results of a large multicentre double-blind comparative trial utilizing intranasal Nafarelin 400–800 mg daily versus Danazol 800 mg daily has recently appeared (Henzl et al 1988). These randomized comparative trials confirm the efficacy of LHRH analogues in the treatment of endometriosis in both their ability to relieve symptoms and induce resolution of endometriotic deposits. The ability of these LHRH analogues to induce resolution of endometriotic deposits was not significantly different in mild to moderate endometriosis when compared to those patients treated with Danazol.

Looking in more detail at the results of our own studies they have shown that LHRH analogues achieve a greater degree of suppression of serum oestradiol 17β than Danazol. The preparation of LHRH analogue, Zoladex, (D Ser (TBu)[6] Aza-Gly[10] LHRH) is more effective than intra-nasally administered preparations, achieving more sustained and improved hypo-oestrogenism.

Symptomatic relief of the main symptoms in groups of patients with endometriosis randomized to Danazol or LHRH analogue is shown in Table 17.3. This data indicates good symptomatic relief by both Danazol and LHRH analogues.

Table 17.3   Symptomatic response during and following treatment for endometriosis with Danazol or Buserelin for 6 months. (Reproduced with permission from Matta & Shaw 1987.)

	Danazol 600–800 mg orally daily			Buserelin 400 µg t.d.s. intranasally		
	Pre-treatment	End of treatment	6 month follow up	Pre-treatment	End of treatment	6 month follow up
Dysmenorrhoea	13	1	7	37	2	10
Pelvic pain	10	2	3	29	3	7
Dyspareunia	8	2	4	25	4	7
Rectal pain/ bleeding	1	0	1	9	1	7

Danazol induces side effects related to its androgenic base structure. Side effects induced by LHRH analogues are those that may be expected from induction of a state of profound hypo-oestrogenism and are similar to those of oestrogen deficiency observed in post-menopausal patients. These side effects are seen in Table 17.4 with their relative frequency.

Ability to induce resolution of endometriotic deposits, as scored using the revised AFS classification, is shown in Figure 17.4. It would seem that LHRH analogues achieve extremely good resolution of deposits in stages 1–2 disease and also induce a significant reduction in AFS scores in stages 3 and 4, with many of these subjects having complete resolution of all their visible deposits. The AFS scores referred to in Figure 17.4 are for points given to endometriotic deposits alone and exclude those related to adhesions, which would not be expected to resolve by medical treatment alone.

The LHRH analogues are thus shown to be a well tolerated and effective

Table 17.4   Principal side-effects experienced in patients randomized to receive Buserelin or Danazol for 6 months. (Reproduced with permission from Matta & Shaw 1987.)

	Buserelin	Danazol
Dose	400 µg t.d.s. intranasally	600–800 mg orally daily
No. of patients	39	18
Symptoms		
Hot flushes	★74%	22%
Breakthrough bleeding	23%	★55%
Headaches	20%	39%
Vaginal dryness	★23%	5·55%
Superficial dyspareunia	★5·2%	Nil
Weight gain (>3 kg)	Nil	★66%
Acne/Oily skin	Nil	39%

SCORE

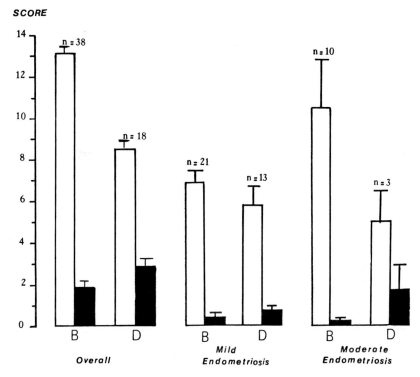

Fig. 17.4   Changes in AFS point scores for endometriotic deposits (excluding adhesion contribution) in randomized patients overall and in patients with mild or moderate endometriosis (severe excluded as too few on each treatment). B, Buserelin 400 µg t.d.s. intranasally. D, Danazol 400 mg–800 mg daily orally.

means of treating endometriosis but continued studies will be needed to evaluate long-term recurrence rates of the disease and fertility rates in patients who have received LHRH analogues to see if they are more beneficial than those achieved with Danazol, Gestrinone or other current medical treatments. Effects of prolonged hypo-oestrogenism induced by LHRH analogues on bone, however, represent a worrying side effect. It has been shown that, as observed in postmenopausal patients, the degree of hypo-oestrogenism achieved with LHRH analogues leads to increased urinary calcium excretion and a significant though reversible reduction, in vertebral trabecular bone density (Matta et al 1988). It may be these induced effects of bone calcium haemostasis which will determine for how long and how frequently LHRH analogues may be administered to treat the chronic debilitating conditions of endometriosis.

It remains a disappointment that as yet there is no definitive medical treatment for endometriosis which eradicates the disease permanently. However, a number of new surgical and medical approaches to treatment provide a choice of treatment modalities. It may require the development of an immunological treatment approach to achieve a permanent cure in what still remains an extensively investigated but poorly understood disorder.

REFERENCES

Acien P, Shaw R W, Irvine L, Burford G, Gardner R L 1989 CA 125 levels in endometriosis patients before, during and after treatment with Danazol or LHRH agonists. Eur J Obstet Gynaecol Reprod Med 32: 241–246

Barbieri R L, Ryan K J 1981 Danazol: endocrine pharmacology and therapeutic applications. Am J Obstet Gynecol 141: 453–463

Barbieri R L, Evans S, Kistner R W 1982 Danazol in the treatment of endometriosis: analysis of 100 cases with a 4-year follow-up. Fertil Steril 37: 737–746

Barbieri R L, Bast R C, Niloff J M, Kistner R W, Knapp R C 1985 Evaluation of a serological test for the diagnosis of endometriosis using a monoclonal antibody OC-125. Presented at the Annual Meeting of the Society for Gynaecological Investigation. 33 pp

Buttram V C 1979 Conservative surgery for endometriosis in the infertile female: a study of 206 patients with implications for both medical and surgical therapy. Fertil Steril 2: 117–123

Coutinho E M, Husson J M, Azadian-Boulanger G 1984 Treatment of endometriosis with Gestrinone—5 years experience. In: Raynaud J D, Ojasoo T, Martin L (eds) Medical management of endometriosis. Raven Press, New York, pp 249–260

Dmowski W P, Cohen M R 1975 Treatment of endometriosis with an antigonadotrophin, danazol: a laparoscopic and histologic evaluation. Obstet Gynecol 46: 147–154

Dmowski W P, Cohen M R 1978 Antigonadotrophin (danazol) in the treatment of endometriosis: evaluation of post-treatment fertility and 3-year follow-up data. Am J Obstet Gynecol 130: 41–48

Dmowski W P, Steele R W, Baker G F 1981 Deficient cellular immunity in endometriosis. Am J Obstet Gynecol 141: 377–383

Fahraeus L, Larsson-Cohn U, Ljungbert S, Wallentin L 1984 Profound alterations of the lipoprotein metabolism during danazol treatment in pre-menopausal women. Fertil Steril 42: 52–57

Feste J 1984 Laser laparoscopy. Fertil Steril 41: 745

Gomel V 1980 The impact of microsurgery on gynecology. Clin Obstet Gynecol 23: 1301–1310

Halme J, Becher S, Wing R 1984 Accentuated cyclic activation of peritoneal macrophages in patients with endometriosis. Am J Obstet Gynecol 148: 85–90

Henzl M R, Corson S L, Moghissi K, Buttram V C, Bergquist C, Jacobson C 1988 Administration of Nafarelin as compared to Danazol for endometriosis. N Engl J Med 318: 485–489

Jeffcoate T N 1975 Principles of gynaecology 4th edn. Butterworth, London, pp 350–364

Kaupilla A, Veli I, Ronnbergh L, Vierikko P, Vikko R 1985 Effect of gestrinone in endometriosis tissue and endometrium. Fertil Steril 44: 466–470

Kistner R W 1975 Endometriosis. In: Sciarra J (ed) Gynaecology and obstetrics, vol 1. Harper & Row, Hagerstown

Lemay A, Maheux R, Faure N, Jean C, Fazekas A 1984 Reversible hypogonadism induced by a luteinizing hormone-releasing hormone (LHRH) agonist (buserelin) as a new therapeutic approach for endometriosis. Fertil Steril 41: 863–871

Low R A, Roberts A D, Lees D A R 1984 A comparative study of various dosages of danazol in the treatment of endometriosis. Br J Obstet Gynaecol 91: 167–171

Matta W H, Shaw R W 1987 A comparative study between Buserelin and Danazol in the treatment of endometriosis. Br J Clin Pract 41 (suppl 48): 69–73

Matta W M, Shaw R W, Hesp R, Evans R 1988 Reversible trabecular bone density loss following induced hypo-oestrogenism with the GnRH analogue Buserelin in premenopausal women. Clin Endocrinol 29: 45–51

Meldrum D R, Chang R J, Lu J, Vale W, Rivier J, Judd H L 1982 'Medical oophorectomy' using a long acting GnRH agonist: a possible new approach to the treatment of endometriosis. J Clin Endocrinol Metab 54: 1081–1083

Sampson J A 1927 Peritoneal endometriosis due to menstrual dissemination of endometrial tissue into peritoneal cavity. Am J Obstet Gynecol 14: 422

Schenken R S, Malinak L R 1982 Conservative surgery versus expectant management for the infertile patient with mild endometriosis. Fertil Steril 37: 183–186

Schifrin B S, Erez S, Moore J G 1973 Teenage endometriosis. Am J Obstet Gynecol 116: 973

Schmidt C L 1985 Endometriosis: a reappraisal of pathogenesis and treatment. Fertil Steril 44: 157–173

Schriock E, Monroe S E, Henzl M, Jaffe R B 1985 Treatment of endometriosis with a potent agonist of gonadotrophin releasing hormone (Nafarelin). Fertil Steril 44: 583–588

Shaw R W, Matta W M 1986 Reversible pituitary ovarian suppression induced by an LHRH agonist in the treatment of endometriosis: comparison of two dose regimens. Clin Reprod Fertil 4: 329–336

Shaw R W, Fraser H M, Boyle H 1983 Intranasal treatment with luteinizing hormone releasing hormone agonist in women with endometriosis. Br Med J 287: 1667–1669

Simpson J L, Elias S, Malinak L R, Buttram V C Jr 1980 Heritable aspects of endometriosis I: genetic studies. Am J Obstet Gynecol 137: 327–331

Steingold K A, Cedars M, Lu J K H, Randle R N, Judd H L, Meldrum D R 1987 Treatment of endometriosis with a long acting gonadotrophin-releasing hormone agonist. J Obstet Gynaecol 69: 403–411

Thomas E J, Cooke I D 1987 Impact of gestrinone on the course of asymptomatic endometriosis. Br Med J 294: 272–274

Tyson J E A 1974 Surgical considerations in gynaecologic endocrine disorders. Surg Clin N Am 54: 425–442

18. Oestrogens and affective disorders

L. Appleby   J. Montgomery   J. Studd

The increased risk of affective illness in the puerperium, as well as the occurrence of depression in menopausal women and premenstrual women has often been attributed to rapid changes in circulating steroid hormone levels. Oestrogens, in particular, have been proposed as aetiological agents in mood disturbance. Supportive evidence, however, is largely indirect and often self-contradictory.

This chapter reviews the link between oestrogens and both postpartum affective disorders and depression at the menopause. It examines the research methods in these fields, suggesting that flaws in methodology have led to the lack of substantial research findings. Premenstrual syndrome has recently been reviewed elsewhere (Magos & Studd 1984). New approaches are described which might lead to a clarification of this presumed association.

POSTPARTUM PSYCHIATRIC DISORDERS

The theoretical link between plasma oestrogens and postpartum mental disorder has been based on three lines of reasoning. First, the rapid postnatal fall in circulating oestrogens might alter brain chemistry, resulting in mental disturbance. Second, the finding that postpartum psychosis frequently begins within the first 2 weeks after delivery (Brockington & Cox-Roper 1988) suggests precipitation by a fixed event, such as postpartum hormonal change. Third, psychiatric morbidity has also been reported at the menopause and in the premenstrual period during which sex steroid levels similarly decline (see section on the menopause).

However, attempts to elucidate the mechanisms by which oestrogen might provoke psychiatric symptoms have produced inconclusive results. These are reviewed below followed by some overall methodological and conceptual criticisms.

Three areas will be examined:

1. The direct relationship between oestrogens and mental symptoms
2. Indirect effects on mental symptoms mediated by other hormones
3. The relationship between oestrogens and neurotransmitter systems implicated in aetiological theories of mental illness.

Relationship between oestrogens and psychiatric phenomena

A link between mental symptoms and oestrogen levels, whether absolute or changing, around the time of delivery has proved difficult to demonstrate. Nott et al (1976) compared pre-delivery oestrogen and other hormone levels in two groups of women: those who developed significant maternity 'blues' and those who did not. Of 76 comparisons made, only 2 reached significance at the 0·05 level, fewer than might be expected by chance. Of 30 correlations, calculated between individual symptoms and levels of oestrogen and progesterone pre- and post-delivery, 5 were significant at the 0·05 level. These included high pre-delivery oestrogen and irritability, and low post-delivery oestrogen and sleep disturbance. These symptoms are not, of course, clinical disorders in themselves so the pathological significance of such findings has yet to be established.

A possible disturbance of oestrogen metabolism has been reported in some patients with postpartum manic depressive illness who showed reversal of the oestradiol:oestrone ratio (normally 2:1 in non-pregnant women) in the follicular phase of the menstrual cycle (Hatotani et al 1979). However, there was no correlation between mental symptoms and total oestrogen levels.

Effect of oestrogens on other hormones

In the absence of a demonstrable direct link with oestrogen, attention has also focused on other hormonal correlations with mood which may be influenced by oestrogen, notably parathyroid hormone (PTH) and endorphins.

Riley & Watt (1985) postulated that elevated ionized serum calcium might provoke postpartum psychosis in patients without pre-existing vulnerability (i.e. personal or family history of psychosis). Their psychotic subjects had higher ionized calcium levels than three comparison groups: those with a positive history, non-puerperal psychotic patients and normal postnatal women. Since high oestrogen opposes parathyroid hormone, their conclusion was that falling oestrogen following delivery leaves unopposed parathyroid hormone activity, which elevates calcium levels. However, the methods behind these results are open to question. First, there is little justification from family or follow up studies for a distinction between puerperal and non-puerperal psychoses. Second, all subject groups showed mean ionized calcium levels above the normal range which raises doubts about the accuracy of the assay. Third, there was a greater time interval between delivery and assay in the positive history group, which might have allowed calcium levels to decline. If a relationship between calcium and psychiatric morbidity does exist, its aetiological significance is uncertain and the contribution of falling oestrogen speculative.

Similarly, the possible link between postpartum psychiatric symptoms and endogenous opioids may be influenced by oestrogen. Newnham et al (1984) speculated that withdrawal of circulating β-endorphins following delivery might underlie symptoms of 'blues' or depression. However, they found no significant correlation between β-endorphin level before, at or after delivery or the rate of fall of β-endorphins and a postpartum 'blues' symptom score. Two studies (Brinsmead et al 1985, George & Wilson 1983) have produced evidence of correlation between β-endorphins and neurotic symptoms, though because there are simultaneous fluctuations in other hormone levels, their aetiological significance is unclear.

There is also evidence of oestrogen influence on hypothalamic β-endorphin activity during the menstrual cycle (Blankstein et al 1981, Quigley & Yen 1980). This has led to the suggestion that high circulating oestrogen increases the opioid mediated inhibition of gonadotrophin releasing hormone in late pregnancy and the early postnatal period (Ishizuka et al 1984).

Although it would be convenient to combine these areas of evidence into one aetiological theory, the influence of oestrogen is observed on a specific CNS region, while the suggested link with psychiatric symptoms concerns endorphins in the systemic circulation.

Effect of oestrogens on neurotransmitter systems

Neurotransmitter theories of psychosis have often focused on dopamine, serotonin or noradrenaline. Although single transmitter theories are probably over-simplified, it has been proposed that underactive 5HT and noradrenergic systems underlie depressive illness while dopaminergic overactivity may occur in schizophrenia.

Noradrenaline. Noradrenaline receptors are classified into subtypes a and b, both of which are further divided into types 1 and 2. Down-regulation of postsynaptic β receptor binding is the most consistent receptor finding following antidepressant administration to rats (Sulser 1984), though this change may require additional serotoninergic neuronal input and α-2 noradrenergic subsensitivity.

Three studies of these crucial receptors in rat cerebral cortex have demonstrated decreased β-adrenergic responses or receptor membrane density following oestrogen treatment, though the mechanism, and the site of oestrogen action remain unclear.

Such results present the possibility that oestrogen withdrawal following childbirth may reverse the antidepressant action of high circulating oestrogens (Biegon et al 1983, Wagner et al 1979, Wagner & Davis 1980).

Postsynaptic α-2 receptors appear to be reduced in depressed patients, as measured by clonidine-induced growth hormone secretion (Checkley et al 1986), indirect measurement of CNS α-2 receptors being obtained by studying platelet α-2 receptors. Since these are reduced postnatally, falling oestrogens in postpartum women may increase vulnerability to mood disturbance by lowering CNS α-2 receptors. However, Metz et al (1983) found that platelet α-2 receptors showed persistent, higher binding capacity in patients with 'blues' and there was no direct relationship to oestrogen or progesterone levels. In addition, there remain doubts about the validity of platelet studies as models of CNS changes.

Serotonin. There is a great deal of evidence linking depression to a deficit in CNS serotoninergic systems. As with noradrenergic β receptors, 5HT-2 receptor down-regulation occurs following long-term antidepressant administration and may explain the delay in mood changes seen following treatment with tricyclic drugs (Peroutka & Snyder 1980). This anti-depressant induced down-regulation of 5HT-2 appears to be oestrogen dependent (Kendall et al 1981).

Studies of oestrogen effects on 5HT binding are few and conflicting. Binding of the tricyclic antidepressant imipramine is often used as a marker of 5HT activity since this drug exerts its action primarily through serotoninergic mechanisms, principally presynaptic re-uptake. Imipramine binding in rat brain has been reported to increase following both oophorectomy (Stockert & de Robertis 1985) and, conversely, oestrogen treatment (Ravizza et al 1985, Rehavi et al 1987), though these reports differed regarding the brain areas studied. A further complication in understanding the influence of oestrogen is that oestrogen administered to oophorectomized rats appears to decrease 5HT-1 receptors but increase 5HT-2 receptors (Biegon et al 1983).

Dopamine. Many studies have examined oestrogen effects on dopaminergic systems but measurements of dopamine receptor binding or turnover have not shown consistent results (Deakin 1988). This has led to the proposal that oestrogen exerts a bi-directional effect on sub populations of CNS dopaminergic neurones, increasing sensitivity to dopamine in some but not others (Chiodo & Caggiula 1983).

Similarly, oestrogen-induced increases and decreases have both been observed in the stereotypes induced in animals by dopamine agonists. A possible explanation is a bi-phasic response in which dopamine binding is initially suppressed by oestrogen but after 48 h (following withdrawal) is enhanced (Gordon 1980). These increased behavioural responses could then represent an oestrogen withdrawal phenomenon. Prolonged oestrogen exposure, as in pregnancy, should therefore suppress dopaminergic function so that on withdrawal after delivery, enhanced dopaminergic activity may lead to psychotic disturbance.

In summary, although oestrogen can be shown to alter central synaptic transmission and neuronal activity, conflicting results suggest a more complex role for oestrogen than is at present apparent. The inconsistent findings, the confounding effects of other hormones, the likely interdependence of neurotransmitter systems and the overall inadequacy of a single transmitter theory of psychosis have made the significance of the above findings to postpartum mental illness unclear.

Methodological problems and solutions

The failure to find a consistent link between oestrogens and postpartum psychiatric disorder has resulted from uncertain responses to three questions.

1. *What is meant by psychiatric disorder?* Conventionally, psychiatric symptoms after parturition are divided into 3 syndromes—maternity 'blues', postnatal depression and postpartum psychosis. Although a degree of overlap exists between these, in their most characteristic form they are distinct. Many studies correlate hormonal changes with maternity 'blues' since it is common. However, 'blues' is clinically insignificant and not linked to psychotic breakdown. Postnatal depression is relatively common (10–15% of newly delivered mothers) but its timing is less closely linked to postpartum endocrine change than is postpartum psychosis. Also, its occurrence is linked to psychosocial risk factors (Kumar & Robson 1984, Watson et al 1984), suggesting that the influence of biological change is less prominent than may be the case for psychotic disorders. So any link between oestrogen and postpartum illness is likely to be strongest in the case of postpartum psychosis but research into this condition is hampered by its relative rarity (0·1–0·2% of deliveries).

2. *What should be assayed?* Research focused on oestrogen itself has measured absolute oestrogen levels or changing levels. However, it seems likely from simple endocrinological observation, that these measurements are too crude to reflect the functional changes which may influence mood. Furthermore, hormone levels may reveal less about function than would target sensitivity. Finally, it seems more likely that central pathway function will be influenced by interacting or antagonistic hormonal change rather than by alterations in single hormone levels.

3. *What is the relationship of oestrogens to neurotransmitter systems?* Many studies have examined the influence of oestrogens on noradrenergic, serotoninergic and dopaminergic synaptic transmission in animals but only rarely have these been correlated with behaviour, let alone translated into equivalent human behaviour and emotion. Studies of human systems have measured platelet enzymes and receptors, the relation of which to CNS equivalents remains in doubt. Many of these studies have had to address single neurotransmitters only, although the interaction of different systems is likely to have more functional relevance. When single systems have been examined, they have not always reflected current theory, e.g. some have examined noradrenergic pathways for evidence of disturbance without focusing on postsynaptic β receptors.

Kumar et al (1983) and Appleby (in press) have proposed a solution to these problems, requiring the study of a clinically homogenous group of high-risk subjects, i.e. with previous affective or postpartum psychosis. These subjects, carrying a substantial risk of postpartum psychosis, should be followed during and after pregnancy, during which time psychosocial and biological variables, including life events and results of biological challenge tests, could be monitored. Thus endocrine hypotheses generated by animal research could be tested in clinically relevant circumstances, comparison samples being drawn from the same high-risk population.

In summary, no relationship between oestrogens and postpartum mental disorder has yet been established despite much investigation and many speculative theories. The complexity of interacting biological changes and the many methodological difficulties leave any such relationship a matter for future, more precise and valid research.

THE MENOPAUSE

Symptoms of depression and irritability occurring in association with classical menopausal symptoms of hot flushes and night sweats are common clinical findings (Bungay et al 1980). However, a specific psychological syndrome linked to the menopause has not been confirmed. Studies of the sex differences in depression indicate that women are two to three times as likely to report symptoms of depression than men at all ages but there is no clear evidence that this ratio increases at the menopause (Shepherd et al 1966) or that a menopausal peak of psychological morbidity occurs (Ballinger 1975).

Attempts to elucidate a link between the menopause and low mood will be examined according to: (1) epidemiological evidence, including case definition and sampling, (2) therapeutic trials, using hormonal treatments.

Epidemiological evidence

Definitions of menopause and menopausal status

The comparability of studies on menopausal mood change is hampered by problems of definition, both of depression and the menopause itself. For the latter, cessation of menstruation has most often been used (Hunter et al 1986, Ballinger 1975, McKinlay et al 1987b), relying on retrospective self-report of subjects' recent menstrual history. Age alone has provided an alternative definition (Bungay et al 1980) on the assumption that the age of menopause in the population occurs within a narrow period of chronological age. Typical menopausal symptoms have also defined the menopause (Chakravarti et al 1979). Different results may well reflect these varying definitions.

Cessation of menses appears to have three clear advantages over the other definitions: first, it is central to the clinical concept of the menopause; second, its timing can be specified; third, it allows subdivision of menopausal subjects according to precise menopausal status. Thus subjects may be classed as postmenopausal, perimenopausal and premenopausal, according to the presence and duration of amenorrhoea.

However, rarely have psychological studies attempted to confirm these subdivisions with FSH estimations, relying instead on retrospectively self-reported symptoms, a potentially inaccurate basis for classification.

Of the alternatives, age is self-evidently a poor means of identifying the menopause precisely, and is equally a poor means of subdividing by menopausal status. Nor can 'typical' menopausal symptoms be used to define the menopause in any study which hopes to examine the prevalence or treatment response of symptoms in relation to the menopause.

Definition and measurement of depression

The difficulty of defining cases of minor psychiatric morbidity may lead to different rates of disorder in prevalence studies. Relatively few studies have used standardized, validated assessment instruments, although Ballinger's studies of the general population and gynaecology clinic attenders did so (Ballinger 1975, 1977) but without an accompanying interview to validate 'caseness'.

Most other studies have used unstandardized self-report of emotional symptoms (Bungay et al 1980, McKinlay et al 1987b, Hallstrom & Samuelsson 1985) without further validation. Hunter et al (1986) devised a questionnaire of menopausal symptoms with some face validity but the problems of self-report and lack of objective validation remained.

Winokur (1973), who did not demonstrate a link between depression and the menopause, used hospital admission to define clinically significant depression. However, by doing so he would have missed the bulk of neurotic conditions which do not lead to admission.

Sampling

Most studies have used samples affected by selection bias. Some samples have responded to newspaper advertisements (i.e. self-selected) while others were attending clinics such as GP surgeries or gynaecology outpatients. These cannot be used in prevalence studies.

Ballinger's general population study (1975) found that 29% of a random sample of women aged 40–55 years were 'cases' of psychological morbidity according to the General Health Questionnaire (Goldberg 1972). 'Cases' reported more family problems than 'non-cases' and more heavy periods. Cases were more likely to be aged 45–49 and currently menopausal (3–12 months since last period). Within the 45–49 year olds, however, the highest morbidity occurred in subjects still menstruating. Ballinger concluded that increased symptoms occurred in those about to stop menstruating and in the first menopausal year, a conclusion similar to that of Greene & Cooke (1980) and Bungay et al (1980). However, a large prospective study, using a multi-stage, random sampling design, found no increase in psychological ill-health related to the menopause (McKinley et al 1987b).

Therapeutic response

An alternative way of examining the impact of falling oestrogens on mood at the menopause is to monitor the effect of oestrogen treatment. Problems of this approach include:

1. The large placebo response (Campbell & Whitehead 1977)
2. The assumption that therapeutic trials can give aetiological information
3. The possible role of confounders such as physical symptoms, which could be improved by oestrogen leading to a secondary decline in depressed mood.

A number of studies have found improved mood in patients on oestrogen hormone replacement therapy compared with placebo, though the above inconsistencies over case definition, measurement and sampling make their results difficult to compare.

Brincat et al (1984) and Cardozo et al (1984), using unstandardized self-report scales, reported an improvement in menopausal women given oestrogen by implant. Campbell & Whitehead (1977) found a similar result using a visual analogue measurement scale for psychiatric symptoms but when using standardized instruments such as the GHQ, they found an equally impressive improvement on placebo, leading them to conclude that standardized methods were insufficiently sensitive to pick up the difference between placebo and active treatment!

Brincat et al (1984) suggested that the return of menopausal symptoms at 4–6 months after hormone replacement therapy may result from falling circulating hormone levels when the HRT impact expires. McKinley et al (1987a), however, did not find depression associated with the analogous transition from the pre- to immediately postmenopausal state. Furuhjelm et al (1984), using unusual measurement instruments, also described an advantage in oestrogen treatment over placebo, though their sample was entirely composed of postmenopausal subjects. Klaiber et al (1979) treated depressed women with oestrogens and found, despite overall improvement, that menopausal status did not influence the result. However, their measure of menopausal status was crude: the mean age of the premenopausal group was only 32 years.

Furuhjelm et al (1984) found no correlation between initial mood or treatment response and hormone estimations, including FSH. Klaiber et al (1979) postulated an influence of oestrogen on monoamine oxidase activity but failed to find a correlation between plasma MAO and improvement in measured depression.

Our own study attempted to use standardized assessment methods for psychological morbidity, validated by standardized interview of a subject subsample (Montgomery et al 1987). It attempted also to support the pre- and postmenopausal distinction with endocrine evidence. Its design was a

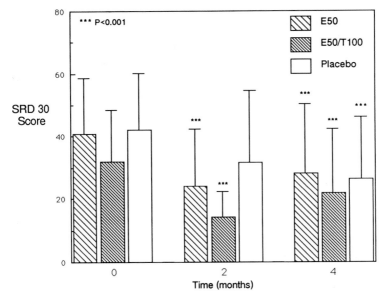

Fig. 18.1 Effect of hormone implants on SRD score: total group of women. Scores at 0, 2 and 4 months ($n = 70$). Significances based on Wilcoxon Matched-Pairs Signed-Ranks Test.

double-blind placebo-controlled trial of hormone replacement therapy in the treatment of psychiatric symptoms at the menopause. The subjects were 84 women referred to a menopause clinic with symptoms of hot flushes but not necessarily symptoms of depression. FSH and oestradiol were measured and a clinical assessment of menstrual cycles made. The women were divided into two groups, perimenopausal, defined as those with irregular cycles and FSH level $> 15\,IU/ml$, and postmenopausal, those with more than 6 months amenorrhoea and FSH $> 40\,IU/ml$. Psychological symptoms were assessed 2-monthly throughout the study using the Symptom Rating Test (Kellner & Sheffield 1973). The women were randomly allocated in a double-blind fashion into one of three treatment groups: oestradiol 50 mg, oestradiol 50 mg plus testosterone 100 mg, and placebo. Each treatment was administered by implant. Data were analysed for the 70 subjects who remained in the study.

The treatment groups had improved significantly at 2 months while the placebo group had not (Fig. 18.1). The difference originated in the response of the perimenopausal women to both implants but not to placebo at 2 months (Fig. 18.2). The postmenopausal women responded to both active and placebo groups (Fig. 18.3). At 4 months both groups had significantly improved, regardless of treatment group. The result indicated that only the perimenopausal women were more responsive to hormonal treatment and, by implication, had been biologically vulnerable to affective disorder. Thus, giving implants of oestradiol or oestradiol plus testosterone may

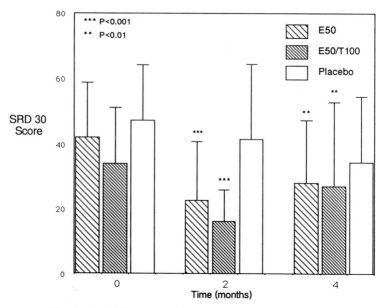

Fig. 18.2 As Fig. 18.1, perimenopausal subjects only ($n = 39$).

counteract biological vulnerability, either by maintaining oestrogen levels or by suppressing FSH.

In our study the mean plasma FSH at baseline in the perimenopausal

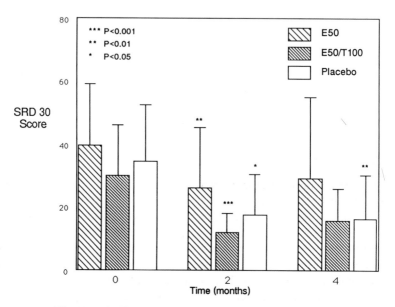

Fig. 18.3 As Fig. 18.1, postmenopausal subjects only ($n = 31$).

women treated with active implants was 15·6 IU/ml, falling to 7·2 IU/ml at 2 months, while in the perimenopausal women treated with placebo implants values were 12·3 IU/ml at baseline and 17·0 IU/ml at 2 months. Oestradiol levels showed little change between baseline and 2 months and appear to be a crude indicator of vulnerability to mood disturbance when compared to FSH level.

Neuroendocrine correlations

The above review of oestrogen-sensitive neuroendocrine findings in postpartum women is also applicable to the menopause. Few studies have directly examined neuroendocrine sensitivity to oestrogens with specific reference to the menopause. Bearn et al (1986) have described how an indicator of central oestrogen sensitivity, i.e. oestrogen-sensitive neurophysin, may be applied to postpartum disorders and we are currently extending this work to perimenopausal and postmenopausal subjects.

Summary

There is a lack of convincing epidemiological evidence to link depression with the menopause itself. Oestrogen treatment of the menopause is often associated with mood improvement but there is in most careful studies a large placebo response. Our own work, as yet unreplicated, suggests that only perimenopausal women have significant biological vulnerability, although the precise neuroendocrine nature of this vulnerability requires further investigation.

Some epidemiological findings have identified a peak of psychological morbidity prior to the mean age of the clinical menopause (Ballinger 1975). This could be explained by a biological vulnerability in those women approaching or beginning the clinical changes of the menopause, i.e. the perimenopausal group.

CONCLUSIONS

Despite considerable circumstantial evidence, the putative link between oestrogens and affective disorder remains undeveloped, largely because of methodological difficulties. In the case of postpartum psychosis, which is usually an affective illness, the likely precipitation by falling oestrogens remains no more than a plausible assumption: no direct evidence has been found despite several possible aetiological theories. Both the involvement of other interacting or mediating hormones and also changes in the sensitivity of interacting neurotransmitter systems seem likely but the details remain obscure. Postnatal depressive neurosis has been associated with several psychosocial factors but not convincingly with oestrogens or other hormones.

Although depression in menopausal women is well known, specific vulnerability to depression occurring at the menopause has not been shown. Our own therapeutic trial suggests that perimenopausal, but not post-menopausal, mood disturbance might be biologically provoked and oestrogen responsive.

REFERENCES

Appleby L 1990 The aetiology of postpartum psychosis: why are there no answers? J Infant and Reproductive Psychol (in press)

Ballinger C B 1975 Psychiatric morbidity and the menopause; screening of general population sample. Br Med J ii: 344–346

Ballinger C B 1977 Psychiatric morbidity and the menopause; survey of a gynaecological out-patient clinic. Br J Psychiatry 131: 83–89

Bearn J, Fairhall S, Checkley S 1986 A new marker for oestrogen sensitivity with potential application to postpartum depression. Presented at the 3rd International Conference of the Marce Society

Biegon A, McEwan B S 1982 Modulation by estradiol of serotonin-1 receptors in brain. J Neurosci 2: 199–205

Biegon A, Reches A, Snyder S L, McEwan B S 1983 Serotonergic and noradrenergic receptors in the rat brain: modulation by chronic exposure to ovarian hormones. Life Sci 32: 2015–2021

Blankstein J, Reyes F I, Winter J S D, Faiman C 1981 Endorphins and the regulation of the human menstrual cycle. Clin Endocrinol 14: 287–294

Brincat M, Magos A, Studd J W W et al 1984 Subcutaneous hormone implants for the control of climacteric symptoms. Lancet i: 16–18

Brinsmead M, Smith R, Singh B, Lewin T, Owens P 1985 Peripartum concentrations of β-endorphin and cortisol and maternal mood states. Aust NZ J Obstet Gynaecol 25: 194–197

Brockington I, Cox-Roper A 1988 The nosology of puerperal mental illness. In: Kumar R, Brockington I F (eds) Motherhood and mental illness 2. Wright, London

Bungay G T, Vessey M P, McPherson C K 1980 Study of symptoms in middle life with special reference to the menopause. Br Med J ii: 181–183

Campbell S, Whitehead M 1977 Oestrogen therapy and the menopausal syndrome. Clin Obstet Gynaecol 4: 31–47

Cardozo L, Gibb D M F, Studd J W W, Tuck S M, Thom M H, Cooper D J 1984 The use of hormone implants for climacteric symptoms. Am J Obstet Gynaecol 148: 336–337

Chakravarti S, Collins W P, Forecast J D, Newton J R, Oram D H, Studd J W W 1976 Hormonal profiles after the menopause. Br Med J ii: 784–786

Checkley S A, Corn T H, Glass I B, Burton S W, Burke C A 1986 The responsiveness of central α-adrenoceptors in depression. In: Deakin J F W (ed) The biology of depression. Gaskell, London

Chiodo L A, Caggiula A R 1983 Substantia nigra dopamine neurones: alterations in the basal discharge rate and autoreceptor sensitivity induced by oestrogen. Neuropharmacology 22: 593–599

Deakin J F W 1988 Relevance of hormone-CNS interactions to psychological changes in the puerperium. In: Kumar R, Brockington I F (eds) Motherhood and mental illness 2. Causes and consequences. Wright, London

Furuhjelm M, Karlgren E, Carlstrom K 1984 The effect of estrogen therapy on somatic and psychical symptoms in postmenopausal women. Acta Obstet Gynaecol Scand 63: 655–661

George A J, Wilson K C M 1983 β-endorphin and puerperal psychiatric symptoms. Br J Pharmacol 80: 493

Goldberg D P 1972 The detection of psychiatric illness by questionnaire. Oxford University Press, London

Gordon J H 1980 Modulation of apomorphine-induced stereotypy by oestrogen: time course and dose response. Brain Res Bull 5: 679–682

Greene J G, Cooke D J 1980 Life stress and symptoms at the climacteric. Br J Psychiatry 136: 486–491

Hallstrom T, Samuelsson S 1985 Mental health in the climacteric. Acta Obstet Gynaecol Scand Suppl 130: 13–18

Hatotani N, Nishikubo M, Kitayama I 1979 Periodic psychosis in the female and the reproductive process. In: Zichella L, Panchevi P (eds) Psychoneuroendocrinology in reproduction. North Holland-Elsevier, Amsterdam

Hunter M, Battersby R, Whitehead M 1986 Relationships between psychological symptoms, somatic complaints and menopausal status. Maturitas 8: 217–228

Ishizuka B, Quigley M E, Yen S S C 1984 Postpartum hypogonadotrophism: evidence for increased opioid inhibition. Clin Endocrinol 20: 573–578

Kellner R, Sheffield B F 1973 Self-rating scale of distress. Psychol Med 3: 88–100

Kendall D A, Stancel G M, Enna S J 1981 Imipramine: effect of ovarian steroids on modification in serotonin receptor binding. Science 211: 1183–1185

Klaiber E L, Broverman D M, Vogel W, Kobayashi Y 1979 Estrogen therapy for severe persistent depressions in women. Arch Gen Psychiatry 36: 550–554

Kuevi V, Carson R, Dixon A F et al 1983 Plasma amine and hormone changes in 'postpartum blues'. Clin Endocrinol 19: 39–46

Kumar R, Robson K M 1984 A prospective study of emotional disorders in childbearing women. Br J Psychiatry 144: 35–47

Kumar R, Isaacs S, Meltzer E 1983 Recurrent postpartum psychosis. A model for prospective clinical investigation. Br J Psychiatry 142: 618–620

McKinlay J B, McKinlay S M, Brambilla D J 1987a The relative contributions of endocrine changes and social circumstances to depression in mid-aged women. J Health Soc Behav 28: 345–363

McKinlay J B, McKinlay S M, Brambilla D J 1987b Health status and utilization behaviour associated with menopause. Am J Epidemiol 125: 110–121

Magos A L, Studd J W W 1984 The premenstrual syndrome. In: Studd W W (ed) Progress in obstetrics and gynaecology vol 4. Churchill Livingstone, Edinburgh

Metz A, Cowen P J, Gelder M G, Stump K, Elliott J M, Grahame-Smith D G 1983 Changes in platelet 2-adrenoceptor binding postpartum: possible relation to maternity blues. Lancet i: 495–498

Montgomery J C, Appleby L, Brincat M et al 1987 Effect of oestrogen and testosterone implants on psychological disorders in the climacteric. Lancet i: 297–299

Newnham J P, Dennett P M, Ferron S A et al 1984 A study of the relationship between circulating β-endorphin-like immunoreactivity and postpartum 'blues'. Clin Endocrinol 20: 169–177

Nott P N, Franklin M, Armitage C, Gelder M G 1976 Hormonal changes in mood in the puerperium. Br J Psychiatry 128: 379–383

Peroutka S J, Snyder S H 1980 Long term antidepressant treatment decreases spiroperidol labelled receptor binding. Science 210: 88–90

Quigley M E, Yen S S C 1980 The role of endogenous opiates on LH secretion during the menstrual cycle. J Clin Endocrinol Metab 50: 427–430

Ravizza L, Nicoletti F, Pozzi O, Barbacia M L 1985 Repeated daily treatments with oestradiol benzoate increase the [3H] imipramine binding in male rat frontal cortex. Eur J Pharmacol 107: 395–396

Rehavi M, Sepcuti H, Weizman A 1987 Upregulation of imipramine binding and serotonin uptake by oestradiol in female rat brain. Brain Res 410: 135–139

Riley D M, Watt D C 1985 Hypercalcaemia in the aetiology of puerperal psychosis. Biol Psychiatry 20: 479–488

Shepherd M, Cooper B, Brown A C, Kalton C W 1966 Psychiatric illness in general practice. Oxford University Press, London

Stockert M, de Robertis E 1985 Effect of ovariectomy and oestrogen on [3H] imipramine binding to different regions of rat brain. Eur J Pharmacol 119: 255–257

Sulser F 1984 Regulation and function of noradrenaline receptor systems in brain. Neuropharmacology 23: 255–261

Wagner H R, Davis J N 1980 Decreased beta-adrenergic responses in the female rat brain are eliminated by ovariectomy: correlation of 3H-dihydroalprenolot binding and catecholamine-stimulated CAMP levels. Brain Res 201: 235–239

Wagner H R, Crutcher K A, Davis J N 1979 Chronic oestrogen treatment decreases beta-adrenergic responses in rat cerebral cortex. Brain Res 171: 147–151

Watson J P, Elliott S A, Rugg A J, Brough D I 1984 Psychiatric disorder in pregnancy and the first postnatal year. Br J Psychiatry 144: 453–462

Weiland N G, Wise P M 1987 Estrogen alters the diurnal rhythm of 1-adrenergic receptor densities in selected brain regions. Endocrinology 121: 1751–1758

Winokur G 1973 Depression in the menopause. Am J Psychiatry 130: 92–93

19. Disorders of female sexuality

F. Reader

CLASSIFICATION

The definition and classification of disorders of female sexuality are open to debate. More than one disorder/dysfunction can coexist, or a woman may move from one dysfunction to another depending on circumstances. It is also important to bear in mind that it is only a disorder to the individual woman, if she herself perceives it as a problem. For example, coital anorgasmia may be a problem for the woman's partner if his belief system leaves him feeling inadequate or rejected if he cannot 'bring his partner to orgasm'. She, on the other hand, may be happy with the situation, experiencing orgasm with self or mutual masturbation and enjoying penetrative sex. This is an example of a problem in that relationship because of different expectations of the female sexual response, but it is not a sexual dysfunction for the woman.

Keeping in mind the importance of recognizing the individual's perception of dysfunction, the classification based on DSM III R is offered in Table 19.1.

This classification is based on the concept of the sexual response cycle described by Kaplan (1974) where she recognized the phase of desire in the

Table 19.1 Classification of female sexual dysfunctions

Phase affected	DSM III R	Dysfunction
1. Desire/appetite	Hypoactive sexual desire disorder 301·71	Impaired sexual desire
2. Arousal/excitement	Female sexual arousal disorder 302·72	Impaired sexual arousal
3. Orgasm	Inhibited female orgasm 302·73	Orgasmic dysfunction
4. Penetration	Dyspareunia 302·76 Vaginismus 306·51	Dyspareunia Vaginismus
5. Other	Sexual aversion disorders 302·79	Sexual phobias

Table 19.2   Frequency of female sexual dysfunctions

Dysfunction	Frequency and comment	Study	Country and numbers
Unspecified sexual dysfunction	59% 'At some time' 23% 'Currently'	Sanders (1985)	UK 4000
Impaired sexual desire	35% 'Disinterest' 42% 'Lack of motivation'	Frank & Rubinstein (1978)	USA 100 'happily married women'
	12% 'Never experienced spontaneous sexual desire'	Garde & Lunde (1980a)	Denmark 225 40-year-old women
Impaired sexual arousal	48% 'Difficulty getting aroused' (n.b. desire and arousal not differentiated)	Frank & Rubinstein (1978)	USA 100 'happily married women'
Orgasmic dysfunction	13% 'Never' 4% Wives 15% Unmarried } 'never' almost never'	Gebhard & Johnson (1979) Sanders (1985)	USA 8000 married women UK 4000
	12% Never 17% 'Rarely or never on sexual intercourse'	Hite (1976)	USA 3000
Vaginismus	2% 'Not consumated relationship'	Kinsey et al (1953)	USA 8000 married women

sexual response cycle. Previously Masters & Johnson (1966) had described the phases of excitement, orgasm and resolution but excluded desire.

All dysfunctions can be primary or secondary, total or situational. For example a woman who has never had interest in sex would be said to have primary total impaired sexual desire (ISD), whereas a woman who has lost interest in sex with her husband whilst having no problems with her lover could be defined as having secondary situational ISD.

FREQUENCY OF DYSFUNCTIONS

Many different methods have been used to look at frequency of the various dysfunctions. Some have a scientific basis such as the General Population surveys of Kinsey et al (1953) refined by Gebhard & Johnson (1979), Frank & Rubinstein (1978) and Garde & Lunde (1980a). Surveys of clients in clinical situations have also been used: psychiatric clinic attenders, Swann & Wilson (1979), gynaecology clinic attenders, Levine & Yost (1976), family planning clinic attenders, Begg et al (1976) and general practice, Golombok et al (1984).

Non-scientific sampling through magazine and other questionnaires have also produced interesting data the most well known being Hite (1976) and Sanders (1985). The latter took 4000 responses as representative from a range of 15 600 women who replied to a questionnaire in *Woman* magazine.

Table 19.2 gives frequencies from some of these studies. The true picture is still far from clear and many studies do not differentiate between the sexual and marital/relationship component of the problem.

Reported frequency of dysfunctions presenting to sexual/marital dysfunction clinics also varies but impaired sexual desire seems to be the most common presentation.

Hawton (1984) looked at 257 women presenting and reported 52% with impaired sexual desire, 19% orgasmic dysfunctions, 18% vaginismus and 4% dyspareunia. Bancroft & Coles (1976) showed similar trends.

Neither study gives data on impaired sexual arousal in women.

CAUSATIVE FACTORS AND THEIR MANAGEMENT

The causes of female sexual dysfunctions are many and various and multiple factors are frequently involved. They may be physiological,

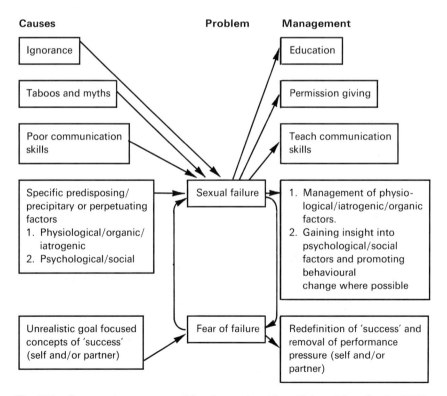

Fig. 19.1   Causes and management of female sexual problems (Adapted from Stanley 1981).

organic, iatrogenic or psychosocial. The psychological component can be either intrapersonal or interpersonal but is usually a mixture of both.

The key factor is that the woman presents with 'sexual failure'. This is either primary, which then leads to 'fear of failure', or else the fear is primary and triggers a self fulfilling prophecy and sexual failure follows. In either event a vicious circle is established.

Management of the problem aims to break this vicious circle and establish acceptable sexual functions as defined by the client or couple.

Figure 19.1 summarizes the general causes of sexual dysfunction and the corresponding management.

Ignorance and education

It is not uncommon for a woman to present with very little knowledge of her body and how it functions sexually. Her hidden internal genitalia remain shrouded in mystery and she may have never used a tampon or dared to look at her own vulva in a mirror.

The Royal Society of Medicine book 'Growing Up, a guide for children and parents' (Doherty 1986) is a very useful resource to help educate women and their partners about female anatomy and physiology. Alternatively the woman can be helped to become familiar with her external genitalia by using the in vivo technique described as the 'guided tour' by Stanley (1981).

It often helps to begin with a relaxation exercise before proceeding to the guided tour. The woman is then encouraged to explore her own external genitalia with the help of a large hand-held mirror which she holds between her legs whilst sitting propped up on the examination couch. The doctor or nurse then assists by pointing out to her the labia majora, labia minora, clitoris, urethral and vaginal openings. The woman's responses also help diagnostically. Involvement of the partner can be beneficial.

For the guided tour to be perceived as both educative and permission giving it is best performed by a female professional.

Myths, taboos and permission giving

Different family, cultural and religious backgrounds can affect the way a woman views her body and her sexuality. The education process outlined previously is also enormously permission giving. However it is important to be wary of appearing to mock a woman's belief system and therefore to work sensitively with her towards change.

Communication problems and teaching communication skills

Many sexual dysfunctions present because of problems in communication either generally, or specifically about sex. Many women find it difficult to ask for what they want sexually and even more difficult to say 'no' to what they don't want.

The existence of bad feelings such as anger, guilt and anxiety can also affect the sexual response cycle. Teaching the individuals within the relationship to recognize, accept and own their own emotions is an important first step.

Good communication also involves learning to say what you mean and mean what you say. It is important to learn to separate the action from the person so that the couple learns that to say 'no' is alright because it is saying 'no' to the action and not a rejection of the person.

Identification and management of specific precipitating and perpetuating factors

General organic factors

Illness affecting any system can affect a woman's sense of wellbeing, self esteem or body image, which in turn may have effect on her sexual responsiveness. A woman with epilepsy may be afraid that the loss of control at orgasm will trigger a fit, and therefore present with anorgasmia. After a coronary a woman may be concerned about returning to sexual activity because of the increase in heart rate that accompanies arousal and orgasm. Surgical procedures are likely to affect body and self image especially mastectomy and hysterectomy which also affect the woman's sense of femaleness. Ostomies, limb amputations, burns and other skin conditions can also affect body and self image and hence sexual responsiveness. The list is endless. In all medical or surgical specialities there will be instances when the disease and/or its treatment can precipitate a sexual dysfunction.

Organic disease can also affect sexual responsiveness directly by hormonal, neurological, or cardiovascular effects on some part of the sexual response cycle.

Table 19.3 lists some of the organic diseases linked to sexual dysfunctions in women.

Sexually transmitted diseases

Sexually transmitted diseases are likely to affect the female sexual response through both psychological, relationship and local genital factors.

Foremost in the 1990s is concern about HIV and AIDS. Any sexually active woman today who is changing partners, uncertain of her partner's sexual history or other current sexual relationships should be thinking about and using safer sex.

Many women find the practice of safer sex very liberating as it focuses on

Table 19.3 Examples of organic disease and female sexual dysfunctions

Disease	Dysfunction

Diabetes	Orgasmic dysfunction
	Arousal phase problems
	e.g. reduced lubrication
	    reduced sensation
	    increased vaginal infections

Pituitary adenoma with hyperprolactinaemia	Impaired sexual desire Impaired sexual arousal
Hypothyroidism	Impaired sexual desire Occasionally secondary anorgasmia
Multiple sclerosis	Orgasmic dysfunction Reduced lubrication Reduced sensation
Spinal injuries	Arousal phase problems Reduced sensation Muscle spasms
Ostomies with surgical sacral nerve damage	Arousal phase problems Reduced sensation Dyspareunia

good communication, full expression of sensuality but without the emphasis on penetrative sex.

For other women however the fear of contracting HIV, AIDS or other sexually transmitted diseases can lead to avoidance and impaired sexual desire.

Genital herpes can have a disastrous affect on female sexual responsiveness both psychologically and because of the episodes of vulval and vaginal soreness. In severe cases long term use of acyclovir for 1 year can reduce attacks. Later this can be modified by taking treatment intermittently at the first signs of an impending attack.

Genital warts may cause local dyspareunia. They may also raise fear in the woman and her partner because of the link with abnormal cervical cytology.

Gynaecological disorders

Gynaecological disorders and surgery are especially likely to affect the woman's sense of herself as a sexual being especially where she also undergoes loss of part of her female organs. Kincey & McFarlane (1984) followed up prospectively on 98 women having hysterectomy and found 19% reported impaired sexual function, 44% improved and 31% reported no change. The effect of dyspareunia on sexual response is dealt with separately at the end of the chapter.

Table 19.4 Drug effects on female sexual response (Kolodny et al 1979)

Drug	Desire	Arousal	Orgasm
CNS effect			
Alcohol	↑ Low dose ↓ High dose	↑ Low dose ↓ High dose	Delayed high dose
Anxiolytics	↑ Low dose ↓ High dose	↑ Low dose ↓ High dose	Delayed high dose
Antidepressants Tricyclics	—	—	? Delayed orgasm
Lithium	↓	—	—
Antipsyalotics Phenothiazines	↓ High dose (↑ prolactin)	—	—
Antiemetics Metachlorpropamide	↓ High dose (↑ prolactin)	—	—
Narcotics	Absent high doses	Absent high doses	Absent high doses
Hormonal effect Testosterone	↑	—	—
Oestrogeg	Some women ↑ Some women ↓	—	—
Progesterone	? Some women ↓	—	—
Cyproterone acetate	↓	—	—
Diuretics/antihypertensives Spironolactone	↓	—	—
B blockers	Sometimes ↓	Sometimes ↓	—
Methyldopa	Sometimes ↓	Sometimes ↓	May be inhibited
Miscellaneous Cimetidine	↓ (Antitesterone)	—	—

Drugs

Table 19.4 lists some common prescribed and non-prescribed drugs and their possible effect on sexual function.

Psychosocial factors

Precipitating or perpetuating factors may be intrapersonal, e.g.

Deprivation in childhood
Unemployment leading to loss of self esteem
Past history of incest or rape
Unresolved grief reaction

Transition to motherhood
Uncertain sexual identity

or interpersonal, e.g.

Loss of trust between partners
Inability to express anger
Transition to parenthood.

Gaining insight into the event or events that precipitated or are perpetuating 'failure' may call for in depth individual psychotherapy or marital/relationship therapy. This should take place before specific therapy for the sexual dysfunction. However for many women the counselling accompanying specific sex therapy will be adequate to overcome the difficulty.

Unrealistic goal focused concepts of success

Unrealistic goals from either the woman or her partner can lead to fear of failure and are best managed by helping to redefine success and remove performance pressures. For example a couple may present concern at their inability to reach simultaneous orgasm. Education about normal sexual response and redefining success to something realistic and mutually acceptable will help remove the fear of failure.

Sensate focus is an ideal behavioural strategy to help remove performance pressures. It is dealt with in detail at the end of the chapter.

MANAGEMENT OF SPECIFIC FEMALE SEXUAL DYSFUNCTIONS

Impaired sexual desire (ISD)

This is the most common presentation in women to sexual dysfunction clinics, 36% was reported by Warner et al (1987).

Primary ISD is likely to be due to intrapersonal problems. Problems of sexual identity may present in this way.

Where the problem is total and secondary it is important to exclude organic factors. Secondary ISD can also be physiological such as when a woman is breast feeding and is subject to high prolactin levels or around the menopause with falling oestrogen levels. ISD at the time of the menopause may respond to hormone replacement therapy especially if poor lubrication is a contributory factor. Added testosterone may also help (Sherwin et al 1985).

The combined oral contraceptive pill has been linked to ISD in some women, but studies are inconclusive and Cullberg (1973) found that any change was probably secondary to mood changes. Whenever there is a possible physiological, organic or iatrogenic component to ISD, it is still important to take a history to check out other intra- and interpersonal factors.

When sexual desire, arousal, or orgasm triggers difficult emotions it is likely to lead to suppression of desire. Fear, guilt and anger are common emotions that may block desire. For example, fear of failure, fear of sexual consequences such as pregnancy, cervical cancer, or sexually transmitted disease, fear of rejection, fear of commitment may be related to an inability to integrate love of another person with the act of sexual intercourse. Other women cannot integrate their role as mother with continuing sexual responsiveness. Loss of sexual desire may be used by a woman as an easier way of expressing her anger and wish to end a relationship or her guilt if she has begun a second relationship.

Impaired sexual arousal

Arousal problems are often linked to inhibited desire but it is quite feasible for either to occur alone. A woman may never experience spontaneous desire but have no problems with arousal when sex is initiated by her partner. Conversely she may desire sex and then not respond with arousal.

During arousal the outer third of the vagina becomes swollen and engorged and the inner two thirds balloons thus lifting the uterus and ovaries up and away from the thrusting penis. The vagina also lubricates by an exudate through the vaginal walls added to by secretions from Bartholin's glands. Thus apart from an awareness of lubrication all the genital signs of arousal in the female are hidden compared to the very obvious sign of erectile problems in the male.

Superficial and deep dyspareunia may be presenting symptoms of arousal problems because of insufficient lubrication and vaginal ballooning. It is important to take a detailed sexual history when dyspareunia is the presenting symptom.

Similar psychological factors as described for ISD can also affect arousability.

Orgasmic dysfunction

Hite (1976) reported 12% of her survey of 3000 women were totally anorgasmic. This situation is sometimes termed 'preorgasmic' assuming that with adequate stimulation all women are potentially orgasmic. However research suggests that nearly half of today's women find orgasm elusive at some time in their lives (Wilson 1981b). It does not appear to be anxiety that is preventing orgasm (Norton & Jehu 1984) nor is it related to a strict religious upbringing (Fisher 1973). Hite's (1976) sample of women reported that intimacy was what women reported as the most enjoyable aspect of a sexual encounter with another person and orgasm to be the 'icing on the cake'. It is not uncommon for women to present with orgasmic problems because it is their partner who wants to 'give them an orgasm' and their failure is seen as rejection or a challenge to his masculinity.

It may be that there are sociobiological reasons why women are less readily orgasmic compared to men. Men need to ejaculate to further the human race whereas women do not need to be orgasmic to be fertile. Rabock & Bartak (1983) found that late menarche was associated with less frequent or absent orgasm in adult life. Chronic constipation has also been linked to orgasmic difficulties (Preston & Lennard-Jones 1986).

Between a third and a half of women never experience orgasm during coitus. This is probably mechanical due to insufficient clitoral stimulation. In some couples this can be overcome with the 'Bridge Technique' (Kaplan 1974, 1981) where the clitoris is stimulated manually by the male or female at the same time as penile containment. The female superior position may also help if this has not been tried before. However despite all these manoeuvres coital orgasms may remain elusive and redefining goals could be the answer particularly if there appear to be no inter- or intrapersonal problems blocking change. An acceptable goal may be to progress from achieving orgasm with solo masturbation, to involving her partner in the stimulation for orgasm to occur. Many women find that manual stimulation either by self or by partner is still insufficient and a vibrator is then useful to take her from the 'edge of orgasm' to 'over the top'.

The self help book 'Becoming Orgasmic—a sexual growth program for women' by Heiman et al (1986) is an extremely useful resource for orgasmic difficulties.

Dyspareunia

Pain on penetration may be superficial or deep. Some of the organic causes are outlined in Table 19.5. However it is not uncommon for dyspareunia to be psychosomatic and a symptom of failure of arousal.

Mira (1988) classified non-organic into Type I (intrapersonal) when the presentation involves guilt, misinformation, previous traumatic experiences, or previous physical factors such as vaginitis or episiotomy, and Type II (interpersonal) where marital problems and poor communication lead to dyspareunia being used as an excuse to avoid sex.

Type I dyspareunia will respond well to education, permission giving and systematic desensitization, whereas Type II needs a marital therapy and communication skills approach.

Women with chronic dyspareunia present as a difficult management problem to many gynaecologists. It is easy to fall into the trap of performing laparoscopy only to find a normal pelvis and confidently pronounce 'I can find nothing wrong'. The implication behind this is that the pain is all in the mind and the patient herself feels frustrated and dissatisfied as she is left with a pain that is real to her and no diagnosis.

Table 19.5 Dyspareunia—common physiological/organic causes

Problem	Common description of pain
Introital/vaginal	
Atrophy/inadequate lubrication	Sharp or low grade superficial/vaginal pain
Hymenal remnants/intact hymen	Sharp introital pain/aware deep penetration impossible
Candida	Superficial soreness/itching
Genital herpes	Severe burning superficial/vaginal pain
Genital warts	Burning superficial/vaginal pain
Allergies (soap, detergents etc.)	Burning superficial/vaginal pain
Poorly healed episiotomy	Sharp introital pain
Acute or chronic abrasions	Sharp introital pain
Bladder/urethra	
Cystitis	Anterior vaginal and lower abdominal pain
Cystocoele	Anterior vaginal pain
Urethral carbuncle	Superficial burning
Bowel	
Inflammatory bowel disease	Posterior vaginal pain or deep pain, maybe left-sided
Chronic constipation	Dull posterior or deep left-sided pain
Uterus	
Cervictis/endometritis/myometritis	Sharp or low grade deep pain induced by thrusting
Adenexae	
Endometriosis/pelvic inflammatory disease	Generalized deep pain often worse premenstrually
Ectopic/ovarian cyst	Sharp deep pain maybe unilateral

Pelvic pain without pathology (PPWOP) and chronic pelvic pain without pathology (CPPWOP) are terms becoming more familiar in recent literature. Black (1988) describes the problems raised by these 'diagnoses' and provides a useful and rational way forward for clinicians and patients. He points out the importance of recognizing the reality of pain for the woman and having the courage to say 'I don't know what the pain is but I can definitely tell you what it isn't'.

Black (1988) also draws attention to the study by Gross et al (1980) when 25 women with CPPWOP were interviewed in depth and 9 (36%) had a past history of incest. This highlights the importance of having time to sensitively take a full sexual history and to establish a relationship between the professional and the patient where she will feel safe to make such a disclosure and begin the healing process essential to moving into incest survival. In this instance the professional could be a psychologist or counsellor working with the gynaecology team.

Vaginismus

Vaginismus is an involuntary contraction of pelvic floor muscles in response to fear or phobia of penetration. Initially therapy aims to help the woman learn to become aware of her pelvic floor muscles and to gain control of their contraction and relaxation. Teaching Kegel's exercises is essential at this stage. Many women also have involuntary spasm of the adductor muscles of their thighs. Relaxation exercises can help the woman to relax generally and to relax these muscles specifically.

The 'guided tour' described earlier is educative, permission giving and also begins the process of desensitization. Following on from the guided tour the woman can be encouraged to explore her own vagina with one finger. She may need the encouragement of the professional gently inserting a finger first but if possible the process of desensitization should be one that empowers the woman to do things herself.

Once the woman has mastered the ability to look at her genitals and to insert a finger into the vagina, she can progress to using vaginal trainers (Stanley 1981).

Vaginal trainers come in 3 sizes of the same length but differing widths, all of them are as long as a fully erect penis. The narrowest trainer is the width of a finger and the largest trainer the width of a fully erect penis. The woman therefore becomes desensitized to the length as well as the width. The plastic containers of varying sized syringes offer an alternative to Stanley trainers.

Another technique to help desensitize the woman is called the 'fantasy trip' (Stanley 1981b, Adler 1989). The woman is asked to imagine herself as very small and to take a trip into her vagina. She then describes what she sees, feels, smells, hears, etc. both as she walks in and out. This can be very illuminating as many women relate a variety of bizarre and frightening misconceptions about their internal genitalia. The professional can work with her to reassure her, educate her and help her find her way to redescribing and defining her vagina in positive, realistic terms.

The book 'Vaginismus' (Vallins 1988) is an excellent resource book to help women with this problem.

The progression from trainers to penile penetration is best achieved initially with the female superior position. Side to side is the next best option. At first the woman is asked to get used to penile containment and then progresses to containment with thrusting.

Sexual phobias

For many women vaginismus is a type of phobia. Other phobias include touching the penis, semen, oral sex, etc. Treatment consists of gradual densitization tailor made to the particular individual and her phobia.

Sensate focus

Sensate focus was first described by Masters & Johnson (1970). It is a behavioural strategy for overcoming sexual problems by removing performance pressure. It is treated as homework for the couple in therapy and is usually adapted to meet their specific needs.

A version of sensate focus can be done by an individual in the form of progressive self discovery and pleasuring exercises. This is useful in the management of vaginismus and type I dyspareunia.

Sensate focus with a couple starts by putting a ban on sexual intercourse thus removing the pressure to achieve this goal.

The couple are asked to set aside two or three separate 1 hour sessions during the week when they can be alone together. Negotiations to achieve this can be very enlightening. Work on communication may be needed before mutually agreeable decisions on when, where and how can be reached. For example, a couple with children may need to look at being assertive about their rights to privacy or a busy working couple may need to look at freeing up time to make sure they can give this homework priority. It is also important to get agreement that when sessions are in progress the phone is off the hook and the doorbell is left unanswered.

The sessions are not goal orientated. The couple are asked to take it in turns to give and receive pleasure. The emphasis is not on arousal but on pleasure. Each individual is asked to practise selfish caring, which means making sure that when receiving pleasure the experience is just that. Thus the receiver needs to be aware of feelings and able to give negative feedback when the giver is touching in a particular way that evokes negative feelings. It is important to ensure the couple understand negative feedback is about the action and does not equate to rejection of the person. The giver should also be focusing on giving pleasure in a way that is pleasing to the giver, not the receiver.

Once a couple are comfortable with negative feedbacks they can progress to negative and positive, but it is important to focus on the negative first as this is usually more difficult.

Sensate focus begins with a ban on touching genitals and breasts as well as the ban on intercourse. The second step is to progress to genital sensate focus.

Sensate focus is useful for the management of ISD. It should be used after teaching communication skills and dealing with any intrapersonal problems. It is particularly useful for arousal and orgasmic problems where inadequate and inappropriate foreplay may have been a causative factor and for vaginismus and type I dyspareunia after the desensitizing process and before progression to penile containment. It helps to ensure good communication about likes and dislikes and to build up trust.

FINAL COMMENT

Individual sexuality is an integral and important part of every human being. It needs to be valued by health professionals and not shied away from because of embarrassment. It is an area of understanding where the health professions should look to improve teaching and training and ensure all staff can talk comfortably about sexual matters with patients thus helping them to value, understand and own their own sexuality.

REFERENCES

Adler E 1989 Vaginismus—its presentation and treatment. Br J Sex Med 16 (11): 420–424
Bancroft J, Coles M 1976 Three years experience in a sexual problems clinic. Br Med J 1: 1575–1577
Begg A, Dickerson M, Loudon N 1976 Frequency of self reported sexual problems in a family planning clinic. J Fam Pl Drs 2: 41–48
Black J S 1988 Sexual dysfunction and dyspareunia in the otherwise normal pelvis. Sex Marital Ther 3 (2): 213–222
Cullberg J 1973 Mood changes and menstrual symptoms with different gestergen/estrogen combinations. Acta Psychiatr Scand (Suppl): 236
Docherty J 1986 The Royal Society of Medicine Growing up: a guide for children and parents. Alcamco/Modus Books, London
Fisher S 1973 The female orgasm. Psychology, physiology, fantasy. Basic Books, New York
Frank E, Rubinstein D 1978 Frequency of sexual dysfunction in 'normal' couples. New Engl J Med 299: 111–115
Garde K, Lunde J 1980a Female sexual behaviour: a study in a random sample of 40 year old women. Maturitas 2: 225–240
Gebhard P H, Johnson A B 1979 The Kinsey data: marginal tabulations of the 1938–1963 interviews conducted by the Institute for Sex Research. Saunders, Philadelphia
Golombok S, Rust J, Pickard C 1984 Sexual problems encountered in general practice. Br J Sex Med 11: 210–212
Gross R J, Doerr H, Caldirola D, Gruzinski G M, Ridley H S 1980 Borderline syndrome and incest in chronic pelvic pain patients. Int J Psychiatry Med 10: 79–96
Hawton K 1984 Sex therapy: a practical guide. Oxford University Press, Oxford
Heiman J, Lopiccolo L, Lopiccolo J 1986 Becoming orgasmic: a sexual growth program for women. Prentice Hall International (UK) Ltd, London
Hite S 1976 The Hite Report: a nationwide study of female sexuality. Dell, New York
Kaplan H S 1974 The new sex therapy. Brunner/Mazel, New York
Kaplan H S 1979 Disorders of sexual desire. Baillière Tindall, London
Kaplan H S 1981 The illustrated manual of sex therapy. Granada, London
Kincey J, McFarlane T 1984 Psychological aspects of hysterectomy. In: Broome A, Wallace L (eds) Psychological and gynaecological problems. Tavistock, London, pp 142–160
Kinsey A C, Pomeroy W B, Martin C E, Gebhard P H 1953 Sexual behaviour in the human female. Saunders, Philadelphia
Kolodny R C, Masters W H, Johnson V E 1979 Textbook of sexual medicine. Little, Brown, Boston
Levine S B, Yost M A 1976 Frequency of sexual dysfunction in a general gynaecological clinic: an epidermiological approach. Arch Sex Behav 5: 229–238
Masters W H, Johnson V E 1966 Human sexual response. Little, Brown, Boston
Masters W H, Johnson V E 1970 Human sexual inadequacy. Churchill, London
Mira J J 1988 A therapeutic package for dyspareunia: a three case example. Sex Marital Ther 3 (1): 77–82

Norton G R, Jehu D 1984 The role of anxiety in sexual dysfunctions: a review. Arch Sex Behav 13: 165–168

Preston D M, Lennard-Jones J E 1986 Severe chronic constipation of young women: idiopathic slow transit constipation. Gut 27: 41–48

Rabock J, Bartak V 1983 Menarche and orgastic capacity. Arch Sex Behav 10: 379–392

Sanders D 1985 The woman book of love and sex. Joseph, London

Sherwin B B, Gelfard M M, Brender W 1985 Androgen enhances sexual motivation in females: a prospective crossover study of sex steroid administration in the surgical menopause. Psychosom Med 47: 339–351

Stanley E 1981a Sex problems in practice: vaginismus. Br Med J 282: 1435–1437

Stanley E 1981b Sex problems in practice: non-organic causes of sexual problems. Br Med J 282: 1042–1044

Swann M, Wilson L J 1979 Sexual and marital problems in a psychiatric out-patient population. Br J Psychiatry 135: 310–314

Valins L 1988 Vaginismus: understanding and overcoming the blocks to intercourse. Ashgrove, Bath

Warner P, Bancroft J and members of the Edinburgh Human Sexuality Group 1987 A regional service for sexual problems: a 3 year study. Sex Marital Ther 2: 115–126

Wilson G 1981 Cross generational stability of gender differences in sexuality. Personality and Individual Differences 2: 254–257

20. Hirsutism

J. A. Eden

Hirsutism may be defined as the presence of excessive coarse (terminal) hair which is socially unacceptable to the patient. The areas commonly involved include the upper lip, chin, sideburn areas, chest, lower abdomen and thighs. Several scoring systems are available, probably the most clinically useful being that of Ferriman & Gallway (1961) which uses a score of 0–4 for each area of the body. The 95% confidence limit for premenopausal women being a score of 8. Hirsutism may or may not be associated with menstrual disturbances.

Virilization is much rarer than hirsutism and is usually secondary to adrenal hyperplasia, androgen producing tumours or the polycystic ovary syndrome (PCOS). As well as acne, hirsutism and amenorrhoea, signs of virilization include clitoromegaly, temporal balding, deepening of the voice, breast atrophy and muscle enlargement.

The true incidence of hirsutism is not known, however it is more common among Mediterranean women who are usually more accepting of their condition. On the other hand, hirsutism is uncommon among Asiatic women. It is important to view hirsutism as both an endocrine and a cosmetic problem. Many women with hirsutism and/or severe acne believe that their problem is incurable and sometimes this is reinforced by ill-informed doctors.

ANDROGEN PRODUCTION

The human menstrual cycle is the result of a complex interaction between the hypothalamic-pituitary-ovarian axis (an *endocrine* system) and local intra-ovarian controls (a *paracrine* system). A *paracrine* mechanism involves a product of one cell influencing an adjacent cell. Pituitary secretion of the gonadotrophins, luteinizing hormone (LH) and follicle stimulating hormone (FSH), is the result of pulsatile release of hypothalamic gonadotrophin releasing hormone (GnRH), modulated by gonadal sex steroids. The granulosa cell is the exclusive target for FSH whereas LH has multiple sites of action including theca, stroma, granulosa and luteal cells (Yen 1987a). The theca is the main source of ovarian androgen which is then converted into oestrogen by the granulosa, if exposed to FSH (Tsang

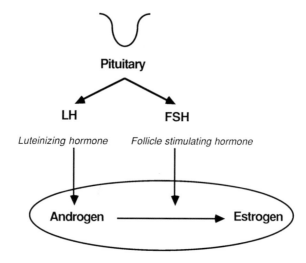

Fig. 20.1   LH acts on the way to produce androgen which is then converted into oestrogen by FSH. (Courtesy of the Department of Medical Illustration, University of New South Wales and Teaching Hospitals.)

et al 1980, Hillier et al 1980, Fig. 20.1). This two-cell cooperation is also influenced by local factors including insulin-like growth factor-1 (IGF1, formerly somatomedin-C). This aspect will be discussed in some detail later.

The ovary secretes three main androgens: testosterone (T), androstenedione (AD) and dehydroepiandrosterone (DHEA). The adrenals, liver, fat and skin also contribute to the production of these androgens (Hillier et al 1980, Eden 1989a, Speroff et al 1989).

The production rate of T in women is 0·2–0·3 mg per day (Speroff et al 1989). About 25% of T production is ovarian, 25% adrenal and the

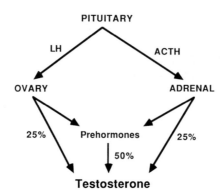

Fig. 20.2   Origin of testosterone in women. (Courtesy of the Department of Medical Illustration, University of New South Wales and Teaching Hospitals.)

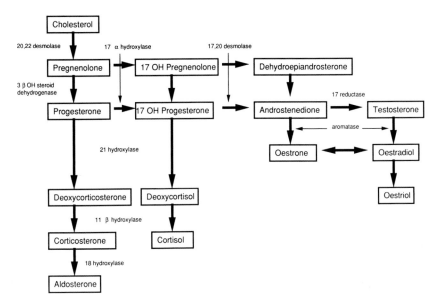

Fig. 20.3   Steroid production in the human. (Courtesy of the Department of Medical Illustration, University of New South Wales and Teaching Hospitals.)

remainder arises from the peripheral conversion of principally AD (Hillier et al 1980, Speroff et al 1989) (Figs 20.2, 20.3). The production of AD is higher in women than men, averaging 3 mg per day and half of this is ovarian derived. The rest is secreted by the adrenal with some peripheral conversion of DHEA. Both AD and T undergo a significant midcycle rise (Kirschner 1987, Eden et al 1988a). DHEA (and DHEA sulphate [DHEAS]) is largely of adrenal origin and its contribution to T production minor (Kirschner 1987).

T (and dihydrotestosterone [DHT]) is avidly bound in serum to sex hormone binding globulin (SHBG) and only the free fraction is biologically active (Anderson 1974, Cunningham et al 1985). Oestradiol (E2) is also bound to SHBG, but T is bound more avidly, so that SHBG is normally saturated with T. Small changes in SHBG will have profound effects on free T (Anderson 1974, Cunningham et al 1985). If SHBG levels fall, T will be liberated and free T rises. If SHBG levels rise, more T is bound and free T falls. The hepatic production of SHBG is inhibited by androgen and increased by oestrogens and thyroid hormone. In other words, androgens and oestrogens potentiate their effect via SHBG. The free androgen index (FAI) may be calculated by using the formula, T (nmol/l) × 100/SHBG (nmol/l), and is a clinically useful index of free T activity (Carlstrom et al 1987, Carter et al 1983, Eden 1988, Eden et al 1989a).

Obesity is associated with a decrease in SHBG levels in women with normal or polycystic ovaries (PCO) (Eden 1989a, 1988). Fat is a site of both androgen and oestrogen metabolism but the main effect is increased conversion of AD to weak oestrogens like oestrone (E1) (Siiteri 1987, Yen 1987b). Obesity is a well known risk factor for oestrogen responsive tumours like endometrial cancer (Jafari et al 1978) but the fall in SHBG has until recently been attributed to a shift to a more androgen milieu (Kirschner 1987, Yen 1987a).

A relationship between hyperinsulinaemia and androgen excess is now well described (Coney 1984, McKenna 1988, Barbieri et al 1988, Bruno & Fabbrini 1985, Smith et al 1987, Shoupe et al 1983, Burgen et al 1980, Chang et al 1983). A strong negative correlation has recently been found between insulin and SHBG (Weaver et al 1989) and since obesity is associated with higher than normal fasting levels of insulin (Conway et al 1988), this offers a more rational explanation for the association between obesity and low SHBG levels. Insulin also stimulates ovarian androgen production (Barbieri et al 1988). Insulin may well be a central player in androgen excess, especially when associated PCO (Bruno & Fabbrini 1985, Smith et al 1987, Shoupe et al 1983, Burgen et al 1980, Chang et al 1983) and hyperinsulinaemia may explain, at least in part, the low levels of SHBG and hyperandrogenism found in the PCO syndrome.

HAIR GROWTH

Hair follicles like neurones and oocytes are not renewed in adult life (Speroff et al 1989). Each single hair is attached to the follicle by a dermal

Table 20.1 Causes of androgen excess in women

Drugs
Androgens
Anabolic steroids
Androgenic progestagens
Phenytoin
Danocrine
Minoxidil
Ovarian causes
Polycystic ovary syndrome
Tumours
Hyperthecosis
Adrenal causes
Congenital adrenal hyperplasia (classical)
Congenital adrenal hyperplasia (late onset)
Cushing's syndrome
Tumour
'Idiopathic hirsutism'
Hyperprolactinaemia
Aggravators
Obesity
Hypothyroidism
Anovulation (per se)

papilla and is associated with a sebaceous gland. Hair growth is cyclical with growing (anagen), involution (catagen) and resting (telogen) phases. Anagen primarily determines the hair length.

The skin and these appendages have an active role in the production of androgens from prehormones as well as being target organs. T in particular binds to androgen receptors and the T-receptor unit is translocated to the nucleus of the cell (Kirschner 1987). Within the skin, T is converted by 5 alpha-reductase into DHT, a very potent androgen. In turn, locally produced DHT is metabolized to androstanediol which also has androgenic properties. Conjugation of androstanediol to glucuronide does not occur in the usual gut or hepatic sites, but rather in skin (and other target tissues) so that circulating levels of this metabolite represent utilization of androgens by target tissues.

Once androgen has stimulated the hair follicle to produce black terminal hair, these changes persist even in the absence of a continuing androgen excess. Androgen excess also stimulates the sebaceous gland to produce its oily sebum, which can block pores thus producing acne.

CAUSES OF ANDROGEN EXCESS

These are summarized in Table 20.1. Many commonly used drugs may cause or worsen hirsutism. These include the anticonvulsant phenytoin, anabolic steroids, danocrine and norethisterone (high dose). These should be stopped, if possible when excess body or facial hair develops.

The commonest endogenous cause of androgen excess is the PCO. This important disorder will be discussed separately later. The term 'idiopathic hirsutism' has been used in the past to describe hirsute women with regular cycles (Yen 1987b). Adams et al (1986) have shown that 90% of these women have ultrasound and biochemical evidence of PCOS and so the term 'idiopathic hirsutism' should be abandoned. Virtually all hirsute women have evidence of increased androgen production (Speroff et al 1989, Kirschner & Jacobs 1971, Kirschner 1987, Yen 1987b) which may not be evident if only a single serum T and DHEAS has been measured (Carter et al 1983).

Androgen secreting tumours are rare and their diagnosis usually straightforward. Their importance has been greatly exaggerated and selective venous catheterization is rarely required to confirm the diagnosis. The presence of a pelvic or abdominal mass will be investigated and treated in the usual manner, however some ovarian masses may be quite small. High resolution ultrasound particularly using vaginal tranducers has greatly improved diagnostic accuracy. Ovarian tumours secreting androgen include arrhenoblastomas, hilar cell tumours, lipoid cell tumours and the pregnancy associated solid luteoma. Some of these may be small and bisection of the ovaries may be necessary. Surgery should be conservative in the younger patient and both ovaries should be inspected and if necessary bisected. Virilization may also be due to theca-lutein cysts found with trophoblastic disease and multiple gestation. Cases of virilized female fetuses have been reported (Hague & Millar 1985).

Most benign adrenal masses are discovered during a workup for Cushing's syndrome (Kirschner 1987). Usually levels of DHEA, DHEAS and AD are very high. Virilization is reasonably common in women with adrenal carcinoma and may be more evident than signs of cortisone excess. Abdominal CT scanning has greatly aided the diagnosis of small adrenal masses.

Cushing's syndrome is a rare but important diagnosis and clinical suspicion should always be high. There are three main causes of this disorder: pituitary overproduction of adrenocorticotrophin hormone (ACTH), ectopic ACTH production by tumours or a cortisol-secreting adrenal adenoma or carcinoma. The most clinically useful initial tests are the 24 hour urinary free cortisol and the 1 mg dexamethasone suppression test. The overnight dexamethasone suppression test is simple and has a low rate of false positive results. Dexamethasone 1 mg is taken orally going to bed and a single plasma cortisol collected at 8 a.m. the next day. The cortisol level should be < 130 nmol/l. The correct diagnosis is usually confirmed by a long dexamethasone suppression test, ACTH measurement and CT scanning of the pituitary and adrenals.

Congenital adrenal hyperplasia can cause hirsutism and is usually diagnosed and treated before puberty. Late-onset adrenal hyperplasia, a milder form of the disease, is increasingly being diagnosed (Speroff et al 1989, Eden 1989b). An asymptomatic variant of the disease is revealed only by an ACTH test. Human leucocyte antigen (HLA) testing suggests that the haplotypes are similar in both the fetal and adult form of the disorder (Speroff et al 1989).

The most common enzyme deficiency is lack of 21-hydroxylase. It is the commonest autosomal recessive disorder, more common than cystic fibrosis (Speroff et al 1989). Many patients with this disorder are asymptomatic. The diagnosis is confirmed by finding an elevated basal plasma level of 17-hydroxyprogesterone (17 OH-P) and may be confirmed by measuring 17 OH-P before and after ACTH stimulation (Rosenfield 1985). It is an important condition to detect because treatment is long term, there is a theoretical risk of cortisol deficiency at times of stress and it may be worthwhile to test partners and siblings for the asymptomatic form of the disorder to permit accurate prenatal counselling. These women will have their androgen and progestogen excess controlled by a small nightly dose of dexamethasone (usually 0·25–0·05 mg).

Hyperthecosis is a rare condition characterized by diffuse luteinization and hyperplasia of ovarian stroma (Yen 1987b). Plasma T is often elevated, sometimes markedly. The aetiology is unknown although it may represent a variant of the PCOS.

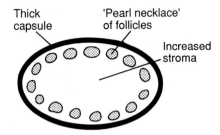

Fig. 20.4 The polycystic ovary. (Courtesy of the Department of Medical Illustration, University of New South Wales and Teaching Hospitals.)

THE POLYCYSTIC OVARY SYNDROME

No other area of reproductive endocrinology remains as controversial as the PCOS. PCO was described well before Stein and Leventhal's paper in 1935 and was linked with dysfunctional uterine bleeding, a point rarely mentioned in modern papers on the subject. They were the first to associate PCO with amenorrhoea. There is little doubt that it represents a heterogenous group of disorders characterized by a particular ovarian morphology. Arguments about the best method of defining the condition (such as ultrasound compared with biochemistry) seem fruitless. Some authors describe patients with the 'PCOS' but with normal ovaries (Kim et al 1979). If this occurs it is rare (Yen 1980, Goldzeiher & Green 1962) and sheds no light on the disorder.

The three main histological features of the PCO are a thick smooth fibrotic pearly white capsule, multiple small (2–8 mm) peripheral placed follicles and theca cell hyperplasia (Goldzeiher & Green 1962, Eden 1989a) (Figs 20.4, 20.5). Ultrasound can be used to diagnose PCO and has a high concordance with a surgical diagnosis (Eden 1988, 1989a, Eden et al 1989a,

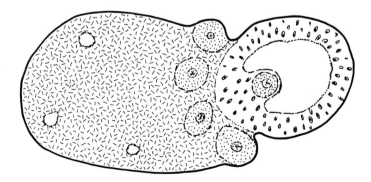

Fig. 20.5 The normal ovary. (Courtesy of the Department of Medical Illustration, University of New South Wales and Teaching Hospitals.)

Adams et al 1986) and biochemical evidence of hyperandrogenism or elevation of LH levels (Eden 1988, Adams et al 1985, Eden et al 1989a). The PCOS or PCO disease may then simply be defined as the presence of PCO and symptoms such as oligo-amenorrhoea, hirsutism, acne, dysfunctional uterine bleeding, infertility and perhaps recurrent miscarriage (Eden 1988, 1989a, Adams et al 1985, Sagle et al 1988, Homberg et al 1988).

It is also clear that the PCOS is underdiagnosed (Eden 1989a). There are many reasons for this, including failure to adequately inspect the ovaries at laparoscopy, failure to collect blood samples at the correct time of the cycle (early follicular phase), poorly established normal ranges for hormone parameters and not measuring appropriate serum androgens, especially free androgen.

About 85% of women with oligomenorrhoea and hirsutism have PCO on ultrasound scan (Eden 1989a, Adams et al 1986) and 90% with 'idiopathic hirsutism' (hirsutism and regular cycles). As many as 23% of 'normal' women may have asymptomatic PCO (Polson et al 1988). It seems likely that PCO may be primary or secondary to a virilizing 'insult' to the ovaries (Eden 1989a) (Fig. 20.6). Hyperandrogenism and high follicular phase levels of LH are the biochemical hallmarks of the PCOS (Eden 1989a, 1988, Yen 1980), however there is considerable confusion over the source of these androgens. This is in part because many authors equate adrenal suppression by dexamethasone or a contraceptive pill with proof of the adrenal or ovarian origin of the disorder. As already mentioned, all androgens undergo significant interconversion.

Around 40–60% of patients with PCOS will have an elevated level of either T, AD or DHEA (S) (Eden 1989a, Speroff et al 1989, Yen 1980). At

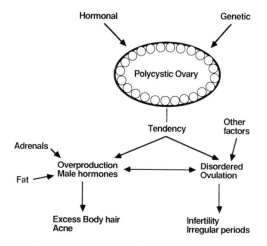

Fig. 20.6   Women with the polycystic ovary have a weight-dependent tendency to overproduce androgen as well as disordered ovulation. (Courtesy of the Department of Medical Illustration, University of New South Wales and Teaching Hospitals.)

least two studies using the combined ovarian and adrenal vein sampling technique have shown that the ovary is the main source of androgen, despite the fact that dexamethasone suppressed the androgens in a third of the patients (Kirschner & Jacobs 1971, Wajchenberg et al 1986). However, patients given exogenous androgens or with specific androgenizing disorders (e.g. Cushing's syndrome) often have PCO, suggesting that PCO can be a secondary disorder (Yen 1980). About 20% of women with PCOS have a mildly elevated prolactin level which may stimulate adrenal androgen production, further aggravating this disorder (Yen 1980, McKenna 1988).

Most authors consider the PCO to be secondary to either an adrenal or hypothalamic-pituitary disorder (Speroff et al 1989, Kirschner 1987, Yen 1980, 1987b). However, another possibility is that the PCOS is a primary ovarian disorder.

Peptide growth factors such as IGF1 are important intra-ovarian regulators of steroid production and cellular growth and differentiation (Eden et al 1988b, 1989c). IGF1 influences both ovarian androgen and oestrogen production (Hernandez et al 1988, Adashi et al 1988). Ovarian follicular fluid (FF) concentrations of IGF1 are probably a composite of serum-derived and locally produced IGF1 (Eden 1989a). Volume matched polycystic follicles contain higher FF levels of IGF1 than normal (Eden et al 1989c) suggesting that a local disorder of regulatory peptides could explain some of the features of the PCOS. It is also possible that the PCOS could result from an excess of inhibitory peptides (Mason et al 1990.) Hyperinsulinaemia, characteristic of the PCOS also stimulates ovarian androgen production (Barbieri et al 1988) and influences IGF1 metabolism. IGF1 has at least four binding proteins which can modulate its activity and one of these appears to be influenced by insulin. This complex interaction is discussed in detail in my review of the PCOS (Eden 1989a) and IGF1 (Eden et al 1989b).

If the PCOS is a consequence of a disorder of these local factors, this would explain why a wedge resection or ovarian diathermy restores ovulation in many women with PCOS. By wounding the ovary, a cascade of stimulatory growth factors is generated to heal tissue and this may also restore the balance of these regulatory growth factors.

Obesity and anovulation (per se) will aggravate the biochemical abnormalities of the PCOS. Free T levels rise with increasing body mass index (BMI), but much more rapidly in the woman with PCO compared with normal (Eden et al 1988a, 1989a). Weight loss is associated with an improvement in the hyperandrogenic state and often the resumption of ovulatory cycles (Pasquali et al 1989). Anovulatory patients with PCOS have lower levels of SHBG than either spontaneously ovulating women with PCO or those with normal ovaries (Eden et al 1988a, 1989d). Restoring ovulation to normal with Clomiphene returns SHBG levels to normal and is associated with a fall in LH levels (Eden et al 1989d). These data suggest that the low SHBG and in part, the high LH levels are a consequence of anovulation, itself. In other words, once rendered anovulatory, the hyperandrogenic state deteriorates, further inhibiting ovulation.

Insulin and IGF1 are also important nutritional hormones and so offer a link between the body mass and nutritional state of the organism and ovarian function. It is possible that women with primary PCO may have inherited a defect of insulin or IGF1 metabolism and the other features of the disorder are secondary. It has been postulated that the PCO may offer species advantages in times of starvation (Eden 1989a).

Why the diagnosis of polycystic ovaries can be missed

If one accepts that the polycystic ovary is common then it is likely that our normal ranges for some sex-hormone measurements have been 'polluted' by these patients. This potential problem was examined in a study performed at Charing Cross Hospital, London (Eden et al 1988a). One hundred and forty consecutive patients with laparoscopically proven normal ovaries and scan proven ovulation were bled in the early follicular phase and had blood levels of LH, FSH, T, SHBG estimated and their free androgen index (FAI) calculated. The upper limit of normal for LH was reduced from 15 U/l to 9·8 U/l and testosterone from 3 nmol/l to 2·5 nmol/l. When these new normal ranges were then applied to the clinical situation it was found that an elevated level of LH, T, FAI or low SHBG concentration were just as likely to predict a laparoscopic diagnosis of polycystic ovaries as a well performed high resolution ultrasound scan (Eden et al 1989a, Eden 1989a). In the same studies it was found that the LH/FSH ratio had higher rates of false negative and false positive results using the newer normal ranges for LH, T, SHBG and FAI. It is strongly recommended that biochemistry laboratories establish normal ranges for these hormone parameters by only using patients with at least scan or surgically proven normal ovaries who are regularly ovulating. It is also important to collect blood samples when possible in the early follicular phase since LH, T, the FAI and androstenedione all undergo a significant mid-cycle rise and both LH and FSH are significantly depressed in the luteal phase.

It is is very easy to miss polycystic ovaries at laparoscopy, particularly if grasping forceps have not been used. The ovaries are usually covered by the Fallopian tubes and it is important, when inspecting the ovaries, to grasp the ovarian ligament and lift the ovary out of the pelvis to allow adequate inspection. With regard to ultrasound, high resolution ultrasound equipment is now widely available and relatively cheap. When training staff to recognize normal or polycystic ovaries it is prudent to intially refer surgically proven cases of either normal or polycystic ovaries to allow staff to gain experience. Vaginal ultrasound is of particular value since it permits the use of high frequency transducers and produces better quality images than is possible using the transabdominal route.

CLINICAL EVALUATION OF HIRSUTISM

The principals involved include:

1. Grade the severity of the hirsutism using a scoring system
2. Exclude serious, potentially life-threatening disease
3. Establish the main source(s) of the androgen excess.

A complete medical history is mandatory with particular attention being paid to the onset and speed of progression of symptoms, a drug history, menstrual irregularities and symptoms suggestive of virilization.

Examination should include a diligent search for abdomino-pelvic masses, signs of virilization (breast atrophy, temporal balding, clitoro-megaly) and the use of a grading system which is clinically useful as a quantitative measure of the success of therapy.

INVESTIGATION OF HIRSUTISM

Patients with mild excess body or facial hair and regular cycles can be treated without extensive investigation. They should be warned to return for reassessment if menses become irregular since androgenized women with severe oligomenorrhoea or amenorrhoea have an increased risk of endometrial hyperplasia and cancer (Siiteri 1987, Jafari et al 1978).

Patients with moderate to severe hirsutism or acne and those with oligo-amenorrhoea should all have at least a few investigations performed.

For the practical clinician, an estimation of plasma levels of T, DHEAS, 17 OH-P, thyroid function, prolactin, the gonadotrophins and perhaps SHBG is a useful start. An early follicular phase serum level of LH > 10 U/l, T > 2·5 nmol/l, SHBG < 35 nmol/l or a FAI > 4·5 strongly suggests a diagnosis of PCO (Eden 1989a, Eden et al 1989a, Adams et al 1986). Free T measurement may be a useful research tool but does not aid the clinician in his selection of therapy. The FAI may be calculated by using T and SHBG levels, as described previously. A serum T level > 6 nmol/l should prompt a search for a tumour or adrenal hyperplasia. An elevated DHEAS suggests an adrenal source of the androgens. If Cushing's syndrome is suspected, then a 24 hour urinary free cortisol or a short dexa-methasone suppression test should be ordered. A marginally elevated 17 OH-P level should be followed up by measuring 17 OH-P before and after ACTH stimulation. It was recently suggested that some patients with late onset hyperplasia may have normal basal levels of 17-hyperoxy-progesterone with the abnormality becoming apparent only after ACTH stimulation (McLaughlin et al 1990).

The virilized woman should have her adrenals and ovaries inspected with CT scanning and/or ultrasound. If an ovarian tumour is suspected then open laparotomy and ovarian bisection, if necessary, is preferable to laparoscopic biopsy which may miss a small tumour.

TREATMENT

The principles of therapy are simple:

1. Suppression of androgen excess
2. Antiandrogens to prevent new hair growth
3. Removal of unwanted hair
4. Weight control.

Suppression of androgen excess alone will *not* cure hirsutism, but must be coupled with an antiandrogen. A contraceptive pill, relatively high in oestrogen and avoiding androgenic progestagens (norethisterone and levonorgestrel) is ideal for ovarian suppression. Dianette (Schering) is useful in this respect as it contains a small amount of cyproterone acetate (CPA). As well as suppressing the ovarian androgen production, the oestrogen will stimulate SHBG production, further lowering free androgen levels.

If DHEAS is elevated then a small nocturnal dose of dexamethasone (0·25–0·5 mg) will control this. These doses rarely, if ever, produce Cushingoid side effects (McKenna 1988, Loughlin et al 1986). Some patients may require both a small dose of dexamethasone and a contraceptive pill to suppress their androgens.

Two antiandrogens have achieved popularity. Spironolactone, in doses of 100 to 200 mg is effective in reducing hirsutism used alone or with a contraceptive pill in 30–60% of cases (Coney 1984, Boiselle & Tremblay 1979, Cumming et al 1982). It is prudent to use this drug with a contraceptive pill because of the theoretical risk of feminizing a male fetus and because it can cause irregular menses. It blocks the androgen receptor, increases the metabolic clearance of T as well as decreasing T production (Coney 1984, Boiselle & Tremblay 1979, Cumming et al 1982, Serafini et al 1985, Helfer et al 1988). Side effects include a transient diuresis, menstrual irregularities and breast enlargement. Women taking the higher doses should have their electrolytes estimated at intervals because of the small risk of hyperkalaemia. There has been some concern, especially in the United Kingdom about a possible carcinogenic effect of Aldactone. A metabolite of Aldactone, canrenone, is theoretically convertible to potassium canrenoate, a carcinogenic substance. However, other sulphated metabolites of Aldactone prevent the production of these mutagenic substances (Cook et al 1988). Also there is no epidemiological evidence that use of Aldactone is associated with an increased cancer risk (Overdiek 1987).

The most effective currently available antiandrogen is cyproterone acetate (Androcur, Schering). It is a competitive inhibitor of DHT binding to its receptor, is a potent progestagen, a potent gonadotrophin inhibitor and has weak corticosteroid effects (Yen 1987b, Chapman et al 1982, Hammerstein et al 1975). Cyproterone has a long half-life and depot-effect and so most patients are given a 'reversed sequential' regime. Ethinyl oestradiol (EE) 30 to 50 mg is given for 21 days out of 28, adding 50–100 mg cyproterone for the first 10 days (Hammerstein et al 1975). As with all antiandrogens, patients should be warned about the theoretical risk of feminizing a male fetus, although taken correctly these treatments are highly contraceptive and by limiting the cyproterone to the first half of the cycle, the fetus should not be exposed to the drug. This theoretical problem may be more of a concern with Aldactone used alone, since it regulates the menstrual cycles of some oligomenorrhoeic women and probably enhances their fertility. It is this author's opinion that Aldactone should therefore generally be used with a contraceptive pill.

Weight control is essential for these women. Increasing obesity will further lower SHBG (and so elevating free T) and aggravate their problem. Obese oligomenorrhoeic women often find that weight loss is associated with a resumption of regular menses and pregnancy. BMI is a useful parameter, being weight (kg)/height (m²). Hirsute women should aim to keep their BMI around 21 kg/m².

Patients should be encouraged to continue with physical removal of the hair, shaving, waxing, bleaching and creams being useful. Properly performed electrolysis is the most satisfactory method of hair removal.

Patients generally require 6 to 12 months of antiandrogen treatment and most will find that the hair will eventually return without some maintenance therapy. Low dose cyproterone (5–10 mg) combined with EE 30–50 mg for 21 out of 28 days or Dianette being useful and contraceptive regimes. Triphasic pills, being relatively oestrogenic, may also be acceptable maintenance therapy. Low dose Aldactone (50 mg) combined with a contraceptive pill is another alternative. Many patients with an elevated serum level of DHEAS will only require 0·25 mg dexamethasone to control symptoms.

CONCLUSION

Hirsutism is a common clinical problem which causes great distress to the patient. Most patients have biochemical evidence of androgen excess. Potentially serious conditions such as Cushing's syndrome or androgen-secreting tumours must be considered but are fortunately rare. Most patients can be successfully treated by using ovarian or adrenal suppression combined with an antiandrogen.

REFERENCES

Adams J, Polson D W, Franks S 1986 Prevalence of polycystic ovaries in women with anovulation and idiopathic hirsutism. Br Med J 293: 355–359

Adashi E Y, Resnick C E, Hernandez E R et al 1988 Insulin-like Growth Factor 1 as an amplifier of follicle stimulating hormone: studies on mechanism(s) and site(s) of action in cultured rat granulosa cells. Endocrinology 122: 1583–1591

Anderson D C 1974 Sex-hormone binding globulin. Clin Endocrinol 3: 69–74

Barbieri R L, Smith S, Ryan K J 1988 The role of hyperinsulinemia in the pathogenesis of ovarian hyperandrogenism. Fertil Steril 50 (2): 197–212

Boiselle A, Tremblay R R 1979 New therapeutic approach to the hirsute patient. Fertil Steril 32 (3): 276–279

Bruno B, Fabbrini A 1985 Insulin resistance and secretion in polycystic ovarian disease. J Endocrinol Invest 8: 443–448

Burgen G A, Givens J R, Kitabchi A E 1980 Correlation of hyperandrogenism with hyperinsulinism in polycystic ovarian disease. J Clin Endocrinol Metab 50: 113–116

Carlstrom K, Gershagen S, Rannevik G 1987 Free testosterone and testosterone/SHBG index in hirsute women: a comparison of diagnostic accuracy. Gynecol Obstet Invest 24 (4): 256–261

Carter G D, Holland S M, Alaghband-Zadeh J, Rayman G, Dorrington-Ward P, Wise P H 1983 Investigation of hirsutism: testosterone is not enough. Ann Clin Biochem 20: 262–263

Chang R J, Nakamura R M, Judd H L, Kaplan S A 1983 Insulin resistance in nonobese patients with polycystic ovarian disease. J Clin Endocrinol Metab 57: 356–359

Chapman M G, Jeffcoate S L, Dewhurst C J 1982 Effect of cyproterone acetate-ethinyl oestradiol treatment on adrenal function in hirsute women. Clin Endocrinol 17: 577–582

Coney P 1984 Polycystic ovarian disease: current concepts of pathophysiology and therapy. Fertil Steril 42 (5): 667–682

Conway G S, Jacobs H S, Holly J M P, Biddlecombe R A, Wass J A H 1988 Insulin resistance and insulin-like growth factor small binding protein (IGF-SBP): comparison of lean and obese women with polycystic ovary syndrome (PCOS). J Endocrinol 119 (suppl): 60

Cook C S, Hauswald C L, Schoenhard G L et al 1988 Difference in metabolic profile of potassium canrenoate and spironolactone in the rat: mutagenic metabolites unique to potassium canrenoate. Arch Toxicol 61: 201–212

Cumming D C, Yang J C, Rebar R W, Yen S S 1982 Treatment of hirsutism with spironolactone. JAMA 247 (9): 1295–1298

Cunningham S K, Loughton T, Cullition M, McKenna T J 1985 The relationship between sex steroids and sex-hormone binding globulin in plasma in physiological and pathological conditions. Ann Clin Biochem 22: 489–496

Eden J A 1988 Which is the best test to detect the polycystic ovary? Aust NZ J Obstet Gynaecol 28: 221–224

Eden J A 1989a The polycystic ovary syndrome. Aust NZ J Obstet Gynaecol 29 (4): 403–416

Eden J A 1989b Two cases of partial 21 hydroxylase deficiency associated with progesterone excess. Aust NZ J Obstet Gynaecol 29: 268–270

Eden J A, Carter G D, Jones J, Alaghband-Zadeh J, Pawson M E 1988a Factors influencing the free androgen index in a group of subfertile women with normal ovaries. Ann Clin Biochem 25 (4): 350–353

Eden J A, Carter G D, Jones J, Alaghband-Zadeh J 1988b A comparison of follicular fluid levels of insulin-like growth factor 1 in normal dominant and cohort follicles, polycystic and multicystic ovaries. Clin Endocrinol 29: 327–336

Eden J A, Place J, Carter G D, Jones J, Alaghband-Zadeh J, Pawson M E 1989a The diagnosis of polycystic ovaries in subfertile women. Br J Obstet Gynaecol 96: 809–815

Eden J A, Carter G D, Jones J, Alaghband-Zadeh J 1989b Insulin-like growth factor 1 as an intra-ovarian hormone—an integrated hypothesis and review. Aust NZ J Obstet Gynaecol 29: 30–37

Eden J A, Jones J, Carter G D, Alaghband-Zadeh J 1989c The polycystic ovary contains higher follicular fluid concentrations of insulin-like growth factor 1 than matched normals. J Endocrinol 121 (suppl): 255

Eden J A, Place J, Carter G D, Alaghband-Zadeh J, Pawson M E 1989d The role of chronic anovulation in the polycystic ovary syndrome—normalisation of sex-hormone binding globulin levels after clomiphene induced ovulation. Clin Endocrinol 30: 323–332

Ferriman D, Gallway J D 1961 Clinical assessment of body hair in women. J Clin Endocrinol Metab 21: 1440–1447

Goldzieher J W, Green J A 1962 The polycystic ovary. I. Clinical and histological features. J Clin Endocrinol Metab 22: 325–338

Hague W M, Millar D R 1985 Excessive testosterone secretion in pregnancy. Case report. Br J Obstet Gynaecol 92: 173–178

Hammerstein J, Meckies J, Leo-Roseberg I, Moltz L, Zielske F 1975 Use of cyproterone acetate (CPA) in the treatment of acne, hirsutism and virilism. J Steroid Biochem 6: 827–836

Helfer E L, Miller J L, Rose L I 1988 Side-effects of spironolactone therapy in the hirsute woman. J Clin Endocrinol Metab 66 (1): 208–211

Hernandez E R, Resnick C E, Svoboda M E et al 1988 Somatomedin C/insulin like growth factor 1 as an enhancer of androgen biosynthesis by rat cultured ovarian cells. Endocrinology 122: 1603–1612

Hillier S G, Van Den Boogaard A M J, Reichert L E, Van Hall E V 1980 Intraovarian sex steroid hormone interactions and the regulation of follicular maturation: aromatization of androgens by human granulosa cells in vivo. J Clin Endocrinol Metab 50: 640–647

Homberg R, Amar N A, Eshel A, Adams J, Jacobs H S 1988 Influence of serum luteinising hormone concentrations on ovulation, conception, and early pregnancy loss in polycystic ovary syndrome. Br Med J 297: 1024–1026

Jafari K, Javaheri G, Ruiz G 1978 Endometrial adenocarcinoma and the Stein-Leventhal syndrome. Obstet Gynecol 51 (1): 97–100

Kim M H, Rosenfield R L, Hosseinian A H, Schneir H G 1979 Ovarian hyperandrogenism with normal and abnormal histological findings of the ovaries. Am J Obstet Gynecol 134: 445–452

Kirschner M A 1987 Hirsutism and virilism in women. In: Gold J J, Josimovich J B (eds) Gynecologic endocrinology, 4th edn. Plenum Medical, New York, pp 468–479

Kirschner M A, Jacobs J B 1971 Combined ovarian and adrenal vein catheterization to determine the site(s) of androgen overproduction in hirsute women. J Clin Endocrinol Metab 33: 199–209

Loughlin T, Cunningham S, Moore A, Culliton M, Smyth P P A, McKenna T J 1986 Adrenal abnormalities in polycystic ovary syndrome. J Clin Endocrinol Metab 62: 42–47

McKenna T J 1988 Pathogenesis and treatment of the polycystic ovary syndrome. N Engl J Med 318 (9): 558–562

McLaughlin B, Barrett P, Finch T, Devlin J G 1990 Late onset adrenal hyperplasia in a group of Irish females who presented with hirsutism, irregular menses and/or cystic acne. Clin Endocrinol 32: 57–64

Mason H D, Margara R, Winston R M L, Beard R W, Reed M J, Franks S 1990 Inhibition of oestradiol production by epidermal growth factor in human granulosa cells of normal and polycystic ovaries. Clin Endocrinol 33 (4): 511–518

Overdiek H 1987 The metabolism and biopharmaceutics of spironolactone in man. In: Drug Metab Drug Interactions 5 (4): 273–302

Pasquali R, Antenucci D, Casimirri F et al 1989 Clinical and hormonal characteristics of obese amenorrheic hyperandrogenic women before and after weight loss. J Clin Endocrinol Metab 68 (1): 173

Plymate S R, Fariss B L, Bassett M L, Matej L 1981 Obesity and its role in polycystic ovary syndrome. J Clin Endocrinol Metab 52: 1246–1248

Polson D W, Wadsworth J, Adams J, Franks S 1988 Polycystic ovaries—a common finding in normal women. Lancet ii: 870–872

Rosenfield R 1985 Congenital adrenal hyperplasia and reproductive function in females. In: Flamigni C, Venturoli S, Givens J R (eds) Adolescence in females. Chicago, pp 373–387

Sagle M, Bishop K, Ridley N et al 1988 Recurrent early miscarriage and polycystic ovaries. Br Med J 297: 1027–1028

Serafini P C, Catalino J, Lobo R A 1985 The effect of spironolactone on genital skin 5 alpha-reductase activity. J Steroid Biochem 23 (2): 191–194

Shoupe D, Kumar D D, Lobo R A 1983 Insulin resistance in the polycystic ovary syndrome. Am J Obstet Gynecol 147 (5): 588–592

Siiteri P K 1987 Adipose tissue as a source of hormones. Am J Clin Nutrition 45 (suppl): 277–282

Smith S, Ravnikar V A, Barbieri R L 1987 Androgen and insulin response to an oral glucose challenge in hyperandrogenic women. Fertil Steril 48 (1): 72–77

Speroff L, Glass R H, Kase N G 1989 In: Speroff L, Glass R H, Kase N (eds) Hirsutism 3rd edn. Williams and Wilkins, Baltimore, pp 583–609

Stein I F, Leventhal M L 1935 Amenorrhoea associated with bilateral polycystic ovaries. Am J Obstet Gynecol 29: 181–191

Tsang B K, Armstrong D T, Whitfield J F 1980 Steroid biosynthesis by isolated human follicular cells in vitro. J Clin Endocrinol Metab 51: 1407–1411

Wajchenberg B L, Achando S S, Okada H et al 1986 Determination of the source(s) of androgen overproduction in hirsutism associated with polycystic ovary syndrome by simultaneous adrenal and ovarian venous catheterization. Comparison with the dexamethasone suppression test. J Clin Endocrinol Metab 63 (5): 1204–1210

Weaver J U, Noonan K, Holly J M P, Wass J A, White N, Kopleman P G 1989 Decreased sex hormone binding globulin and insulin-like growth factor binding protein in obesity. J Endocrinol 121 (supplement): 254

Yen S S C 1980 The polycystic ovary syndrome. Clin Endocrinol 12: 177–208

Yen S S C 1987a The human menstrual cycle. In: Gold J J, Josimovich J B (eds) Gynecologic endocrinology. 4th edn. Plenum Medical, New York, pp 200–236

Yen S S C 1987b Chronic anovulation caused by peripheral endocrine disorders. In: Gold J J, Josimovich J B (eds) Gynecologic endocrinology. 4th edn. Plenum Medical, New York, pp 441–499

21. Medical treatment of menorrhagia

J. M. Higham

Menorrhagia is a benign yet debilitating condition. Excessive menstrual bleeding can cause considerable embarrassment and inconvenience; one does not have to take a history from many women with this complaint before realizing the problems it can generate. Lives may have to revolve around a menstrual calendar, with social and work commitments being cancelled during the menses. In addition to the difficulty in containing the blood flow, chronic anaemia may result if a woman's diet fails to compensate for her loss of iron.

Women of today may experience as many as nine times the number of menses in a lifetime as compared with their female ancestors (Short 1976). Factors contributing to this increase include the smaller family size (with consequent reduction in pregnancy and lactational amenorrhoea), the occurrence of an earlier menarche and later onset of the menopause. In addition, the changing role of women in society has resulted in many being employed outside the home, a place where episodes of flooding are even less tolerable. Consequently, the problem of menorrhagia is a very common one presenting to gynaecologists and one requiring adequate treatment with a minimum of adverse sequelae.

DEFINITION

Menorrhagia is objectively defined as a loss of 80 ml or more per period, derived from the findings of population studies (Hallberg et al 1966, Cole et al 1971). The incidence of anaemia significantly increases when losses exceed 80 ml. Most methods of measurement rely on a woman's ability to make a complete collection of all menstrual blood and therefore are likely to be minimal estimates. In addition, this blood volume is only part of total menstrual discharge, the percentage contribution of blood to this fluid varying from 2 to 82% (Fraser et al 1985).

Facilities to measure menstrual blood loss are not widely available, and consequently the diagnosis is made from the patient's history alone. This subjective diagnosis is unfortunately unreliable. The measured blood volume frequently bears little relation to that which would have been anticipated, given a convincing history (Chimbira et al 1980b, Haynes et al

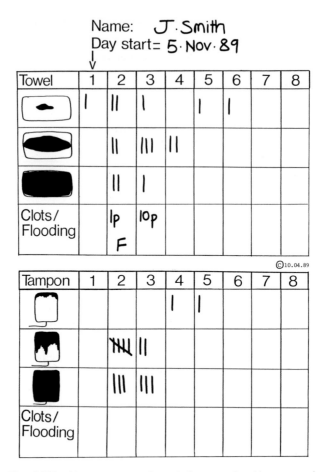

Fig. 21.1   Pictorial blood loss assessment chart. A chart completed by a menorrhagic patient, giving a score compatible with a menstrual blood loss in excess of 80 ml. (Reproduced with permission from Higham et al 1990.)

1977). This means that many women are given treatment for a condition from which they do not actually suffer. This highlights the importance of performing objective assessments of menstrual loss, especially as some women are reassured by the knowledge that their bleeding is normal, and would decline any unnecessary treatment. A recently developed pictorial chart, if reliably completed, may prove helpful in diagnosis and the monitoring of treatment (see Fig. 21.1, Higham et al 1990).

AETIOLOGY

Menorrhagia has been attributed to a number of different causes (see Table 21.1).

Table 21.1   Commonly quoted organic causes of menorrhagia

General	Thyroid dysfunction
	Coagulation disorder
Local	Fibroids
	Intra-uterine contraceptive devices
	Pelvic inflammatory disease
	Endometriosis
	Endometrial polyps
	Endometrial hyperplasia/carcinoma

Systemic conditions

Thyroid dysfunction appears in much of the literature concerning the aetiology of menorrhagia, but little published research exists to support this. A study of 15 women found to have 'mild' hypothyroidism stated that on administration of corrective thyroxine, the complaint of menorrhagia disappeared; blood loss however was not measured (Wilansky & Greisman 1989). When 50 hypothyroid women were questioned, abnormal menstrual patterns were present in 56%. Amongst these, menorrhagia was the most common complaint. One woman who had her loss measured was found to be losing 135 ml (Scott & Mussey 1964).

Data concerning the quantity of menstrual blood lost by women with coagulation disorders is also limited. A study where objective measurements were made on 15 women, found that some demonstrated menorrhagia of a most dramatic kind (losses of between 750 and 1000 ml). This however was not invariably the case; with blood loss in others being well within the normal range (Fraser et al 1986).

Local pathology

Fibroids are a common finding, and those of the sub-mucosal type in particular have been associated with menorrhagia. The blood loss of 18 women with fibroids was measured: 15 of them had recorded losses in excess of 80 ml. Furthermore, surgical removal of leiomyomata resulted in a dramatic reduction in menstrual blood loss (Fraser et al 1986).

Blood loss measurements in women with other pelvic pathology such as endometriosis, pelvic inflammatory disease and endometrial polyps were reported by Fraser in the same paper. The results varied and he concluded that these conditions were not always associated with excessive blood loss.

The insertion of an inert intra-uterine device has been shown to increase the measured menstrual blood volume (Guillebaud et al 1976), and is the most common iatrogenic cause of menorrhagia. Sterilization has previously been associated with the development of menorrhagia. In the short term at least, this has not been substantiated. A study which included four differing methods of tubal occlusion found no significant changes in the objectively quantified menstrual blood loss up to a year following the procedure (Sahwi et al 1989).

As so few women with either local or systemic abnormalities have been studied to date, further research in this area is overdue.

ASSESSMENT OF PATIENTS COMPLAINING OF MENORRHAGIA

Women presenting with the complaint of menorrhagia need to be evaluated by taking a comprehensive history, to include details of the quantity, rhythm and duration of bleeding. The method of contraception used should be noted and the possibility that symptoms could be due to an accident of pregnancy should not be forgotten. Both a general and gynaecological examination (to include cervical cytology) is required.

Investigation of menorrhagia should include a full blood count. Although this exhibits a negative correlation with increasing blood loss, it can be within the normal range with quite grossly excessive loss (see Fig. 21.2). Pelvic ultrasound, luteal phase progesterone and thyroid function studies are also often performed. The incidence of coagulation disorders has been found to be almost 20% in adolescents who required acute medical intervention to treat their menorrhagia (Claessens & Cowell 1981). Analysis of clotting ability is particularly recommended in such cases, but the detection of coagulation disorders in the adult population is small.

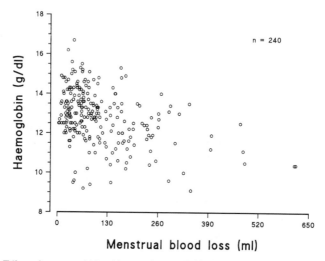

Fig. 21.2   Effect of menstrual blood loss on haemoglobin levels. The haemoglobin (g/dl) at presentation with menstrual blood loss (ml) (as estimated by the alkaline haematin technique, Hallberg & Nilsson 1964), found in 240 women attending the Royal Free Hospital Gynaecology Clinic. (Higham unpublished observations.)

Table 21.2   Drugs prescribed to treat menorrhagia

1. Non-steroidal anti-inflammatory drugs
2. Anti-fibrinolytics/haemostatics
3. Combined oral contraceptives
4. Danazol
5. Progestogens
6. LHRH analogue

It is necessary to perform an endometrial biopsy where there is any suspicion of abnormality such as hyperplasia or carcinoma. Often, this can be performed as an outpatient procedure, without the need for general anaesthetic (Grimes 1982). Hysteroscopy is a more useful investigation for the detection of polyps and submucous fibroids (Loffer 1989).

Where pathology which may be responsible for menorrhagia is identified, it should be treated in the appropriate medical or surgical manner. In more than half of patients however, no obvious abnormality is found either on examination or by routine investigation. In such instances, the bleeding has variously been described as dysfunctional in nature, or as menorrhagia that is unexplained, essential or primary. This chapter concerns the medical treatment of this group of women. Our understanding

Table 21.3   Some recognized potential side effects with medical treatment. *rarely occur; **Rydin & Lundberg (1976), Agnelli et al (1982)

Drug	Side effects
NSAIDs	Nausea, vomiting, gastric discomfort, diarrhoea, headache, dizziness, rashes, bronchospasm, *haemolytic anaemia, *thrombocytopenia
Tranexamic acid	Nausea, vomiting, diarrhoea, dizziness, *transient colour vision disturbance, ?intracranial thrombosis**
Ethamsylate	Headaches, rashes, nausea
Oral contraceptives	Headaches, migraine, weight gain, breast tenderness, nausea, cholestatic jaundice, hypertension, thrombotic episodes, *hepatomas
Danazol	Headaches, weight gain, acne, rashes, hirsutism, mood and voice changes, flushes, muscle spasm, reduced HDL cholesterol, diminished breast size, *cholestatic jaundice
Progestogens	Weight gain, nausea, bloating, oedema, headaches, acne, depression, exacerbation of epilepsy and migraine, loss of libido, ?lipid effects
LHRH analogues	Hot flushes, sweats, headaches, irritability, loss of libido, vaginal dryness, lethargy, reduced bone density

of the various mechanisms which control normal menstruation (being those which potentially could be defective in cases of menorrhagia) is increasing (for more details see Vol. 5 of 'Progress', Ch. 19, by S K Smith). It is likely, therefore, that an explanation as to the mechanism involved in at least some of these cases will eventually be elucidated.

MEDICAL TREATMENT OF UNEXPLAINED MENORRHAGIA

A number of drugs can be prescribed in an attempt to reduce excessive menstrual bleeding (Table 21.2). This list however, is not exhaustive. For example, the use of such agents as vitamin A, tamoxifen and a cotton plant derivative gossypol have been described. The drugs listed here do, however, comprise those most commonly employed in the treatment of menorrhagia. An assessment has been made of their potential benefits and possible side effects (summarized in Table 21.3). In addition, as a negative iron balance and consequent anaemia may be present, this should also be corrected.

Non-steroidal anti-inflammatory drugs (NSAIDs)

Much research in recent years has concentrated upon the potential role of prostaglandins and leukotrienes in menstruation (Smith et al 1981, Rees et al 1987). The ability of NSAIDs to reduce objectively measured blood loss was first reported by Anderson and colleagues using the most commonly prescribed NSAID for this purpose, mefenamic acid at a dosage of 500 mg three times daily (Anderson et al 1976). Since then, a variety of NSAIDs have been shown to reduce menstrual blood loss. They act mainly by inhibiting the cyclo-oxygenase enzyme system, which is a controlling step in the production of cyclic endoperoxides from arachidonic acid.

The fenamates (mefenamic acid, sodium meclofenamate) may have an additional effect, inhibiting the binding of the vasodilator prostaglandin E to its receptor in the myometrium (Rees et al 1988). These drugs are often prescribed as the drug of first choice in the treatment of menorrhagia, their efficacy having been evaluated in a number of controlled trials (see Table 21.4).

Unfortunately not all women respond to treatment with NSAIDs, and in some, blood loss remains unchanged or even increases. This variability in response is also demonstrated by the fact that some women experience a much greater than average reduction in blood loss (reductions of up to 80% have been reported). An improvement has been demonstrated in approximately 75% of women treated with NSAIDs. It is also noteworthy that although blood loss may be lessened by treatment, it may remain in the menorrhagic range. Treatment is unlikely to benefit women whose blood loss is normal, overall response being greater in women with excessive bleeding (Fraser et al 1981). Most studies concern themselves with

Table 21.4   The average % reduction in menstrual blood loss experienced by menorrhagic women when treated with a variety of NSAIDs. *Key:* MBL, menstrual blood loss; pre, pre-treatment value; on Rx, blood loss taking medication; n = no. of patients

Drug	n	Average % reduction MBL	Blood loss (ml) pre	on Rx	Ref
Mefenamic acid	5	37·3	107	67	Anderson et al (1976)
	22	44·5	137	76	Haynes et al (1980)
	35	47·0	—	—	Hall et al (1987)
	30	30·3	111	77	Fraser (1983)
	15	29·7	182	128	Muggeridge & Elder (1983)
	20	20·0	160	127	Dockeray et al (1989)
Naproxen	14	35·7	151	97	Ylikorkala & Pekonen (1986)
Naproxen sodium	35	46·0	—	—	Hall et al (1987)
Ibuprofen	13	24·7	146	110	Makarainen & Ylikorkala (1986)
Meclofenamate sodium	29	51·3	142	69	Vargyas et al (1987)

short-term efficacy, but the beneficial effects of mefenamic acid have been shown to persist when treatment is continued for over a year (Fraser et al 1983).

The NSAIDs may also reduce the dysmenorrhoea and headaches which can be an additional burden during menstruation (Fraser et al 1981, Dockeray et al 1989). They are taken only for the duration of the menses, which is preferable to daily medication for many patients, especially for those experiencing side effects. Treatment for menorrhagia may need to be continued for some considerable time, and this intermittent therapy also reduces prescribing costs.

Anti-fibrinolytics and haemostatics

The anti-fibrinolytic tranexamic acid is given in an attempt to lessen the excessive fibrinolytic activity found in the endometrium of women with heavy menstrual bleeding (Bonnar et al 1983). A study concerning 85 women treated with this drug found a mean reduction in blood loss of 54% (182 to 84 ml) (Nilsson & Rybo 1971). A dosage of 6 g was given daily for the first 3 days of bleeding and reduced thereafter, a minimum total dose of 22 g being given per period. More recently, another study described a reduction of similar magnitude (a mean of 295 ml lessened to 155 ml), in the treatment of 15 women (Andersch et al 1988). Both these reports originate from Sweden, where anti-fibrinolytic agents are more widely prescribed for menorrhagia. Treatment with tranexamic acid produces a slight depression of the fibrinolytic activity in peripheral blood, which may have contributed to the 3 cases of intracranial thrombosis reported in women taking this drug (see Table 21.3).

The potential of introducing anti-fibrinolytic medication directly into the uterine cavity by the means of an intra-uterine device has also been explored (Burns et al 1982).

The haemostatic agent ethamsylate is thought to help maintain capillary integrity, having anti-hyaluronidase activity and possibly an inhibitory effect on prostaglandins. There has been only one small objective study published to date, where patients were instructed to take 500 mg of ethamsylate 4 times daily, starting 5 days before the anticipated onset of menstruation, and continued for 10 days. A 50% reduction in volume was reported (125 ml to 67 ml) in 9 women (Harrison & Campbell 1976). More objective data to substantiate or refute this finding are needed.

Combined oral contraceptive pill

The combined oral contraceptive pill has claim to a variety of beneficial effects, other than being a highly reliable method of birth control (Mishell 1982). When taken in a cyclical fashion, it induces regular shedding of a thinner endometrium and inhibits ovulation. A study of 164 women demonstrated an overall reduction in mean blood loss of 53% when comparing withdrawal bleeds with menstruation (Nilsson & Rybo 1971). The 'pill' preparations used in this study of some 20 years ago employed greater quantities of hormone than are found in contemporary formulations. A controlled trial of these newer preparations is still awaited, but the beneficial effect on menstrual blood loss reported in 8 women would seem encouraging (Dockeray 1988).

Using this method good cycle control can be achieved and, together with the provision of contraception, makes this a most acceptable longer term remedy for some women with menorrhagia. The side effects of therapy restrict its use, especially in smokers, to the younger patient.

Danazol

This synthetic steroid with mild androgenic properties, is known to have a number of effects on the hypothalamic pituitary ovarian axis. Pulsatile gonadotrophin release and the mid-cycle gonadotrophin surge are altered and ovulation inhibited at higher doses (Wood et al 1975). At dosages of 600 mg daily, the endometrium rapidly becomes atrophic, although it is as yet uncertain exactly how danazol brings about a reduction in blood loss (Jeppsson et al 1984). The use of danazol in the treatment of menorrhagia was initially at a dosage of 400 mg daily given to 18 women for 12 weeks (Chimbira et al 1979). Danazol was highly effective, reducing blood loss from a pre-treatment mean of 231 ml to 135 ml, 21 ml and 3 ml in the successive 3 months following the commencement of therapy, amenorrhoea being common. A year later the same group looked at dosages of 200 mg and 100 mg daily (Chimbira et al 1980a) and compared this with the results previously found. The dosage of 200 mg daily was the most acceptable dosage, significantly reducing blood loss: a pretreatment mean of 183 ml was reduced to 38 ml and 26 ml in the second and third months of treatment respectively. In addition, these bleeding episodes tended to be regular which was preferred to both the more frequent menstruation at 100 mg and the amenorrhoea at 400 mg daily. Dysmenorrhoea was also reduced by treatment. Similar patterns of blood loss reduction, down to well within the normal range, have been reported by others (Fraser 1985, Dockeray et al 1989). In the more recent comparative study with mefenamic acid, Dockeray and colleagues found danazol effective (a 60% reduction in blood loss in comparison to a 20% one achieved by the NSAID) but commented that more unacceptable side effects were experienced by the danazol treated group.

Danazol would appear to have a carry-over effect, such that losses do not always return to pretreatment levels until some months following the cessation of therapy. This means that 3 months of relatively expensive therapy can have up to 6 months of beneficial effect.

Progestogens

Progestogens are compounds which can induce secretory change and cause withdrawal bleeding from an oestrogen primed endometrium (Greenblatt 1958). For the past 30 years, progestogens have been widely prescribed, often as the drug of first choice, for a variety of menstrual disorders including menorrhagia (Bishop & de Almeida 1960). Endocrine studies performed on women with proven menorrhagia were found to be similar to those in women with normal loss (Haynes et al 1979). A study of 81 women with no recent changes in menstrual frequency and aged between 40 and 55, found that 95% of them ovulated regularly (Metcalf 1979). The need for any luteal phase progestogen supplementation can thus be questioned in this group of patients.

Only in recent years have studies which included assessment of blood volume been made. A non-significant reduction in median blood loss from 131 to 110 ml was described, when norethisterone was given at a dosage of 5 mg twice daily from days 15–25 of the cycle to 8 ovulatory women (Cameron et al 1987). A similar dosage of the same drug given on days 19–26 of the cycle to 15 ovulatory women produced a median blood loss reduction of 109 ml to 92 ml (Cameron et al 1990). In spite of a diminished flow, 67% of the women remained menorrhagic. A more useful approach in the ovulatory patient may be prolonged cyclical regimens, such as prescribing for 3 weeks out of 4 (Fraser 1990). Progestogen therapy offers additional benefits which are likely to have contributed to their popularity.

They increase the predictability of the onset of bleeding (especially important if contingency plans need to be made in order to cope with menstruation), and also reduce premenstrual spotting.

Progestogens are useful if given to the anovulatory patient with irregular cycles to coordinate regular uterine shedding. We still await the results of clinical trials to see if total blood loss is lessened.

Medicated intra-uterine devices which release progesterone (Bergqvist & Rybo 1983) or levonorgestrel (Thiery et al 1989) have been shown to substantially reduce blood loss and in addition, are a reliable form of contraception. Often, some months after insertion, only irregular spotting of blood occurs. For this reason, counselling as to anticipated bleeding pattern will influence the patients' perception of treatment success. In comparison to orally administered progestogen, fewer side effects are anticipated owing to limited systemic drug absorption. This method may offer a safe long-term medical solution for menorrhagia.

LHRH analogues

Luteinizing hormone releasing hormone (LHRH) analogues are a recent addition to the therapeutic armamentarium, effectively suppressing pituitary ovarian function. An initial study using buserelin nasal spray in 4 women noted how it significantly reduced measured menstrual blood loss, 2 patients becoming amenorrhoeic by the third month of administration (Shaw & Fraser 1984). Depot LHRH preparations are now available, which consistently produce amenorrhoea, and hence are extremely effective in the temporary eradication of menorrhagia and dysmenorrhoea (Higham, Gardner & Shaw, unpublished observations). The effect of LHRH analogues on bone mineralization limits its long term use. Potentially, concurrent administration LHRH with a bone-sparing agent offers an additional (expensive!) therapeutic approach to menorrhagia.

RELATIVE COSTS OF PRESCRIBING

Treatment expenses vary considerably and will depend on the source and the amount of drug prescribed. If one considers the cost of 3 months of treatment, given to a woman that bleeds, on average, for 5 days per cycle, then the combined oral contraceptive, the NSAIDs and the progestogens are the most economic choice. Ethamsylate and tranexamic acid are more expensive, but still cost less than daily medication with danazol. LHRH preparations are the most costly form of treatment of those described here.

SURGICAL SOLUTIONS

Medical treatment can benefit many women with menorrhagia, and is preferred to surgery by a substantial proportion of patients. It may however only be partially successful, both in terms of the reduction in menstrual blood loss achieved and the side effects encountered. For those women who have completed their family, surgery in the form of either an endometrial ablative technique (see Ch. 22) or hysterectomy can provide a permanent and satisfactory cure.

CONCLUSION

A range of therapies are prescribed in an attempt to reduce excessive menstrual blood loss. Objective data has shown that, at least in the short term, a considerable reduction in the volume of the menses is achievable. The choice of drug depends upon its appropriateness and likely acceptability to an individual. Should the initial choice of therapy fail, prescription of one of the alternatives may prove successful. Menorrhagia, unfortunately however, is often a chronic condition, the problem of recurrence on stopping treatment being common to all the medical therapies. This means that medication frequently needs to be continued for years, and therefore the eradication or at least minimization of unacceptable side effects becomes vital.

REFERENCES

Agnelli G, Gresele P, De Cunto M, Gallai V, Nnenci G 1982 Tranexamic acid, IUCD and fatal cerebral arterial thrombosis (case report). Br J Obstet Gynaecol 89: 681–682

Andersch B, Milsom I, Rybo G 1988 An objective evaluation of flurbiprofen and tranexamic acid in the treatment of idiopathic menorrhagia. Acta Obstet Gynecol Scand 67: 645–648

Anderson A B, Haynes P J, Guillebaud J, Turnbull A C 1976 Reduction of menstrual blood-loss by prostaglandin-synthetase inhibitors. Lancet i: 774–776

Bergqvist A, Rybo G 1983 Treatment of menorrhagia with intrauterine release of progesterone. Br J Obstet Gynaecol 90: 255–258

Bishop P M F, de Almeida J C 1960 Treatment of functional menstrual disorders with norethisterone. Br Med J i: 1103–1105

Bonnar J, Sheppard B L, Dockeray C J 1983 The haemostatic system and dysfunctional uterine bleeding. Res Clin Forums 5(3): 27–36

Burns J W, Goodpasture J C, Friel P, Wheeler R, Zaneveld L J 1982 Development and evaluation of an inhibitor-releasing matrix for intrauterine devices. Contraception 26: 521–533

Cameron I T, Leask R, Kelly R W, Baird D T 1987 The effects of danazol, mefenamic acid, norethisterone and a progesterone-impregnated coil on endometrial prostaglandin concentrations in women with menorrhagia. Prostaglandins 34: 99–110

Cameron I T, Haining R H, Lumsden M A, Thomas V R, Smith S K 1990 The effects of mefenamic acid and norethisterone on measured menstrual blood loss. Obstet Gynecol 76: 85–88

Chimbira T H, Cope E, Anderson A B, Bolton F G 1979 The effect of danazol on menorrhagia, coagulation mechanisms, haematological indices and body weight. Br J Obstet Gynaecol 86: 46–50

Chimbira T H, Anderson A B, Naish C, Cope E, Turnbull A C 1980a Reduction of menstrual blood loss by danazol in unexplained menorrhagia: lack of effect of placebo. Br J Obstet Gynaecol 87: 1152–1158

Chimbira T H, Anderson A B, Turnbull A C 1980b Relation between measured menstrual blood loss and patient's subjective assessment of loss, duration of bleeding, number of sanitary towels used, uterine weight and endometrial surface area. Br J Obstet Gynaecol 87: 603–609

Claessens E A, Cowell C A 1981 Acute adolescent menorrhagia. Am J Obstet Gynecol 139: 277–280

Cole S K, Billewicz W Z, Thomson A M 1971 Sources of variation in menstrual blood loss. J Obstet Gynaecol Br Commwlth 78: 933–939

Dockeray C J 1988 The medical treatment of menorrhagia. In: Chamberlain G (ed) Contemporary obstetrics and gynaecology, Butterworths, London, pp 299–314

Dockeray C J, Sheppard B L, Bonnar J 1989 Comparison between mefenamic acid and danazol in the treatment of established menorrhagia. Br J Obstet Gynaecol 96: 840–844

Fraser I S 1983 The treatment of menorrhagia with mefenamic acid. Res Clin Forums 5 (3): 93–99

Fraser I S 1985 Treatment of dysfunctional uterine bleeding with danazol. Aust NZ J Obstet Gynaecol 25: 224–226

Fraser I S 1990 Treatment of dysfunctional uterine bleeding with oral, intramuscular or intrauterine progestogens. In: Shaw R W (ed) Advances in reproductive endocrinology 2: Dysfunctional uterine bleeding, Parthenon, Carnforth, Lancs, pp 139–148

Fraser I S, Pearse C, Shearman R P, Elliott P M, McIlveen J, Markham R 1981 Efficacy of mefenamic acid in patients with a complaint of menorrhagia. Obstet Gynecol 58: 543–551

Fraser I S, McCarron G, Markham R, Robinson M, Smyth E 1983 Long-term treatment of menorrhagia with mefenamic acid. Obstet Gynecol 61: 109–112

Fraser I S, McCarron G, Markham R, Resta T 1985 Blood and total fluid content of menstrual discharge. Obstet Gynecol 65: 194–198

Fraser I S, McCarron G, Markham R, Resta T, Watts A 1986 Measured menstrual blood loss in women with menorrhagia associated with pelvic disease or coagulation disorder. Obstet Gynecol 68: 630–633

Greenblatt R B 1958 A new clinical test for the efficacy of progesterone compounds. Am J Obstet Gynecol 76: 626–628

Grimes D A 1982 Diagnostic dilation and curettage: a re-appraisal. Am J Obstet Gynecol 142: 1–6

Guillebaud J, Bonnar J, Morehead J E, Matthews A 1976 Menstrual blood-loss with intrauterine devices. Lancet i: 387–390

Hall P, Maclachlan N, Thorn N, Nudd M W, Taylor C G, Garrioch D B 1987 Control of menorrhagia by the cyclo-oxygenase inhibitors naproxen sodium and mefenamic acid. Br J Obstet Gynaecol 94: 554–558

Hallberg L, Nilsson L 1964 Determination of menstrual blood loss. Scand J Clin Lab Invest 16: 244–248

Hallberg L, Hogdahl A M, Nilsson L, Rybo G 1966 Menstrual blood loss, a population study. Acta Obstet Gynecol Scand 45: 320–351

Harrison R F, Campbell S 1976 A double-blind trial of ethamsylate in the treatment of primary and intrauterine-device menorrhagia. Lancet ii: 283–285

Haynes P J, Hodgson H, Anderson A B, Turnbull A C 1977 Measurement of menstrual blood loss in patients complaining of menorrhagia. Br J Obstet Gynaecol 84: 763–768

Haynes P J, Anderson A B, Turnbull A C 1979 Patterns of menstrual blood loss in menorrhagia. Res Clin Forums 1 (2): 73–78

Haynes P J, Flint A P, Hodgson H, Anderson A B, Dray F, Turnbull A C 1980 Studies in menorrhagia: (a) mefenamic acid, (b) endometrial prostaglandin concentrations. Int J Gynaecol Obstet 17: 567–572

Higham J M, O'Brien P M S, Shaw R W 1990 Assessment of menstrual blood loss using a pictorial chart. Br J Obstet Gynaecol 97: 734–739

Jeppsson S, Mellquist P, Rannevik G 1984 Short-term effects of danazol on endometrial histology. Acta Obstet Gynecol Scand Suppl 123: 41–44

Loffer F D 1989 Hysteroscopy with selective endometrial sampling compared with D&C for abnormal uterine bleeding: the value of a negative hysteroscopic view. Obstet Gynecol 73: 16–20

Makarainen L, Ylikorkala O 1986 Primary and myoma-associated menorrhagia: role of prostaglandins and effects of ibuprofen. Br J Obstet Gynaecol 93: 974–978

Metcalf M G 1979 Incidence of ovulatory cycles in women approaching the menopause. J Biosoc Sci 11: 39–48

Mishell D R Jr 1982 Noncontraceptive health benefits of oral steroidal contraceptives. Am J Obstet Gynecol 142: 809–816

Muggeridge J, Elder M G 1983 Mefenamic acid in the treatment of menorrhagia. Res Clin
    Forums 5 (3): 83–88
Nilsson L, Rybo G 1971 Treatment of menorrhagia. Am J Obstet Gynecol 110: 713–720
Rees M C P, DiMarzo V, Tippins J R, Morris H R, Turnbull A C 1987 Leukotriene release
    by endometrium and myometrium throughout the menstrual cycle in dysmenorrhoea and
    menorrhagia. J Endocrinol 113: 291–295
Rees M C P, Canete-Soler R, Lopez Bernal A, Turnbull A C 1988 Effects of fenamates on
    prostaglandin E receptor binding. Lancet ii: 541–542
Rydin E, Lundberg P O 1976 Tranexamic acid and intracranial thrombosis. Lancet ii: 49
Sahwi S, Toppozada M, Kamel M, Anwar M Y, Ismail A A 1989 Changes in menstrual
    blood loss after four methods of female tubal sterilization. Contraception 40: 387–398
Scott J C, Mussey E 1964 Menstrual patterns of myxedema. Am J Obstet Gynecol 90:
    161–165
Shaw R W, Fraser H M 1984 Use of a superactive luteinizing hormone releasing hormone
    (LHRH) agonist in the treatment of menorrhagia. Br J Obstet Gynaecol 91: 913–916
Short R V 1976 The evolution of human reproduction. Proc R Soc Lond 195: 3–24
Smith S K, Abel M H, Kelly R W, Baird D T 1981 Prostaglandin synthesis in the
    endometrium of women with ovular dysfunctional uterine bleeding. Br J Obstet Gynaecol
    88: 434–442
Thiery M, Van der Pas H, Delbarge W, Van Kets H 1989 The levonorgestrel intrauterine
    device. Geburtshilfe Frauenheilkd 49: 186–188
Vargyas J M, Campeau J D, Mishell D R Jr 1987 Treatment of menorrhagia with
    meclofenamate sodium. Am J Obstet Gynecol 157: 944–950
Wilansky D L, Greisman B 1989 Early hypothyroidism in patients with menorrhagia. Am J
    Obstet Gynecol 160: 673–677
Wood G P, Wu C H, Flickinger G L, Mikhail G 1975 Hormonal changes associated with
    danazol therapy. Obstet Gynecol 45: 302–304
Ylikorkala O, Pekonen F 1986 Naproxen reduces idiopathic but not fibromyoma-induced
    menorrhagia. Obstet Gynecol 68: 10–12

22. Screening for ovarian cancer

A. Prys Davies   D. Oram

The concept of earlier diagnosis in epithelial ovarian cancer has become a real possibility during the last decade. Towards the end of the century, it may be possible to assess whether screening for epithelial ovarian cancer should be offered as a routine service, along the lines of cervical and breast cancer screening. The World Health Organization has established requirements for prospective screening programmes (Table 22.1) (Wilson & Junger 1968) and these recommendations form the basis of the report of the UK Co-ordinating Committee on Cancer Research on ovarian cancer screening (UKCCCR 1989). Ovarian cancer screening programmes are still in relative infancy and further research is needed to ensure that such programmes can fulfill these criteria prior to their widespread implementation.

There is general agreement that ovarian cancer poses an important health problem. In the UK, ovarian cancer is the fourth most common cancer causing death in females. In 1990 5000 women will be registered with the Cancer Registry as having ovarian cancer, and over 4000 women will die from the disease (OPCS 1983). The poor survival rate for women with epithelial ovarian cancer can be directly correlated with the stage distri-

Table 22.1 World health criteria for screening. Reproduced with permission from Scott et al 1990 and originally adapted from Wilson & Jungner (1968)

1. The condition should pose an important health problem.
2. The natural history of the disease should be well understood.
3. There should be a recognizable early stage.
4. Treatment of the disease at an early stage should be of greater benefit than treatment started at a later stage.
5. There should be a suitable test.
6. The test should be acceptable to the population.
7. There should be adequate facilities for the diagnosis and treatment of the abnormalities detected.
8. For disease of insidious onset, screening should be repeated at intervals determined by the natural history of the disease.
9. The chance of physical and psychological harm to those screened should be less than the chance of benefit.
10. The cost of the screening programme should be balanced against the benefit it provides.

Table 22.2 Five-year survival rates by stage at presentation for epithelial ovarian cancer. Reproduced from Kottmeier 1982

Stage	% Incidence	5-year survival (%)
Ia	17·9	69·7
Ib	4·3	63·9
Ic	3·0	50·3
Total for stage I	25·2	67·1
IIa	4·8	51·8
IIb + c	12·8	42·4
III	39·5	13·3
IV	17·7	4·1
Total for stages III and IV	57·2	10·4
Total for all stages	100·0	30·6

bution of the disease at presentation (Table 22.2). At diagnosis, the vast majority of women have advanced disease (Kottmeier 1982). Despite continuing improvements in surgical, chemotherapeutic and immunological techniques, which may give rise to longer periods of remission, the overall 5-year survival for women with epithelial ovarian cancer has altered little during the past 30 years. It is noteworthy, however, that the 5-year survival rates for women with properly staged, well-differentiated stage I (FIGO) epithelial ovarian tumours may be as high as 98%, with complete cure possible after surgery alone (Dembo et al 1990). Hence the rationale behind screening to detect early disease, ideally at stage Ia, when treatment is of greater benefit than treatment started at a later stage. There may also be other benefits—in terms of improved operability, length of remission—from diagnosing more advanced, stage II or III disease, earlier. These are more difficult to quantify, and would need to be balanced against the adverse side-effects of any adjuvant chemotherapy prescribed for women diagnosed with stage II or III disease.

The natural history of pre-clinical disease is less well documented. A pre-invasive condition—along the lines of cervical dysplasia or atypical endometrial hyperplasia—has not so far been identified. Uncertainty still remains over the malignant potential of benign ovarian cysts (Fox 1990). Methods of screening for ovarian cancer are therefore directed at detecting asymptomatic invasive disease. The duration of the quiescent but screen-detectable stage of ovarian cancer is unknown. Were this duration found to be short with rapid progression to advanced, symptomatic disease, the opportunity for screening and treatment to be effective would be too small for interval screening programmes to be of value (Fig. 22.1). However, it is likely that heterogeneity exists, and that whilst rapidly progressing ovarian

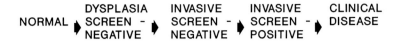

Fig. 22.1 Phases in tumourigenesis.

cancers will not lend themselves to traditional interval screening programmes other cancers, more slowly growing, which constitute the
majority, will do so. Data exist to support the hypothesis that certain
epithelial ovarian cancers may be detectable up to two years prior to their
clinical presentation (Jacobs & Oram 1990). It is probable that the inter-
screen interval of a programme would need to be of one to two years, but
this remains to be confirmed (Campbell et al 1989).

A screening test detects an abnormality that may—or may not—be
cancer. Histological examination of the suspicious ovary is necessary for the
definitive diagnosis, and using currently accepted procedures this requires
an operation under general anaesthesia. To minimize the number of women
undergoing an 'unnecessary' operation, it is important that a prospective
screening test is specific for ovarian cancer. It is unlikely that a test with a
positive predictive value of less than 10% (which would lead to no less than
10 surgical interventions per case of ovarian cancer diagnosed) would be
acceptable to either clinician, patient or state. Neither would it be in
keeping with the spirit of the WHO criteria for screening, i.e. that the
benefit to those screened should be greater than any physical or psychological harm that might arise as a result of screening.

The demand for high specificity is compounded by the relatively low
incidence of ovarian cancer in the general population. To illustrate:
screening 10 000 women (of all ages) using a test with 100% sensitivity and
99% specificity for early ovarian cancer would identify one case of ovarian
cancer—and 100 women with false positive results needing further
investigation (Smith & Ol 1984b). The positive predictive value of the same
test may be improved, without altering the test, by directing screening to
high-risk groups, where the incidence of disease is higher. With respect to
ovarian cancer, environmental (Muir & Mectoux 1978), genetic (Hildreth
et al 1981, Lynch et al 1981) and reproductive (Casagrande et al 1979,
Cramer et al 1982) risk factors have been identified. However these are not
of immediate practical value when selecting a high-risk group for a screening programme, e.g. familial cases of ovarian cancer account for only 3–5%
of all cases of the disease. Age is probably the most useful criterion for
selecting an at-risk population for ovarian cancer. The UK annual
incidence of ovarian cancer in women over 45 years is 4:10 000, and by
directing screening at women of this age, a test with 100% sensitivity would
require 99·6% specificity to achieve a positive predictive value of
10%.

There should be a suitable test

Methods of screening for ovarian cancer

Over the past 20 years or so, various techniques for detecting ovarian cancer have been explored (Smith & Ol 1984a).

Malignant ovarian cells have been detected on Papanicolaou smears. However only 10–30% of advanced cases of ovarian cancer are associated with such abnormalities, rendering cervical smears insufficiently sensitive as a method of screening for ovarian cancer (Shapiro & Nunez 1983). Peritoneal cytology is also of insufficient sensitivity and specificity for early ovarian cancer to be used as a screening test (Keetal et al 1974). Moreover the technique is prohibitively invasive. Although immunoscintigraphy (Epenetos et al 1982), CAT scans (Brenner et al 1983) and magnetic resonance imaging (MRI) (Powell et al 1987) may detect small-volume ovarian cancer and have been used in the detection and monitoring of established disease, their invasiveness and expense precludes their use as primary screening tests for the general population.

Methods currently being evaluated as screening tests include:

1. Bimanual pelvic examination
2. Ultrasound
3. Tumour markers.

Each will be considered in turn with reference to their suitability as a screening test in terms of sensitivity and specificity.

BIMANUAL PELVIC EXAMINATION

The main advantages of pelvic examination as a screening test for ovarian cancer are its relatively low cost, the ease with which it may be performed, and that it does not require specialized equipment. However, neither the specificity nor the sensitivity of pelvic examination for early ovarian cancer is known. A tumour volume of 1 cm³, which is probably the smallest mass detectable on clinical examination, contains about a billion cancer cells and may already be associated with widespread intra-abdominal seeding (Barber 1979).

The specificity of an abnormal pelvic examination for ovarian cancer is dependent on the woman's age and menstrual state. The diameters of a normal postmenopausal ovary are approximately $2 \times 1 \times 0\cdot5$ cm, rendering it impalpable on bimanual physical examination. Any ovary palpable in a woman more than 3–5 years after the menopause must be considered pathological, and an indication for prompt investigation. The management of an adnexal mass in the younger, menstruating woman is more complex as cystic enlargements are more common with a large differential diagnosis. Most cysts in this age group are functional or benign (Spanos 1973).

Studies evaluating bimanual physical examination and the detection of ovarian cancer are few, and their significance for screening a healthy population unclear. Reeves et al (1980) compared pelvic examination with preoperative ultrasound in 72 women undergoing laparotomy for a pelvic mass. They found that there was no significant difference in the accuracy of ultrasound over pelvic examination in the detection, estimation of size or determination of bilateral position of the pelvic mass. However, ultrasound was significantly more accurate in determining the solid or cystic nature of the mass—a feature which is considered important for differentiating benign from malignant disease pre-operatively. Four of the women in the study had ovarian cancer, although the stage of the disease was not stated. Thus, although the Reeves paper credits pelvic examination with accuracy of location of a pelvic mass, the ability of pelvic examination to distinguish benign from malignant disease, and the sensitivity of detection in the general population remain unresolved.

Andolf et al (1986) performed both a bimanual examination and a trans-abdominal pelvic ultrasound scan on 805 women between 40 and 70 years of age attending a gynaecology outpatients clinic. The person performing the scan was unaware of the findings on physical examination, and in some instances up to 12 weeks had lapsed between the examination and the scan. In 12 cases the bimanual examination was considered abnormal, whilst 83 women had an abnormal first scan. (Ten had abnormalities detected on both examinations.) Thirty-nine women underwent surgical exploration, including eight in whom the physical examination was considered to be abnormal. These eight cases were associated with benign ovarian pathologies. The bimanual examination of two women diagnosed as having borderline ovarian cancer (maximum diameters of 6 cm and 4 cm respectively) and one woman found to have invasive ovarian cancer (stage III) had been passed as normal or as not suspicious of malignancy. The conclusion drawn by Andolf was that ultrasound was superior to bimanual pelvic examination for the detection of ovarian cancer.

In an earlier population-based study involving 1319 women aged 30–80 years, MacFarlane et al (1955) discovered only six ovarian cancers having performed 18 753 routine pelvic examinations over a 14-year period.

In summary, bimanual physical examination is probably neither sufficiently sensitive nor specific for asymptomatic ovarian cancer. However, the ease with which it may be performed, and integrated into the cervical cytology programme, means that it is currently the most widely practised method of screening for ovarian cancer and certainly remains the most frequent way in which established ovarian cancer is diagnosed.

ULTRASOUND

Throughout the 1970s and 1980s improvements in ultrasound technology and scanning skills have meant that visualizing ovaries has become possible.

The feasibility of screening for ovarian cancer using this technique has therefore been explored.

Ultrasound features of ovarian malignancy

The ultrasound findings indicative of ovarian cancer have been described and include semi-solid, semi-cystic masses with thick septa and surface papillary growths, bilateral lesions and ascites (Moyle et al 1983, Herrmann et al 1987). Using the above characteristics as indicators of malignancy, DeLand et al (1979) correctly identified 13 of 14 women with ovarian cancer out of a total of 60 women with an adnexal mass undergoing a preoperative ultrasound scan. More than 70% of lesions with complex or solid patterns were malignant, although the stage of the cancer was not recorded. However, the above characteristics are not exclusive to malignant ovarian disease. A study by Herrmann et al (1987) of 404 women with suspicious pelvic masses or histories suggestive of ovarian cancer showed that up to 58% of benign ovarian tumours presented with some solid element. Tumour or papillary growth on the outer ovarian surface, described in almost half the cases of carcinoma, were also found in approximately 10% of benign ovarian adenomas (Beck et al 1988). Ascites and matted bowel loops are usually associated with advanced disease—and may be the only ultrasound findings suggestive of ovarian cancer (Herrmann et al 1987).

Ovarian volume

Ultrasound features of early ovarian cancer may be more difficult to detect—and are still being defined. The view of Timor-Tritsh et al (1988) that 'if the ovaries are visualized in the postmenopausal patient ... a work up of the case is advisable' may still be the guideline for some gynaecologists. However, the ovaries of postmenopausal women are being visualized increasingly frequently and other definitions of abnormality have been compiled, e.g. based on ovarian size. Moyle et al (1983) gave $2 \times 1.5 \times 0.5$ cm as the maximum diameters of the normal postmenopausal ovary as measured by trans-abdominal ultrasonography.

The pelvic findings of 31 postmenopausal women undergoing a trans-abdominal ultrasound examination were reported by Campbell et al in 1982. Both ovaries were identified in 26 patients, and the calculated ovarian volumes ranged from 1.47 to 10.43 ml (mean 4.33 ml). The ovarian sizes were confirmed at subsequent laparotomy. They also found that an ovary with a volume more than twice that of the overall mean and also more than twice that of its pair should be regarded with some suspicion. Later, having calculated the ovarian volumes of 2221 women, the King's College Hospital group (Goswamy et al 1988) produced a nomogram of mean ovarian

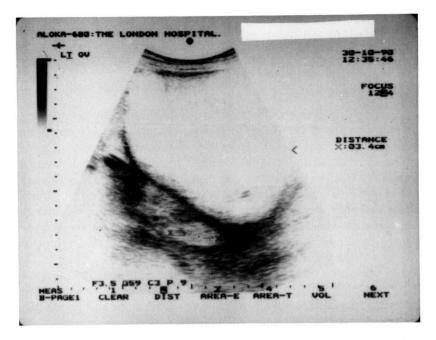

Fig. 22.2   Ultrasound and ovarian cancer. Trans-abdominal ultrasonography for assessing ovarian volume and morphology.

volume according to years since menopause. It was concluded that a woman with a mean ovarian volume above the 99·5th centile should be considered at risk of having ovarian cancer, and subject to further investigation (Fig. 22.2). In addition to the length of menopause, they also found that a woman's weight, parity, age at menopause, history of taking hormone replacement therapy or of previously diagnosed breast cancer could influence the ovarian volume. These factors should therefore be taken into consideration when using ovarian volume as an indicator of potential ovarian disease.

Other features of a normal postmenopausal ovary include uniform echogenicity, an ovoid shape and a smooth echogenic outline (Goswamy et al 1988).

Ultrasound for the early detection of ovarian carcinoma

Women attending gynaecology outpatient departments or admitted for assessment of an adnexal mass have formed the subjects of many of the earlier studies on the detection of ovarian pathology using ultrasound. In the Andolf study of physical and ultrasound pelvic examinations previously mentioned, the subjects were 805 women between 40 and 70 years of age attending an outpatients clinic (Andolf et al 1986). The scan findings were considered adequate for analysis:

1. If both ovaries could be identified, or
2. If the ovarian vessels were normal, or
3. If 'nothing pathological could be seen in their vicinity'.

Aspects of this definition of a 'normal ovarian scan' may be considered inadequate as the diagnosis of normality rests on exclusion rather than positive identification. Results from 795 women were analysed. The first scan was considered abnormal in 85 cases (10·3%), but in 33 of these, the abnormality had resolved by a second scan. Thirty-nine of the 50 women with an abnormal repeat ultrasound scan underwent surgical exploration. In four cases the operative findings were normal. Abnormalities included one ovarian carcinoma, two ovarian carcinomas of borderline malignancy and one cancer of the caecum. Other pathologies included serous and mucinous cystadenomas, a dermoid cyst, endometriosis, fibroids. The positive predictive value of a single abnormal scan for ovarian cancer was 1·2%, increasing to 2% with a repeat scan. Including the cases of borderline malignancy, the positive predictive values of single and paired ultrasound examinations for malignant ovarian disease increased to 3·6% and 6% respectively.

Using healthy self-selected volunteers (aged 18–78 years, mean age 52) as subjects, Campbell et al (1989) also reported a low positive predictive value of an abnormal scan for primary ovarian cancer. Countrywide advertisements for volunteers (ideally over 45 years) to undergo three annual screening tests for ovarian cancer using trans-abdominal ultrasonography produced 5479 participants. Ovarian features considered to be abnormal included an irregular outline, hypo- or hyper-echogenicity or a volume >20 ml. Women found to have such an abnormality either underwent a repeat scan after 6 weeks or were referred directly for surgical exploration. Seventy-seven per cent of the volunteers completed the three screening tests, giving a total of 15 977 scans. Abnormal ultrasound findings indicating the need for surgical exploration were detected in 326 of the volunteers (5·6%). These included five patients with primary ovarian cancer (two stage Ia borderline, one stage Ib borderline and two stage Ia) giving a positive predictive value for primary ovarian cancer of 1·5%. Four other patients at laparotomy had metastatic ovarian cancer. Interestingly no advanced primary ovarian cancer was detected in the course of the prevalence screen.

Other pathologies at operation included benign ovarian cysts, endometrioid cysts, and sex-cord stromal and germ cell tumours. Even though these volunteers did not have cancer, they may have benefited from undergoing surgery before the potential development of complications necessitating emergency laparotomy. However, in the case of 29% of the volunteers who underwent surgery either no abnormality was detected or the mass was not ovarian in origin, or the surgeon did not consider the ovarian mass to be malignant, requiring no further treatment or investigation. It is not apparent, apart from peace of mind, what benefit these volunteers gained from undergoing surgery.

Sensitivity of ultrasound for ovarian cancer

It appears that ultrasonography is very sensitive for the detection of asymptomatic, early ovarian cancer—a detection rate of 100% (within the confines of the study) has been cited by the authors of the King's College Hospital study.

In this study a very high proportion of ovaries were visualized (98–99%). This ability to identify postmenopausal ovaries on ultrasound examination has not been universal. Fleischer (1988) reported being able to identify only 20% of 'normal' postmenopausal ovaries on examining 30 patients awaiting hysterectomy and bilateral salpingo-oophorectomy for endometrial cancer. Further studies are therefore needed, in other ultrasound centres, to confirm the sensitivity—and indeed specificity—of ultrasound for early ovarian cancer.

Improving the positive predictive value of ultrasound

In order to decrease the number of 'unnecessary' laparotomies (i.e. to enhance the odds ratio for primary ovarian cancer at operation of 1:65), methods of improving the specificity of ultrasound for ovarian cancer are being considered. One such method may be to confine screening to high-risk groups, e.g. to postmenopausal women where the incidence of malignant disease is higher and the incidence of 'physiological' pathologies lower. Of the volunteers in the above study, 45·1% were premenopausal and a further 12·1% artificially postmenopausal.

Using the same study population, Campbell et al (1990) have calculated an improved odds ratio (1:50) for primary ovarian cancer by considering temporal changes in ovarian volume in addition to the absolute ovarian volume.

Trans-vaginal ultrasonography

Since the mid-1980s, with technical advances in instrumentation and imaging, trans-vaginal ultrasonography has gained in popularity. The advantages of this approach are two-fold:

1.   The ultrasound transducer is closer to the objects of interest and not separated from them by layers of fat and muscle. The pelvic organs can therefore be studied with higher ultrasound frequencies, producing images of greater resolution and enhanced quality.
2.   The need for a full bladder is obviated.

On the other hand there are some disadvantages to trans-vaginal ultra-sonography. It is more invasive and postmenopausal vaginal atrophy may limit access and patient acceptability. The ultrasound frequencies used improve resolution, but decrease penetration to 10 cm. Thus ovaries situated high or lateral in the pelvis, or greatly enlarged so that they are no longer in the pelvis, may not be seen on scan. Co-incident abdominal palpation or bimanual pelvic examination (or a trans-abdominal scan) should ensure that such ovaries are detected (Timor-Tritsh et al 1988).

Studies are currently being undertaken to evaluate trans-vaginal ultrasound as a means of screening for ovarian cancer. Such studies will need to assess whether the increased resolution leads to reliable identification of postmenopausal ovaries (Fleischer 1988) and the changes associated with early ovarian cancer.

Doppler

Whilst ultrasound imaging has provided a non-invasive method of studying ovarian morphology, pulsed Doppler combined with real-time ultrasound (the duplex method) has the potential to examine patterns of blood flow and hence of identifying functional changes. The duplex technique has been used to track changes in ovarian artery blood flow during the menstrual cycle (Taylor et al 1985). The artery supplying the ovary containing the dominant follicle or corpus luteum shows a lower pulsatility index (PI)—which reflects vascular impedance—than its pair, implying increased blood flow.

Tumours are also associated with changes in vascularization. In animal experiments, pulsed Doppler has been used to identify tumours on finding high-peak velocities, increased mean velocities and a low pulsatility index in supplying vessels (Rubin et al 1987).

It has recently become possible to obtain colour Doppler signals using a trans-vaginal probe. Colour combined with pulsed Doppler has been used to investigate the pelvic circulation under various physiological and patho-logical conditions (Kurjak et al 1989). Changes in vascularity (which may be an indication of malignancy) can be identified as fluctuating areas of colour. Applying pulsed Doppler to these areas gives a measurement of blood flow and impedance. Two studies have shown that ovarian cancers may be distinguished from benign adenomas using this technique (Kurjak et al 1989, Bourne et al 1989). The intra-ovarian pulsatility index in all 5 women with ovarian cancer in the Yugoslav study and 7 of the 8 women in the King's College Hospital study was significantly lower than in women with benign ovarian pathology.

It is probable that the techniques of pulsed and colour Doppler will play an increasingly important role in the differential diagnosis of a pelvic mass, and will serve to improve the specificity of ultrasound for ovarian cancer. It is yet to be shown that their use as a secondary test, having found a pelvic abnormality in a postmenopausal woman participating in an ovarian cancer screening programme, will lead to a significant decrease in the surgical intervention rate. Many gynaecologists—and patients themselves—may feel uneasy leaving an ovarian mass or cyst in a postmenopausal woman. Flow studies may however modify the type of surgery employed and indeed the place of surgery, with women considered to have malignant disease being referred to a gynaecologist with an interest in oncology. Although currently controversial, trans-vaginal or trans-abdominal cyst aspiration with cytological examination of the cyst fluid may prove to be an alternative method of managing women found to have an ovarian cyst considered to be benign (on its ultrasonographic and flow-study appearance, and serum tumour marker expression) (DeCrespigny et al 1989, Diernaes et al 1987).

TUMOUR MARKERS

Quantitative and qualitative changes in numerous circulating substances have been associated with epithelial ovarian cancer. These may reflect an alteration in ovarian function or surface molecular structure, or a 'general' response to malignancy (Smith & Ol 1984b, Bast & Knapp 1987).

Changes in circulating enzymes (van Kley et al 1981, Awais 1978, Gauduchon et al 1983, Cramer et al 1989), hormones (Heinonen et al 1982, Backstrom et al 1983), non-specific inflammatory proteins (Lukomska et al 1981), placental and fetal antigens (Donaldson et al 1980, Nouwen et al 1985, Doellgast & Homesley 1984) have all been identified in women with ovarian cancer (Fig. 22.3). Apart from the association of alpha-feto protein (AFP) with germ cell ovarian cancer (especially endodermal sinus and embryonal tumours) (Gallion et al 1983) and human chorionic gonado-trophin (beta HCG) with choriocarcinoma (Bagshawe 1976), these markers have not shown sufficient sensitivity or specificity for early epithelial ovarian cancer to be of value as screening tests (Oram & Jacobs 1987).

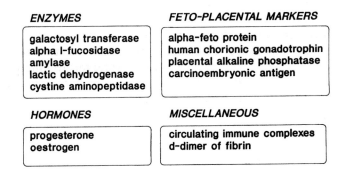

ENZYMES

galactosyl transferase
alpha l-fucosidase
amylase
lactic dehydrogenase
cystine aminopeptidase

FETO-PLACENTAL MARKERS

alpha-feto protein
human chorionic gonadotrophin
placental alkaline phosphatase
carcinoembryonic antigen

HORMONES

progesterone
oestrogen

MISCELLANEOUS

circulating immune complexes
d-dimer of fibrin

Fig. 22.3   Serum markers for ovarian cancer.

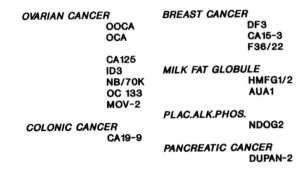

Fig. 22.4 Antigens associated with ovarian cancer.

Monoclonal antibodies

Advances in monoclonal antibody techniques have resulted in the improved definition of antigens expressed on the malignant cell surface (Old 1981). Antigens expressed by ovarian cancers may enter the circulation by one of two routes; either via the lymphatics or vessels supplying the ovarian stroma, or through the diaphragmatic lymphatics having been shed from the ovarian surface into the peritoneal cavity (Bast et al 1990). The anatomical position of the ovaries may therefore mean that quantification of shed tumour antigens in serum would form an effective way of detecting and monitoring malignant disease.

To date, the antigens defined on malignant ovarian epithelial cells have been tumour-associated rather than tumour-specific. Antigen expression may therefore be a feature of other tissues or pathologies, thus lowering specificity for ovarian cancer (Fig. 22.4). Amongst the first ovarian cancer antigens to be detected in serum (using rabbit polyclonal hetero-antiserum) were OCC and OCA (Bhattacharya & Barlow 1973, 1978, Knauf & Urbach 1980). They reported serum OCA levels to be raised in 70% of women with stage I and II epithelial ovarian cancer. As raised serum OCA levels are also detected in 10% of healthy women the positive predictive value of an abnormal test would be prohibitively low for serum OCA to be used as a screening test in the general population.

Using monoclonal antibody techniques, antigens with improved specificity and sensitivity for epithelial ovarian cancer have been defined— though the ultimate tumour-specific antigen remains elusive. The most extensively studied ovarian tumour-associated antigen is CA 125 (Bast et al 1983).

CA 125

CA 125, a high molecular-weight glycoprotein, is recognized by a murine monoclonal antibody, OC 125 (Bast et al 1983). Immunohistochemical studies have demonstrated CA 125 expression to be a feature of cells derived from the embryonal coelomic epithelium and Mullerian duct (Kabawat et al 1983), and both benign and malignant pathologies affecting tissues with these embryological origins have been associated with increased CA 125 expression (Niloff et al 1984). Neither the normal fetal nor adult ovary expresses CA 125. However, serum CA 125 levels measured by radioimmunoassay are greater than 35 U/ml in over 80% of women with epithelial ovarian cancer (especially of the non-mucinous types) (Bast et al 1983, Hawkins et al 1989). Bast et al have also shown that only 1% of healthy female blood donors have serum CA 125 levels of > 35 U/ml.

A population-based, retrospective study—The JANUS study—showed that it was possible, in a proportion of cases, to detect raised serum CA 125 levels months (even years) prior to the clinical diagnosis of ovarian cancer (Zurawski et al 1988). Study subjects comprised women who had agreed to undergo repeat venepuncture, and the serum was frozen and stored. Ovarian cancer was later diagnosed in 105 women. The stored sera from these women were assayed for CA 125 quantification, and the levels compared with those detected in serum from 323 apparently healthy matched controls. Although cases had a higher median serum CA 125 concentration than controls (18 U/ml *cf* 10 U/ml), this is probably of little practical significance. However, serum CA 125 levels of > 35 U/ml were measured in 50% of cases within 18 months of diagnosis, and a third of cases had serum CA 125 levels > 65 U/ml within 18 months of diagnosis. This has been confirmed by prospective studies of screening for ovarian cancer using serum CA 125.

CA 125 and screening for ovarian cancer

In view of the high specificity demanded of a prospective ovarian cancer screening programme and the association of CA 125 with pathologies other than ovarian cancer, the positive predictive value of a single raised serum CA 125 level for the disease would be too low for serum CA 125, in isolation, to be acceptable as a screening method. Methods of improving the specificity of a screening programme incorporating serum CA 125 estimation are therefore being investigated.

Improving specificity

CA 125 and ultrasound.   At The Royal London Hospital, a multimodal or stepwise screening programme for ovarian cancer has been in operation since 1985 (Jacobs et al 1988). The study population consists of apparently healthy, postmenopausal women of 45 years or above, recruited through advertisements in 'women's magazines' or by general practitioners located throughout the UK who recognized eligible women through their age–sex registers. On recruitment, all women underwent venepuncture. Women

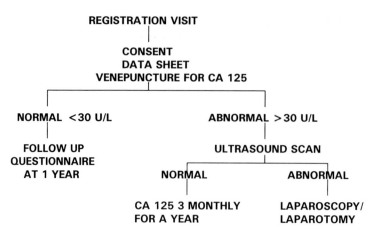

Fig. 22.5   Study design.

with a serum CA 125 level of greater than 30 U/ml were recalled for a pelvic examination and ultrasound scan. (In the first years of the study the ultrasound scans were performed trans-abdominally, latterly the trans-vaginal route has also been employed.) Participants found to have a per-sistent pelvic abnormality on ultrasound were further investigated by laparoscopy or laparotomy. Women with normal ultrasound findings were monitored by three-monthly serum CA 125 levels for the remainder of the year. All women were contacted 12 months following recruitment with a questionnaire enquiring into the occurrence of any illnesses during the year (Fig. 22.5).

   To date almost 23 000 women have been recruited into the screening programme but as not all of the women have completed a year since recruitment the results are incomplete. Nevertheless interim data indicates that a combination of a raised serum CA 125 level and abnormalities on a pelvic ultrasound examination is highly specific for ovarian cancer (Table 22.3) (Jacobs & Oram 1990). A review of the first 20 000 women screened shows that approximately 1–2% of participants were found to

Table 22.3   Specificity for ovarian cancer of vaginal examination, CA 125 and ultrasound. The London Hospital ovarian cancer screening project in post menopausal women. $n = 4000$. (Reproduced with permission from Jacobs & Oram 1990)

Test	Specificity (%)
CA 125	97·0
Vaginal examination	97·3
Vaginal examination and ultrasound	99·0
CA 125 and ultrasound	99·8
CA 125 and vaginal examination	100·0
CA 125, vaginal examination and ultrasound	100·0

Table 22.4 Study results (incomplete one year follow up)

Screen negative				Screen positive
CA 125 < 30 u/l				CA 125 > 30 u/l
				Abnormal USS
$n = 19\,719$				$n = 22$
3 False negatives:				11 True positives
Stage	Histology	CA 125	Interval	11 False positives
III	Granulosa	10	8/12	CA 125 > 30 ul
III	Serous	22	13/12	Normal USS
III	Clear cell	85	6/12	$n = 259$

have an elevated serum CA 125 level and were recalled for an ultrasound scan. This is in keeping with the distribution of CA 125 in healthy female blood donors as described by Bast et al (1983). For 22 women the ultrasound scan was also abnormal, indicating the need for operative intervention. At laparotomy, eleven were diagnosed as having ovarian cancer whilst the others were found to have various benign pathologies, giving an odds-ratio for ovarian cancer at laparotomy of 1:2 (Table 22.4).

CA 125 and other tumour markers. The use of a panel of monoclonal antibodies directed against a spectrum of tumour-associated antigens is also being reviewed as a method of improving the specificity of serum CA 125 for ovarian cancer. These antigens may be different epitopes on the same complex or totally separate antigens.

At Duke University Medical Centre, USA, Bast et al (1990) looked for CA 125, CA 15-3, TAG 72, PLAP, HMFG1, HMFG2 and NB/70K expression in serum from patients with known ovarian cancer and from women with a 'false positive' elevation of CA 125. His findings indicate CA 15-3 and TAG 72 to be the more useful antigens for differentiating benign from malignant disease. Serum levels of all three antigens were elevated in 77% of women with ovarian cancer compared with only 5% of women with benign disease. The improved specificity for ovarian cancer using the combination of serum CA 125, CA 15-3 and TAG 72 has been confirmed by others. Einhorn et al (1989) found 98% specificity for malignancy when serum levels of all three antigens were raised, compared with 83% for CA 125 used as a single test.

A highly specific ovarian cancer screening programme may therefore be achieved by using a panel of antigens as an initial test, and investigating further only those women with raised serum levels of multiple antigens. The increase in specificity using such a method may however occur at the expense of sensitivity, for ultimately the overall sensitivity of the screening programme would be dependent upon the sensitivity of the least sensitive marker. A fall in sensitivity for ovarian cancer to 53% has been documented using a combination of serum CA 125, CA 15-3 and TAG 72 (Jacobs et al 1991).

CA 125—sensitivity of a screening programme

The sensitivity of CA 125 for detecting early ovarian cancer has been questioned. A meta-analysis of studies of preoperative serum CA 125 levels in women undergoing laparotomy to investigate a pelvic mass confirms that over 80% of women with ovarian cancer have elevated levels (Table 22.5); however, analysis by stage shows a skewed distribution, with elevated serum CA 125 levels being detected in 90% of women with stage II, III and IV disease, but in only 50% of women with stage I ovarian cancer. Although with a disease as fatal as ovarian cancer, improvements in mortality figures may well be achieved by detecting just 50% of cases with disease confined to the ovaries, it is possible that this degree of sensitivity would not be acceptable to women with false-negative results, who feel that they have been misleadingly reassured. It is also highly probable that this degree of sensitivity would adversely affect the cost–benefit analysis of the screening programme. While maximum improvement in mortality from ovarian cancer would be achieved by detecting all cases at stage Ia, improvements in quality of life may still result from diagnosing more advanced disease earlier. For example, at one end of the spectrum of FIGO

Table 22.5   The proportion of women with ovarian cancer with an elevated pre-operative serum CA 125 level in relation to FIGO stage (* = upper limit 25 u/ml, remaining studies 35 u/ml; # = not included in total as this was a study of stage I and II disease). (Reproduced with permission from Jacobs & Oram 1990)

Author	FIGO stage				
	I	II	III	IV	Total
Bast et al (1983)	1/1	2/2	15/16	3/3	21/22
Brioschi et al (1987)	4/13	3/3	29/30	22/23	58/69
Canney et al (1984)	—	—	—	—	48/58
Crombach & Wurtz (1984)	3/5	5/6	13/19	10/10	31/40
Cruickshank et al (1987)	3/12	2/3	15/16	10/10	31/42
Fuith et al (1987)	4/6	4/5	16/18	8/10	32/39
Heinonen et al (1985)	0/3	←9/9 stages II–IV→			9/12
Kaesemann et al (1986)	←31/46→		←135/153→		166/199
Kivinen et al (1986)	3/3	10/10	15/15	1/1	29/29
Krebs et al (1986)	3/4	8/8	25/25	7/8	43/45
Li-juan et al (1986)	1/2	3/3	22/23	—	26/28
Ricolleau et al (1985)	—	—	—	—	35/38
Schilthuis et al (1987)	6/8	5/5	20/20	13/13	44/46
Zanaboni et al (1987)	8/15	3/4	29/34	3/4	43/57
Zurawaski et al (1988b)	12/24	10/12	—	—	#
Total	48/96	55/61	199/216	77/82	615/723
%	50·0	90·0	92·1	93·9	85·1

stage III disease are women with cancer grossly limited to the true pelvis but with isolated foci of cancer in the omentum or a solitary lymph node metastasis. This is in contrast to women classified as having stage IIIc ovarian cancer who have massive and diffuse disease. The prognosis for women with small volume stage III disease is better than that for women in the latter category (taking into account tumour grade). Further follow-up studies are needed to investigate potential benefits that may result following the earlier diagnosis by screening (e.g. smaller volume disease, improved operability, longer period of remission).

An assessment of the sensitivity of serum CA 125 as part of a screening programme for ovarian cancer may be obtained from The Royal London Hospital study. At the 20 000 women screened review, the 12-month following recruitment questionnaire had been returned by almost all participants contacted. To date, this has identified three other women with ovarian cancer—false negatives (see Table 22.4). One of them had a granulosa cell tumour—tumours that are not normally associated with CA 125 expression. In a second case, a serous adenocarcinoma of the ovary was diagnosed 8 months following the detection of an elevated serum CA 125, the patient having declined an ultrasound scan. The apparent sensitivity of the programme for ovarian cancer is therefore 78%. With longer follow up, the sensitivity will probably fall as more screen negative women are diagnosed as having ovarian cancer.

A screening programme may also be evaluated in terms of the number of interval cancers prevented. In a year, 8 cases of ovarian cancer would be expected in 20 000 postmenopausal women. Referring to The Royal London Hospital study (20 000 women screened), three cases of ovarian cancer were diagnosed in the year following screening, i.e. interval cancers. The screening programme had therefore decreased the expected number of interval cancers by 60%.

Analysis of the stage distribution of the cancers detected by the screening programme (Table 22.6) shows that approximately 63% of women had stage III or IV disease at diagnosis. A follow-up re-screening study is in progress to assess whether, having eliminated the prevalent cancers, interval or incidence screening will alter the stage distribution and the extent of disease at diagnosis.

Table 22.6 Stage at diagnosis. The London Hospital study

FIGO stage	No.
I	3
II	1
III	5
IV	2

Methods of improving the sensitivity of a screening programme are also being assessed.

Improving sensitivity

CA 125 and other tumour markers. As a panel of tumour-associated antigens may improve the specificity of serum CA 125 for ovarian cancer, a combination of other markers, directed at different epitopes, may improve sensitivity. Serum CA 125 and NB/70K (Knauf et al 1985) together achieve a higher sensitivity for ovarian cancer than either when used as single tests. Other antibodies that have been shown to improve the detection rate in conjunction with CA 125 include MOV 2 (Miotti et al 1985), DF 3 (Sekine et al 1985), PLAP (Dhokia et al 1986, Ward et al 1987a) and HMFG 2 (Dhokia et al 1986, Ward et al 1987a, b). However, the improvement in sensitivity may occur at the expense of specificity.

Temporal changes in serum CA 125 levels. Serial measurements of serum CA 125 are also under evaluation as a method of improving the detection rate while preserving specificity. Progressive elevations with rapid doubling of the serum CA 125 level have been associated with a subsequent diagnosis of ovarian cancer (Zurawski et al 1990). In a case report, a woman with a raised serum CA 125 level was subject to intensive clinical follow up, including pelvic examination and ultrasonography (which were considered normal) and repeat serum CA 125 assays. Twenty one months following the initial raised serum CA 125 level and normal scan, and 15 months after the first measured doubling in CA 125, ovarian cancer was diagnosed (stage III). The value of progressively elevating serum CA 125 levels in the identification of women with ovarian cancer is under review at The Royal London Hospital, where similar cases have been reported (Fig. 22.6).

Future developments in tumour markers

New ovarian cancer-associated antigens are being identified, which may have importance for screening. It has been suggested that antigens of low molecular-weight (e.g. alpha-feto protein) may have greater relevance for screening than antigens of higher molecular-weight, as their detection in serum may occur at an earlier stage of tumourigenesis as a consequence of improved permeability across cellular basement membranes (Duffy 1989).

ONCOGENES, PROTO-ONCOGENES AND GROWTH REGULATORY FACTORS

Recent research has led to an improved understanding of the fundamental abnormalities of cancer cells; the molecular pathways leading to

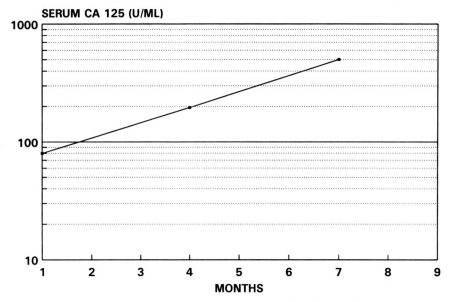

SERUM CA 125 (U/ML)

MONTHS

Fig. 22.6 Progressively elevating serum CA 125 prior to diagnosing ovarian cancer.

carcinogenesis and the promoters of abnormal cell growth. It is now accepted that specific genes are involved in the regulation of cell division and differentiation. The aberrant expression of these genes (oncogenes and proto-oncogenes) is thought to be responsible for the uncontrolled growth which characterizes cancer cells. Oncogenes may be 'switched on' to produce cancers (Chan & Sikora 1987) either by:

1. Transduction by viruses
2. Chromosome translocations
3. Gene amplification
4. Gene mutation.

Studies of oncogenes in ovarian epithelial tumours have shown variable qualitative and quantitative alterations in *c-fos*, *c-myc*, *n-myc*, *v-fms*, *c-Ha-ras* and *c-erb* expression, but not of *l-myc*, *c-myb*, *c-erbB* or *c-mos* expression (Tyson et al 1988). Oncogene amplification and rearrangements may be identified using specific gene probes on DNA and RNA taken from tissue specimens.

The effector molecules of oncogenes are their protein products (oncoproteins) which may be released into the circulation. The detection of serum oncoproteins, e.g. using monoclonal antibodies, may prove to be a method of detecting and monitoring cancer. To illustrate, *c-myc*—which may have a role in controlling cell division and differentiation—is amplified in a proportion of ovarian cancers. *c-myc* expression has also been associated with a serum protein of 40 000 dalton molecular weight, p40 (Chan &

Sikora 1987). Further research is needed to establish the clinical relevance of serum p40 levels, *c-myc* expression and the detection and monitoring of ovarian cancer.

Another oncogene that may be expressed by epithelial ovarian cancer cells is *c-fms*, which has been shown to share many features of macrophage colony stimulating factor (M-CSF). M-CSF may stimulate the proliferation of macrophages and endothelial cells and it has been suggested that *c-fms* expression may be important for the regulation of growth of ovarian cancer. *C-fms* and M-CSF may have potential as markers for the disease—either alone or in association with serum CA 125 (Bast et al 1990). Although Xu et al (1991) demonstrated increased M-CSF in 57% of women with clinical ovarian cancer its value as a potential marker for asymptomatic ovarian cancer has yet to be assessed. Other growth factors that may be implicated in tumour initiation and growth include transforming growth factors -alpha and -beta (TGF-alpha, TGF-beta) (Yeh & Yeh 1989). TGF-alpha has been shown to be a structural and functional analogue of epidermal growth factor (EGF). By binding to EGF receptors, TGF-alpha may trigger a signal for cell proliferation.

The HER-2/*neu* oncogene encodes a cell surface glycoprotein that is similar in structure to the epidermal growth factor receptor itself (Berchuck et al 1990). It has been postulated that the HER-2/*neu* gene product may function as a receptor for some as yet unidentified growth factor. Using immunohistochemical techniques involving a monoclonal antibody reactive with HER-2/*neu*, 32% of epithelial ovarian cancers tested showed over-expression of HER-2/*neu* compared with normal ovarian tissue (Berchuck et al 1990). Patients whose tumours had a high HER-2/*neu* expression were found to have a worse prognosis than those with 'normal' levels, and were less likely to have a complete response to primary therapy or have a negative second-look laparotomy when preoperative serum CA 125 levels were normal. The significance of this oncogene with respect to screening remains as yet unexplored.

The study of tumour-specific allelic loss may have particular importance for screening or identifying those at risk of developing cancer in hereditary ovarian cancer families. A possible consequence of the allelic loss may be the loss of a growth regulatory gene (proto-oncogene), which in turn would lead to uncontrolled cell division and differentiation—i.e. cancer. In ovarian cancers, allelic loss has been variously described on chromosone 1, 6q, 11p and 17p (Lee et al 1990). More work however is needed to identify a consistent allelic loss (or losses) that may be a marker for a predisposition for ovarian cancer and hence may be of value in screening for susceptible individuals in ovarian cancer prone families.

CONCLUSION

Ovarian cancer screening programmes, using ultrasound and tumour markers, are currently being developed. To date, the most specific and sensitive programme involves the combining of methods in a step-wise manner. However, none of the current screening programmes has an adequate follow-up period or a sufficient number of women screened for an evaluation of the benefits that might accrue from screening to be made. The adverse effects—anxiety, further investigation, potential risks from surgery—must also be part of the cost–benefit evaluation. A large, population-based, randomized controlled study of a suitable screening programme is needed to make an assessment of benefit and harm—as was the recommendation of the report of the UKCCCR (1989). As mortality rates from ovarian cancer are roughly a third those of breast cancer, the randomized trials of ovarian screening would need to be three times as large if the same degree of effect were to be detected.

The financial implications of screening for ovarian cancer have not been addressed in this chapter. It is highly unlikely, with the low incidence of the disease, that such screening will be cost-effective. Decisions pertaining to such cost implications will be evaluated by health-planners and the public. Nevertheless, there is a broad consensus that, in the absence of effective treatment for established disease, the quest for early diagnosis is of vital importance. In spite of the aforementioned obstacles to screening, and a not insignificant amount of clinical scepticism, the direction of future research should be to emulate, and indeed to improve upon, the success of screening programmes for other lethal tumours.

ACKNOWLEDGEMENT

Ann Prys Davies is funded by a grant from Birthright.

REFERENCES

Andolf E, Svalenius E, Astedt B 1986 Ultrasonography for early detection of ovarian carcinoma. Br J Obstet Gynaecol 93: 1286–1289

Awais G M 1978 Carcinoma of the ovary and serum lactic dehydrogenase levels. Surg Gynecol Obstet 146: 893–895

Backstrom T, Mahlck C G, Kjellgren O 1983 Progesterone as a possible tumour marker for 'nonendocrine' ovarian malignant tumours. Gynecol Oncol 16: 129–138

Bagshawe K D 1976 Risk and prognostic factors in trophoblastic neoplasia. Cancer 38: 1373–1385

Barber H R K 1979 Ovarian Cancer, Part 1. Cancer J Clinicians 29: 341

Bast R C, Knapp R C 1987 Humoral markers for epithelial ovarian carcinoma. In: Piver (ed) Ovarian malignancies. Churchill Livingstone, Edinburgh, pp 11–25

Bast R C, Klug T L, St John E et al 1983 A radioimmunoassay using a monoclonal antibody to monitor the course of epithelial ovarian cancer. N Engl J Med 309: 883–887

Bast R C, Boyer C M, Olt G J et al 1990 Identification of markers for early detection of epithelial ovarian cancer. In: Sharp F, Mason W P, Leake R E (eds) Ovarian cancer: biological and therapeutic challenges. Chapman & Hall, London, pp 265–275

Beck D, Deutsch M, Bronshtein M 1988 The ovary. In: Timor-Tritsch I E, Rottem S (eds) Transvaginal sonography. Heinemann Medical, London, pp 59–86

Berchuck A, Kamel A, Whitaker R et al 1990 Overexpression of HER-2/*neu* is associated with poor survival in advanced epithelial ovarian cancer. Cancer Res 50: 4087–4091

Bhattacharya M, Barlow J J 1973 Immunologic studies of human serous cystadenocarcinoma of the ovary. Demonstration of tumor-associated antigens. Cancer 31: 588–595

Bhattacharya M, Barlow J J 1978 Ovarian tumor antigens. Cancer 42: 1616–1620

Bourne T, Campbell S, Steer C, Whitehead M I, Collins W P 1989 Transvaginal colour flow imaging: a possible new screening technique for ovarian cancer. Br Med J 299: 1367–1370

Brenner D E, Grosh W W, Jones H W 1983 An evaluation of the accuracy of computed tomography in patients with ovarian carcinoma prior to second look laparotomy. ASCO Proceedings 2: 149

Brioschi P A, Irion O, Bischoff P, Bader M, Forni M, Krauer F 1987 Serum CA 125 in epithelial ovarian cancer. A longitudinal study. Br J Obstet Gynaecol 94: 196–201

Campbell S, Goessens L, Goswamy R, Whitehead M 1982 Real-time ultrasonography for determination of ovarian morphology and volume. Lancet i: 425–426

Campbell S, Bhan V, Royston P, Whitehead M I, Collins W 1989 Transabdominal ultrasound screening for early ovarian cancer. Br Med J 299: 1363–1367

Campbell S, Royston P, Bhan V, Whitehead M I, Collins W P 1990 Novel screening strategies for early ovarian cancer by transabdominal ultrasonography. Br J Obstet Gynaecol 97: 304–311

Canney P A, Moore M, Wilkinson P M, James R D 1984 Ovarian cancer antigen CA 125: a prospective clinical assessment of its role as a tumour marker. Br J Cancer 50: 765–769

Casagrande J T, Louie E W, Pike M C, Roy S, Ross R K, Henderson B E 1979 'Incessant ovulation' and ovarian cancer. Lancet ii: 166–172

Chan S, Sikora K 1987 The potential of oncogene products as tumour markers. Cancer Surveys 6: 185–207

Cramer D W, Hutchison G B, Welch W R, Scully R E, Knapp R C 1982 Factors affecting the association of oral contraceptives and ovarian cancer. N Engl J Med 307: 1047–1051

Cramer D W, Harlow B L, Willet W C et al 1989 Galactose consumption and metabolism in relation to the risk of ovarian cancer. Lancet i: 66–71

Crombach G, Wurz H 1984 CA 125 & PA & CEA in ovarian cancer—a critical evaluation of single and contained determinants of serum markers. In: Getean H, Klapdor R (eds) New tumour-associated antigens. George Viene Verland, Stuttgart, p. 134

Cruickshank D J, Fullerton W T, Klopper A 1987 The clinical significance of preoperative serum CA 125 in ovarian cancer. Br J Obstet Gynaecol 94: 692–695

DeCrespigny L C L, Robinson H P, Davoren R A M, Fortune D 1989 The 'simple' ovarian cyst: aspirate or operate? Br J Obstet Gynaecol 96: 1035–1039

DeLand M, Fried A, van Nagell J R, Donaldson E S 1979 Ultrasonography in the diagnosis of tumors of the ovary. Surg Gynecol Obstet 148: 346–348

Dembo A J, Davy M, Stenwig A E, Berle E J, Bush R S, Kjorstad K 1990 Prognostic factors in patients with stage I epithelial ovarian cancer. Obstet Gynecol 75: 263–273

Dhokia B, Canney P A, Pectasides D, Munro A J, Moore M, Wilkinson P M, Self C, Epenetos A A 1986 A new immunoassay using monoclonal antibodies HMFG1 and HMFG2 together with an existing marker CA 125 for the serological detection and management of epithelial ovarian cancer. Br J Cancer 54: 891–895

Diernaes E, Rasmussen J, Soerensen T, Hasch E 1987 Ovarian cysts: management by puncture? Lancet i: 1084

Doellgast G J, Homesley H D 1984 Placental-type alkaline phosphatase in ovarian cancer fluids and tissues. Obstet Gynecol 63: 324–329

Donaldson E S, van Nagell J R, Pursell S, Gay E C, Meeker W R, Kashmiri R, van de Voorde J 1980 Multiple biochemical markers in patients with gynecologic malignances. Cancer 45: 948–953

Duffy M J 1989 New cancer markers. Ann Clin Biochem 26: 379–387

Einhorn N, Knapp R C, Bast R C, Zurawski V R 1989 CA 125 assay used in conjunction with CA 15-3 and TAG-72 assays for discrimination between malignant and non-malignant diseases of the ovary. Acta Oncol 28: 655–657

Epenetos A A, Britton K E, Mather S, Shepherd J, Granowska M, Taylor-Papadimitriou J 1982 Targeting of iodine-123-labelled tumour-associated monoclonal antibodies to ovarian, breast and gastrointestinal tumours. Lancet ii: 999–1005

Fleischer A C 1988 Transvaginal sonography helps find ovarian cancer. Diagn Imaging 10: 124–128

Fox H 1990 The pathology of early malignant change. In: Sharpe F, Mason W P, Leake R E (eds) Ovarian cancer: biological and therapeutic challenges. Chapman and Hall, London, pp. 165–167

Fuith L C, Daxenbichler G, Dapunt O 1987 CA 125 in the serum and tissue of patients with gynaecological disease. Arch Gynecol Obstet 241: 157–164

Gallion H, van Nagell J R, Donaldson E S 1983 Immature teratoma of the ovary. Am J Obstet Gynecol 146: 361–365

Gauduchon C, Tillier C, Guyonnet C, Heron J-F, Bar-Guilloux E, Le Talaer J Y 1983 Clinical value of serum glycoprotein galactosyltransferase levels in different histological types of ovarian carcinoma. Cancer Res 43: 4491–4496

Goswamy R K, Campbell S, Roystone J P et al 1988 Ovarian size in postmenopausal women. Br J Obstet Gynaecol 95: 795–801

Hawkins R E, Roberts K, Wiltshaw E, Munday J, McCready V R 1989 The clinical correlates of serum CA 125 in 169 patients with epithelial ovarian carcinoma. Br J Cancer 60: 634–637

Heinonen P K, Tuimala R, Pyykkok K, Pystynen P 1982 Peripheral venous concentrations of oestrogens in postmenopausal women with ovarian cancer. Br J Obstet Gynaecol 89: 84–86

Heinonen P K, Tontti K, Koivula T, Pystynen P 1985 Tumour associated antigen CA 125 in patients with ovarian cancer. Br J Obstet Gynaecol 92: 528–531

Herrmann U J, Locher G W, Goldhirsch A 1987 Sonographic patterns of ovarian tumours. Prediction of malignancy. Obstet Gynecol 69: 777–781

Hildreth N G, Kelsey J L, LiVolsi V A et al 1981 An epidemiologic study of epithelial carcinoma of the ovary. Am J Epidemiol 114: 398–405

Jacobs I, Oram D 1990 Potential screening tests for ovarian cancer. In: Sharpe F, Mason W P, Leake R E (eds) Ovarian cancer: biological and therapeutic challenges. Chapman and Hall, London, pp. 197–205

Jacobs I, Stabile I, Bridges J, Kemsley P, Reynolds C, Grudzinskas J, Oram D 1988 Multimodal approach to screening for ovarian cancer. Lancet i: 268–271

Jacobs I, Oram D, Bast R C 1991 Approaches to improve the specificity of screening for ovarian cancer with tumour-associated antigens CA 125, CA 15-3, TAG-72. (in prep)

Kabawat S E, Bast R C, Welch W R, Knapp R C, Calvin R B 1983 Immunopathologic characterization of a monoclonal antibody that recognizes common surface antigens of human ovarian tumours of serous, endometrioid and clear cell types. Am J Clin Pathol 79: 98–104

Kaesemann H, Caffier H, Hoffmann F J et al 1986 Monoklonale Antikorper in diagnostik und verlaufskontrolle de ovarialkarzinomas. CA 125 als tumormarker. Klin Wochenschr 64: 781–785

Keetel W C, Pixley E E, Buchsbaum H J 1974 Experience with peritoneal cytology in the management of gynecologic malignancies. Am J Obstet Gynecol 120: 174–182

Kivinen S, Kuoppala T, Leppilampi M, Vuori J, Kauppila A 1986 Tumor-associated antigen CA 125 before and during the treatment of ovarian carcinoma. Obstet Gynecol 67: 468–472

Knauf S, Urbach G I 1980 A study of ovarian cancer patients using a radioimmunoassay for human ovarian-associated antigen OCA. Am J Obstet Gynecol 138: 1222–1223

Knauf S, Anderson D J, Knapp R C, Bast R C 1985 A study of the NB/70K and CA 125 monoclonal antibody radioimmunoassays for measuring serum antigen levels in ovarian cancer patients. Am J Obstet Gynecol 152: 911–913

Kottmeier H (ed) 1982 Annual report on the results of treatment in gynaecological cancer 18. FIGO, Stockholm

Krebs H B, Goplerud D R, Kilpatrick S J, Myers M B, Hunt H 1986 Role of CA 125 as tumour marker in ovarian carcinoma. Obstet Gynecol 67: 473–477

Kurjak A, Zalud I, Jurkovic D, Alfirevic Z, Miljan M 1989 Transvaginal color doppler for the assessment of pelvic circulation. Acta Obstet Gynecol Scand 68: 131–135

Lee J H, Kavanagh J J, Wildrick D M, Wharton J T, Blick M 1990 Frequent loss of heterozygosity on chromosomes 6q, 11 and 17 in human ovarian carcinomas. Cancer Res 50: 2724–2728

Li-juan L, Xiu-feng H, Wen-shu L, Ai-ju W 1986 A monoclonal antibody radioimmunoassay for an antigenic determinant CA 125 in ovarian cancer patients. Clin Med J 99: 721–726

Lukomska B, Olszewski W L, Engeset A 1981 Acute phase reactive proteins and complement components and inhibitors in patients with ovarian cancer. Gynecol Oncol 11: 288–298

Lynch H T, Albano W, Black L, Lynch J F et al 1981 Familial excess of cancer of the ovary and other anatomic sites. JAMA 245: 261–264

MacFarlane C, Sturgis M C, Fetterman F S 1955 Results of experiment in control of cancer of female pelvic organs and report of 15 year research. Am J Obstet Gynecol 69: 294–298

Miotti S, Aguanno S, Canevari S, Diotti A et al 1985 Biochemical analysis of human ovarian cancer-associated antigens defined by murine monoclonal antibodies. Cancer Res 45: 826–832

Moyle J W, Rochester D, Sider L, Shrock K, Krause P 1983 Sonography of ovarian tumors: predictability of tumour type. Am J Radiol 141: 985–991

Muir C S, Mectoux J 1978 Ovarian cancer: some epidemiological features. World Health Statistics 31: 51

Niloff J M, Knapp R C, Schaetzl E, Reynolds C, Bast R C 1984 CA 125 antigen levels in obstetric and gynecologic patients. Obstet Gynecol 64: 703–707

Nouwen W J, Pollet D E, Schelstraete J B et al 1985 Human placental alkaline phosphatase in benign and malignant ovarian neoplasia. Cancer Res 45: 892–902

Old L J 1981 Cancer immunology: the search for specificity. Cancer Res 41: 361–375

OPCS 1983 Registrations. Cases of diagnosed cancer registered in England and Wales. HMSO, London

Oram D, Jacobs I 1987 Improving the prognosis in ovarian cancer. In: Studd J (ed) Progress in obstetrics and gynaecology. Churchill Livingstone, Edinburgh, pp. 399–432

Powell M C, Worthington B S, Symonds E M 1987 The application of magnetic resonance imaging (MRI) to ovarian carcinoma. In: Sharp F, Soutter W P (eds) Ovarian cancer—the way ahead. Royal College of Obstetricians and Gynaecologists, London, pp. 141–158

Reeves D, Drake T S, O'Brian I F 1980 Ultrasonographic versus clinical evaluation of a pelvic mass. Obstet Gynecol 55: 551–554

Ricolleau G, Chatal J F, Fumoleau P et al 1985 Radioimmunoassay of the CA 125 antigen of ovarian carcinomas: advantages compared with CA 19-9 and CEA. Tumour Biol 5: 151–159

Rubin J M, Carson P L, Zlotecki R A, Ensminger W D 1987 Visualization of tumor vascularity in a rabbit VX2 carcinoma by Doppler flow mapping. J Ultrasound Med 6: 113–120

Schilthuis M S, Aalders J G, Bouma J et al 1987 Serum CA 125 levels in epithelial ovarian cancer: relation with findings at second-look operations and their role in the detection of tumour recurrence. Br J Obstet Gynaecol 94: 202–207

Scott I V, Milford Ward A, Selby C, Whitehead S, Wilcox M 1990 Development of population based studies of ovarian cancer screening. In: Sharpe F, Mason W P, Leake R E (eds) Ovarian cancer: biological and therapeutic challenges. Chapman & Hall, London, p 245

Sekine H, Hayes D F, Ohno T et al 1985 Circulating DF3 and CA 125 antigen levels in serum from patients with epithelial ovarian carcinoma. J Clin Oncol 3: 1355–1363

Shapiro S P, Nunez C 1983 Psammoma bodies in the cervicovaginal smear in association with a papillary tumour of the peritoneum. Obstet Gynecol 61: 130–134

Smith L H, Ol R H 1984a Detection of malignant ovarian neoplasms: a review of the literature. I. Detection of the patient at risk; clinical, radiological and cytological detection. Obstet Gynecol Surv 39: 313–328

Smith L H, Ol R H 1984b Detection of malignant ovarian neoplasms: a review of the literature. II. Laboratory detection. Obstet Gynecol Surv 39: 329–345

Spanos W J 1973 Preoperative hormonal therapy of cystic adnexal masses. Am J Obstet Gynecol 116: 551–556

Taylor K J W, Burns P N, Wells P N T, Conway D I, Hull M G R 1985 Ultrasound Doppler flow studies of the ovarian and uterine arteries. Br J Obstet Gynecol 92: 240–246

Timor-Tritsh I E, Rottem S, Sarit E 1988 How transvaginal sonography is done. In: Timor-Tritsh I E, Rottem S (eds) Transvaginal sonography. Heinemann, London, pp. 15–25

Tyson F L, Soper J T, Daly L 1988 Over expression and amplification of the c-erbB2 (HER 2?neu) proto-oncogene in epithelial ovarian tumours and cell lines. Proc Am Assoc Cancer Res 29: 471–474

UK Co-ordinating Committee on Cancer Research 1989 Ovarian Cancer Screening, London.

van Kley H, Cramer S, Burns D E 1981 Serous ovarian neoplastic amylase (SONA). Cancer 48: 1444–1449

Ward B G, Cruickshank D J, Tucker D F, Love S 1987a Independent expression in serum of three tumour-associated antigens: CA 125, placental alkaline phosphatase and HMFG2 in ovarian cancer. Br J Obstet Gynecol 94: 696–698

Ward B G, Lowe D G, Shepherd J H 1987b Patterns of expression of a tumour-associated antigen, defined by the monoclonal antibody HMFG2, in human epithelial ovarian cancer. Cancer 60: 787–793

Wilson J M G, Jungner G 1968 Principles and practice of screening for disease. (Public health papers 34.) World Health Organization, Geneva

Xu F J, Ramakrishans S, Daly L 1991 M-CSF as a serum marker for ovarian cancer (in preparation)

Yeh J, Yeh Y-C 1989 Transforming growth factor—alpha and human cancer. Biomed Pharmacother 43: 651–660

Zanaboni F, Vergadoro F, Presti M et al 1987 Tumor antigen CA 125 as a marker of ovarian epithelial carcinoma. Gynecol Oncol 28: 61–67

Zurawski V R, Orjaseter H, Andersen A, Jellum E 1988 Elevated serum Ca 125 levels prior to diagnosis of ovarian neoplasia: relevance for early detection of ovarian cancer. Int J Cancer 42: 677–680

Zurawski V R, Sjovall K, Schoenfeld D A et al 1990 Prospective evaluation of serum CA 125 levels in a normal population, phase I: the specificities of single and serial determinations in testing for ovarian cancer. Gynecol Oncol 36: 299–305

23. Endometrial ablation for menorrhagia

A. L. Magos

Menorrhagia is a common gynaecological complaint and one which is often managed by the ultimate cure, hysterectomy (Studd 1989). Although there are considerable national and international variations (Coulter et al 1988), hysterectomy has become one of the most frequently performed major operations for women of reproductive age in the Western world; for instance, in the period 1970–1978 a total of 3·5 million non-radical hysterectomies were carried out in the USA (Dicker et al 1982b), and experience shows that about a third of such procedures are carried out for menstrual disorders (DHSS 1985). While hysterectomy is a relatively safe operation with a low mortality rate of only 6/10 000 for benign indications (Wingo et al 1985), operative morbidity can be as high as 42·8/100 when the abdominal route is used (Dicker et al 1982a). In recent years concern has also been expressed about the possible long-term complications of hysterectomy such as premature ovarian failure (Siddle et al 1987), cardio-vascular disease (Centerwall 1981), intestinal and urinary dysfunction (Taylor et al 1989) and vault prolapse; earlier descriptions of psychosexual problems and a 'post-hysterectomy syndrome' have not been borne out by prospective studies (Iles & Gath 1989).

Menorrhagia can develop secondary to pathologies such as endometriosis and fibroids, but several audits have shown that in about half the cases the uterus removed at hysterectomy is histologically normal (Grant & Hussein 1984). In other words, many patients are being subjected to major surgery to remove an apparently normal organ. It is no wonder that gynaecologists have been searching for a less radical surgical solution to abnormal menstruation.

TRAUMATIC INTRAUTERINE ADHESIONS AND ASHERMAN'S SYNDROME

The medical basis of most attempts to surgically improve menorrhagia without resorting to hysterectomy is the syndrome formally detailed by Asherman in a series of reports and which bears his name. In 1948 he first described a specific type of amenorrhoea, amenorrhoea traumatica, secondary to cervical stenosis in the region of the internal os following endometrial 'interference', typically endometrial curettage after pregnancy (Asherman 1948). Despite ovulation, the endometrium remained in a state of inactivity, and a haematometra did not develop behind the stenosis. Treatment was simply by cervical dilatation. Two years later, he described a further consequence of uterine curettage, that is partial or complete obliteration of the uterine cavity due to conglutination of opposing uterine walls by traumatic adhesions in the uterine body itself (Asherman 1950). Symptoms associated with intra-uterine adhesions included infertility and recurrent abortions. In contrast to isthmic adhesions, Asherman advocated digital adhesiolysis of the uterine cavity at laparotomy to restore uterine function.

Studies since have shown that partial or total obliteration of the uterine cavity may result not only from the formation of mucoid, fibrous or muscular adhesions as described by Asherman (1950), but also simply from the adherence of opposing walls (Louros et al 1968). Whatever the nature and site of trauma, the two common aetiological denominators in the majority of cases remain puerperal or postabortal trauma, particularly when performed at what appears to be a critical time of 1–4 weeks after the pregnancy, and endometritis (Carmichael 1970).

It is now evident that the menstrual manifestations of Asherman's syndrome are also protean and depend on the site and extent of any stenosis or adhesions (Klein & Garcia 1973). The spectrum extends from incidental findings of minor changes at hysterosalpingography or hysteroscopy to any combination of menstrual dysfunction and pelvic pain associated with more severe abnormalities (Table 23.1). Intrauterine adhesions themselves appear to be remarkably common with a reported incidence of almost 25% following post-partum dilatation and curettage carried out within 2 months of delivery (Eriksen & Kaestel 1960). In the longer term, the frequency of

Table 23.1   Abnormal menstrual outcomes of Asherman's syndrome

Partial cervical/isthmic stenosis	Hypomenorrhoea Amenorrhoea Dysmenorrhoea
Total cervical/isthmic stenosis	Amenorrhoea Haematometra Haematosalpinx Lower abdominal pain
Partial corporeal obliteration	Hypomenorrhoea Menorrhagia Adenomyosis Dysmenorrhoea
Total corporeal obliteration	Amenorrhoea Adenomyosis Lower abdominal pain

synechiae as judged by hysterosalpingography can range from 1·5% to 39% depending on risk factors (Dmowski & Greenblatt 1969). Hysterograms may however be misleading as appearances suggestive of intrauterine filling defects can result solely from abnormal neuromuscular contractions (Zondek & Rozin 1964). Asherman indeed postulated in 1948 that the amenorrhoea that sometimes followed cervical stenosis was the result of an inhibitory neural reflex acting on endometrial development despite normal ovarian function.

Typically, amenorrhoea occurs if there is total atresia of either the cervico-isthmic area or the uterine cavity, the latter being characterized by absence of functional endometrium. Hypomenorrhoea is a more common outcome of uterine damage and is associated with scattered areas of fibrosis. Cyclical lower abdominal pain and dysmenorrhoea are features in a quarter of patients secondary to either the development of a haematometra or haematosalpinx in the presence of cervical stenosis and functional endometrium, or to adenomyosis in cases of endometrial trauma (Bergman 1961). On theoretical grounds, therefore, the induction of a therapeutic type of Asherman's syndrome can lead to both beneficial and detrimental effects ranging from menstrual improvement to pelvic pain.

EARLY TECHNIQUES OF ENDOMETRIAL DESTRUCTION

Real interest in endometrial destruction started in the late 1960s and early 1970s, impetus in the main being the search for a transuterine non-surgical mode of tubal occlusion as a means of female sterilization. The intrauterine application of a large variety of highly toxic physical and chemical agents were investigated (Table 23.2) and almost incidentally, the endometrial and menstrual effects of these treatments became evident and hence the possibility of a new line of management for 'functional menorrhagia'. The most promising of these was cryocoagulation and particularly the experiments of Droegemueller (Droegemueller et al 1970, 1971), but by the late 1970s, these techniques were generally abandoned due to their unreliability both in terms of tubal blockage and menstrual suppression.

The reason for the failure of these early attempts at endometrial ablation were two-fold. First, some approaches were associated with unacceptable short-term or long-term sequelae including malignancy or even death (e.g. radiotherapy, iodine tincture). Secondly, with rare exceptions (e.g. ethanol, 10% formalin) other techniques failed to produce full-thickness necrosis or left untreated skip areas. Both these eventualities meant that any menstrual improvement tended to be temporary, treatment being eventually followed by endometrial regeneration and a recurrence of symptoms. Not only that, but some treatments such as cryocoagulation could be followed by complications such as haematometra and uterine abscess formation (Burke et al 1973). Although it is uncertain whether endometrium regenerates from

Table 23.2 Methods of endometrial destruction

Chemical
Iodine tincture
Iodoacetate
Podophylline
Colchicine
Sodium chloride solution (10%)
Phenol
Cadmium
Thio-tepa
Ethanol (100% and 50%)
Formalin (2%) in ethanol
Quinacrine
Silver nitrate
Zinc chloride
Cyanoacrylate + zinc chloride
Methyl cyanoacrylate
Formalin (10%)
Copper sulphate pentahydrate pellets
Talc suspension
Sodium lauryl sulphate

Physical
External irradiation
Intracavitary radium
Superheated steam
Cryocoagulation (freon, nitrous oxide)
Autologous fibroblasts
Homologous fibroblasts
Radiofrequency-induced thermal ablation

Surgical
Laser (ablation, coagulation)
Electrocautery (resection, coagulation)

residual stromal or glandular elements (Baggish et al 1967; Schenker et al 1971), there is no doubt that the endometrium has a tremendous capacity for regeneration (Schenker & Polishuk 1973); for instance, there are signs of endometrial regeneration within three hours of curettage and the endometrial surface is completely lined by regenerating cells after 48 hours (Schenker et al 1971). Furthermore, and relevant to the potential value of hormonal modulation around the time of endometrial ablation, pretreatment with neither oestrogen nor progesterone has been shown to influence the rate of endometrial regrowth after curettage (Schenker et al 1973a, b). Whether postoperative suppression of endogenous oestrogen concentrations would result in inhibition of endometrial regeneration long enough for intrauterine fibrosis to establish itself remains to be proven but it has been found that Asherman's syndrome is most likely to develop if curettage is performed between the second and fourth weeks postpartum or postabortion, at a time of relative hypo-oestrogenaemia (Eriksen & Kaestel 1960).

RADIOFREQUENCY-INDUCED THERMAL ABLATION

The common denominator to the early attempts at tubal blockage and endometrial ablation was that in all cases treatment was applied to the uterine cavity without direct visualization. Recently another 'blind' technique has been developed which, in contrast to the conceptually similar experiments of Cahan and Brockunier (1967) employing cooling, relies on heating the endometrium to cytotoxic levels by means of radiofrequency electromagnetic thermal energy delivered by a probe placed inside the uterine cavity (Phipps et al 1990a, b). Although the temperature at the endometrial surface may be as high as 66°C, there is minimal heating of the uterine serosa. Treatment is performed under general anaesthesia and involves dilating the cervix to 10 mm, fully inserting the 1 cm diameter angled probe into the uterine cavity via a vaginal guard, and slowly rotating it 360° over 20 minutes. Postoperative lower abdominal pain is usual over the first 6–48 hours particularly following higher energy doses, but treatment can usually still be performed as a day-case.

As this approach is new, there is no long-term follow-up information, but there does appear to be a dose–response relationship between menstrual results and the energy applied such that in the short term at least, amenorrhoea is achieved in 0–30% of patients, with overall menstrual improvement in 30–85%. Therapy has so far been reserved for cases of dysfunctional uterine bleeding and has the advantages of technical simplicity and the need for minimal surgical skills. The operative time is comparable to hysteroscopic methods of endometrial destruction. On the debit side, distortion of the uterine cavity by endometrial polyps and submucous fibroids are contraindications to this approach making preoperative hysteroscopy an essential part of the pre-treatment assessment. Inadvertent heating of the vagina resulting in vesicovaginal fistulae has been reported, and even more worrying is the potential for unrecognized intraoperative uterine perforation with consequent thermal necrosis of intra-abdominal contents. In the longer term, it remains to be seen whether thermal ablation will share the same problems of incomplete treatment as the earlier chemical and physical methods of years ago.

HYSTEROSCOPIC INTRAUTERINE SURGERY

In total contrast to the above 'blind' methods, the last decade has seen the emergence of hysteroscopic techniques of endometrial destruction, surgery being performed under visual control. The dawn of modern hysteroscopy began in the early 1970s with the development of better optics, illumination and above all safe means of uterine distension (Lewis 1989). Initially used for diagnosis, technical advances led to the possibility for surgical manoeuvres inside the uterine cavity under direct vision such as directed endometrial biopsy, polypectomy and even myomectomy. Endometrial ablation and resection represented the logical progression from these 'focal' procedures to more extensive intrauterine surgery for patients with abnormal bleeding. These methods hold out more promise partly because they are carried out under direct vision thus making the assessment of the depth of tissue damage easier and skip lesions less likely, and also because of their versatility in dealing with not only the normal cavity but also those which are enlarged or distorted by submucous fibroids.

Laser ablation

Despite the introduction of the resectoscope for the excision of submucous myomas as early as 1978 by Neuwirth (Neuwirth 1978), the first hysteroscopic technique used to destroy the endometrium in cases of menorrhagia employed laser rather than electrical energy. In what has now become a historic study, Goldrath and his co-workers from Detroit in the USA reported the first series of 22 hysteroscopic Nd:YAG laser photovaporizations of the endometrium in 1981 with very encouraging results: short hospitalization of only one or two days, minimal postoperative problems, and most importantly amenorrhoea or hypomenorrhoea in 21 (95·5%) of the cases, there being only one treatment failure (Goldrath et al 1981). Two patients did require retreatment and there were two cases of uterine perforation, but nonetheless the scene was set for a totally new approach to the management of the common problem of menorrhagia. Numerous publications, mostly from the USA, have since confirmed the efficacy of this approach to endometrial ablation.

Of the currently available sources of laser energy the neodymium: yttrium-aluminium-garnet laser as used by Goldrath has remained optimal for intrauterine surgery; it can be delivered along a narrow 0·6 mm diameter flexible fibre (an advantage with the awkward shape of the endometrial cavity), it can be transmitted through liquid media (as used for uterine distension in operative hysteroscopy), and the depth of tissue penetration can be controlled (a relative protection against uterine perforation). There have however been technical advances in instrumentation with the design of a dual channel hysteroscope for easier irrigation and a better operative view (Baggish & Baltoyannis 1988), and even the adaptation of a narrow flexible endoscope for laser intrauterine surgery (Cornier 1986).

The target effects of laser energy include the sequence of warming, coagulation, evaporation and carbonization, tissue destruction typically occurring to a depth of 4–5 mm. This means that surgery must be performed either immediately after menstruation or following endometrial suppression with agents such as danazol, progestogens or LHRH agonists (Goldrath 1990). At the typical power settings used for endometrial ablation of 20–100 watts depending on the technique employed, heat transmission through the myometrium is not clinically important, additional protection being afforded by the continuous flow of cool irrigation fluid as well as circulating blood flow (Goldrath et al 1981, Davis 1989).

Three techniques are available: touch technique, non-touch technique, and a combination of the two. The touch technique, originally described by Goldrath et al (1981), involves dragging a bare, or less often sapphire-tipped, quartz fibre across the endometrium with resultant vaporization and the production of deep furrows down to myometrium. In the non-touch technique, first described by Lomano (1986), the endometrium is merely coagulated, an effect that is characterized by blanching and swelling. Whatever the surgical method, most gynaecologists treat the entire endometrial cavity down to the endocervix. The non-touch technique appears superior in terms of per-operative fluid overload or postoperative bleeding but is generally considered not as effective in improving menstrual flow as the touch technique (Loffer 1988), although this has been disputed (Lomano 1988). All three methods are followed by bleeding and sero-sanguineous discharge for a number of weeks while the cavity heals. The duration of surgery is variable, but the figures of 55 minutes (40–120) published by Baggish & Baltoyannis (1988) is probably representative.

Goldrath (1981) has shown with hysterosalpingography and biopsy that treatment is followed by progressive scarring, deformity and contraction of the cavity, leading to eventual obstruction of the uterotubal junction by $1-1\frac{1}{2}$ years. For this reason, elective tubal sterilization is no longer practised routinely (Baggish & Baltoyannis 1988). Biopsy of the new cavity up to 4 months after surgery typically reveals necrotic myometrium with little or no endometrium, while later only minute fragments of normal endometrial fragments can be obtained even after vigorous curettage. Incidental hysterectomy 10 months after successful surgery with resultant amenorrhoea showed myometrium covered with a single layer of cuboidal epithelium showing minimal inflammation or carbonization.

As for the longer term results of laser ablation, there is general agreement that a large proportion of patients derive significant menstrual benefit from this mode of intervention, the only question remaining is exactly how much. The reason for some confusion is difficulty in the interpretation of the currently published series because of differences in patient selection (e.g. some include postmenopausal women), surgical technique and experience, the use of pre- and particularly postoperative endometrial suppressants, and definition as to what is considered 'improvement'. Nonetheless, the data show that 12–71% of patients become amenorrhoeic (Davis 1989, Baggish & Baltoyannis 1988), and only 1·6–22% appear not to be helped by a single treatment (Daniell et al 1986, Lomano 1988). As demonstrated by most authors, laser ablation can be repeated, usually with benefit, should the first attempt fail. It has also been suggested that endometrial ablation improves the premenstrual syndrome (Lefler 1989).

The range of therapeutic results reveals another aspect of laser ablation, namely that the learning curve is quite shallow; Loffer (1988) estimated that between 20 and 25 patients have to be treated before one can be confident about the results of surgery. Learning curve aside, considerably better results seem to be obtained with higher power settings (Davis 1989), and conversely, poorer results are associated with younger patients, the presence of submucous fibroids, enlarged uterine cavity > 10 cm in length, and perhaps adenomyosis (Goldrath 1986).

Endometrial electrocautery and resection

The dawn of endometrial surgery using electrocautery was the publication in 1978 by Neuwirth of the resection of the intracavity portion of sessile submucous fibroids in women with abnormal bleeding by means of a urological resectoscope. In a subsequent review article of 1983, Neuwirth gave brief details of more extensive surgery in women with menorrhagia, namely electrocautery destruction of the entire uterine cavity by systematically shaving the endometrium as far as the isthmus using the cutting loop of the resecting hysteroscope (Amin & Neuwirth 1983). At the same time, and also from the USA, DeCherney and Polan (1983) published their experience with emergency resectoscopic electrocoagulation of the endometrium in 11 women with intractable and life-threatening uterine haemorrhage resistant to other therapies who were unfit for hysterectomy. Their series was updated 4 years later to include 21 patients followed for a maximum of 6 years, all but three suffering from blood dyscrasias or other serious illnesses, and treated with either endometrial diathermy or resection as originally described by Amin and Neuwirth (DeCherney et al 1987). The results were impressive, 18 of the 19 patients who survived their primary illness having no bleeding and only one requiring retreatment.

The story then moved to Europe where Jacques Hamou, a master hysteroscopist, introduced endometrial resection to Paris in 1985 and made a number of important modifications to the technique. Drawing from the experience of urologists who have been performing the conceptually similar procedure of transurethral resection of the prostate (TURP) on men for several years, he recommended non-viscous fluids such as 1·5% glycine solution as a more manageable alternative to the Dextran 70 used by both Neuwirth and DeCherney for uterine distension and irrigation, coupled this to the use of a continuous flow resectoscope sheath for easier and safer fluid control as developed by Hallez, and suggested what has come to be known as *partial endometrial resection* as an alternative to hysterectomy in otherwise healthy women with dysfunctional menorrhagia, the aim of surgery being not to stop periods but to make them light enough to be acceptable. In 1988, Hamou demonstrated his operation to a spell-bound audience in Oxford, UK, from which was born the more extensive procedure of *total endometrial resection* (Magos et al 1989b). Fittingly, because of the parallels with endoscopic prostate surgery, the term 'trans-cervical resection of the endometrium' (TCRE) was coined by Smith, senior urological surgeon in Oxford, to describe what in effect is the gynaecologist's version of the TURP.

TCRE is generally performed with a 26 French gauge unmodified continuous flow resectoscope fitted with a 4 mm forward-oblique telescope and 24 French gauge cutting loop. The uterus is distended via the inner inflow sheath and irrigation is achieved by continuous suction of the outer sheath of the resectoscope. We prefer a passive as opposed to an active handle mechanism with the cutting loop sitting inside the sheath at rest as there is no obstruction to the endoscopic view when the uterine cavity is being inspected and accidental trauma is less likely than with a permanently exposed loop. The depth of cut of the loop of 3–4 mm means that, as with laser ablation, surgery should ideally be performed immediately post-menstrually when the endometrial thickness is about 3 mm or after endometrial suppression. As a further consideration, Reid and Sharp (1988) have shown that glandular elements are almost invariably present deep in the myometrium and resection (or ablation) should therefore include 2·5–3 mm of myometrium as well. For logistic reasons we routinely treat our patients with danazol at a dose of 200 mg t.d.s. for 6 weeks prior to surgery, a regimen which has been shown to produce a thin, atrophic endometrium (Jeppsson et al 1984); such preparation has the added advantage of making the endometrium less 'fluffy' and so small debris are less likely to block the out-flow holes of the outer sheath and thus impede clear vision. As with all endoscopic procedures, surgery is also facilitated by video monitoring with advantages in terms of operator comfort, magnification of the operative field, maintenance of the interest of nurses and other theatre staff, and not least teaching.

Submucous myomectomy is easily performed first, if indicated, followed by the systematic excision of the endometrium down to the superficial layer of myometrium using a blended cutting and coagulating current of 75–125 watts. The depth of resection is judged by the obvious landmark of the circular myometrial fibres, care being taken not to continue surgery deeper with risk of haemorrhage. The fundus is resected with a slightly forward-angled loop and the remainder of the cavity with the conventional loop. Depending on the patient's wishes for amenorrhoea or hypomenorrhoea, the endometrium is resected either over the entire cavity (total resection) or to within 0·5–1 cm of the isthmus (partial resection). At the end of surgery the resected tissue is removed with a flushing curette or polyp forceps and sent for histological examination. Surgery can be performed under either general or local anaesthesia combined with sedation. The autonomic nerve supply of the uterus means that the uterus is relatively insensitive to touching, cutting or burning. Minor hysteroscopic procedures using relatively narrow instruments have already been described under these conditions (Cornier 1986, Hallez et al 1987), but we have found that extensive intrauterine surgery such as TCRE can also be carried out using a wider instrument without recourse to general anaesthesia (Magos et al

1989a). Our current protocol involves admitting the patient in time for pre-medication with temazepam 20 mg and mefenamic acid 500 mg one hour before surgery. In the endoscopy suite or operating room, anxiolysis and light sedation are achieved with small doses of intravenous midazolam, systemic analgesia with incremental doses of intravenous fentanyl, and finally local anaesthesia with a combination of para- and intracervical and intrauterine lignocaine/adrenaline mixture, the latter injected under direct vision around the pericornual regions using the resectoscope. Heart rate, electrocardiogram and arterial oxygen saturation are monitored continuously, facial oxygen being given if there is evidence of hypo-ventilation. Patients remain full co-operative during surgery, some even choosing to watch their operation 'live' on the video monitor.

Postoperative recovery is fast and most women are fit for discharge from hospital within 3–4 hours. Patient acceptance of this technique is good, and as proof almost all women who have required retreatment have agreed to the second procedure also being carried out under sedation. It should be little surprise that we prefer sedation and now employ general anaesthesia for only about half of our procedures. This system, which combines intrauterine surgery with sedation and local anaesthesia, avoids the two most important hazards of hysterectomy, namely major surgery and general anaesthesia. A further advantage is the possibility of treating patients with menorrhagia for whom hysterectomy is considered un-desirable, dangerous or impossible (Lockwood et al 1990).

There has only been one detailed prospective report of total and partial TCRE in cases of menorrhagia showing the short-term efficacy of treatment in 15 women, 11 undergoing total and four partial TCRE (Magos et al 1989b). We have now treated over 250 patients chosen according to the criteria outlined in Table 23.3 and would estimate that about 75% or so of women with menorrhagia would be suitable for this approach, including those with a normal uterus or a uterus enlarged by moderately sized fibroids. TCRE cannot guarantee against pregnancy, but the risk is very small and we no longer insist on tubal sterilization, advising instead the use

Table 23.3 Criteria for endometrial resection

—Menorrhagia resistant to medical
   therapy
—Uterine size no greater than the
   equivalent of 12 weeks pregnancy (or
   uterine cavity no greater than 10 cm in length)
—Submucous fibroids no greater than
   5 cm in diameter
—Endometrial histology showing
   normal or low-risk hyperplasia
—Family complete
—Careful counselling

of barrier methods of contraception. As with all ablation techniques, thoughtful counselling with respect to the likely menstrual results, and possible short- and long-term complications is essential.

I have summarized details of our first 100 patients in Table 23.4. The

Table 23.4 Endometrial resection: the first 100 patients over the first year (results expressed as average and range, or number of cases, or as percentage)

Preoperative characteristics

Number of patients	100
Age (years)	41·9 (15–54)
Parous	87
Length of periods (days)	8·4 (4–30)
Length of cycle (days)	26·5 (14–37)
Perious medical treatment	74

Surgery

Procedure:	
Total TCRE	85
Partial TCRE (patient request)	10
Partial TCRE (total TCRE not possible)	2
Simultaneous myomectomy	16
Failed (laparotomy)	3
Anaesthesia:	
GA	55
Sedation with LA	45
Glycine balance (ml)	350 (0–4350)
Procedure time (mins)	38·8 (10–100)
Complications	
Unable to dilate cervix > 8 mm	1
Fluid absorption > 1500 ml	5
Uterine perforation	3
Haemorrhage	1
Urinary retention	1
Pyrexia	1
Severe nausea	1

Recovery

Postoperative hospital stay (days)	0·9 (0–13)
Duration of postoperative bleeding (days)	11·9 (0–42)
Duration of postoperative discharge (days)	10·4 (0–42)
Return to normal domestic activities (weeks)	2·4 (0·5–21)
Return to work (weeks)	3·6 (0·5–28)

Menstrual results at 12 months and patient satisfaction

Total resection	
Amenorrhoea	53·8%
Menstrual improvement	38·5%
No improvement in menstruation	7·7%
Partial resection	
Amenorrhoea	20·0%
Menstrual improvement	80·0%
No improvement in menstruation	0·0%
Patient attitude	
Satisfied	94
Request for repeat TCRE	4
Request for hysterectomy	1
Medical treatment	1

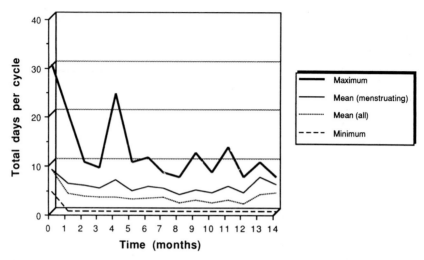

Fig. 23.1   Effect of total endometrial resection on the duration of menstruation.

data include the learning curve of several operators and teaching sessions, and hence the range of operative times, occasional use of large volumes of irrigant, and not least three uterine perforations which all occurred early in our series. They are worthy of comment from the educational point of view: one patient had an acutely retroflexed uterus which made insertion of the rigid hysteroscope difficult, the other an incompetent cervix which prevented adequate uterine distension, and the third was the first solo

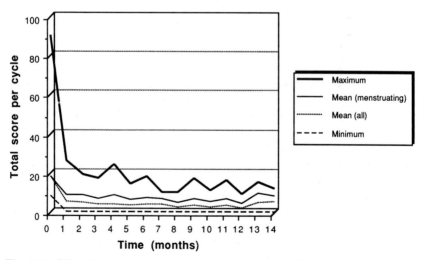

Fig. 23.2   Effect of total endometrial resection on total amount of menstrual bleeding each month. Blood loss scored daily on a scale of 0–3 (none to heavy).

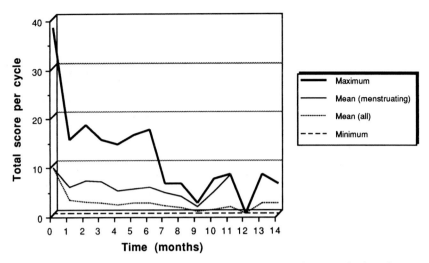

Fig. 23.3 Effect of total endometrial resection on total amount of menstrual pain each month. Pain scored daily on a scale of 0–3 (none to heavy).

procedure of one of us with inadvertent cornual perforation. As a result of these experiences, our safety protocol includes ensuring that the tubal ostia are identified before proceeding with resection, the insertion of a cerclage in cases of excessive fluid leakage from the cervix, and the use of a forward-angled loop for the fundus and cornual regions. Despite these early problems, the menstrual results of TCRE are comparable to those achieved with laser ablation with amenorrhoea in over 50% of patients undergoing total TCRE after one year of follow up. Our data also highlight how quick recovery is after surgery both in terms of short hospitalization and speedy return to normal activities in most cases, a feature of all forms of 'minimally invasive surgery'.

More detailed analysis of the effects of TCRE involved the use of daily menstrual calenders and menstrual blood loss measurements in a subgroup of women. Both confirmed the retrospective report of our patients showing that generally even those who continued to bleed after total TCRE developed relative hypomenorrhoea with a reduction in not only the duration of bleeding and amount of blood loss, but also the amount of pain experienced during menstruation (Figs 23.1–23.3). These subjective impressions have been confirmed by objective measures of menstrual blood loss (MBL) using the alkaline haematin method, analysis showing that 24 of the 25 (96%) patients monitored after total TCRE had measurements well within the normal range (MBL < 80 ml/cycle) following surgery, with only one patient seeming to get worse (13 ml/cycle preoperatively, 15 ml/cycle postoperatively!) (Fig. 23.4). The MBL results of partial TCRE were not as impressive despite the favourable reports of our patients (Fig. 23.5). As an explanation for these menstrual outcomes, hysteroscopy 3 and 12

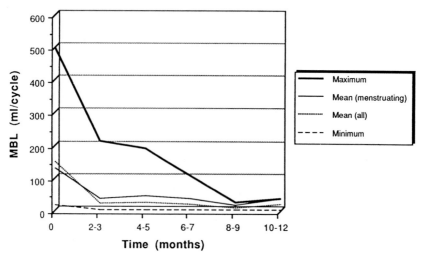

Fig. 23.4   Menstrual blood loss after total endometrial resection ($n = 25$).

months after resection typically showed extensive fundal fibrosis of the uterine cavity with occasional cases of total obliteration. Interestingly, even in women who are amenorrhoeic, microscopic deposits of endometrium can often be found in biopsies taken from the new cavity. Uterine ultrasound 3 months after surgery revealed that it was only the cavity that had shrunk from an average 3 ml to 1 ml and not the whole uterus. The menstrual benefits were not associated with significant changes in gonadotrophins even in the amenorrhoeic cases. The fear expressed by Hamou relating to

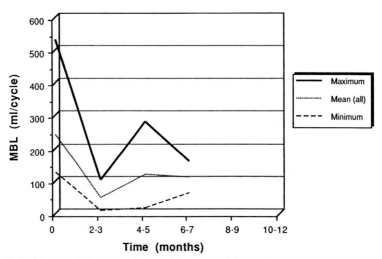

Fig. 23.5   Menstrual blood loss after partial endometrial resection ($n = 5$).

Table 23.5 Complications of
hysteroscopic intrauterine surgery

Uterine perforation
Haemorrhage
Gas embolism
Fluid overload
Infection

the development of haematometra after total TCRE has not been borne out by clinical experience, although we have had two cases with fundal collections of blood causing cyclical pain in women who were otherwise amenorrhoeic.

A variant on the technique of endometrial resection is electrocoagulation using a 2 mm roller-ball electrode fitted to the resectoscope instead of a cutting loop (Vancaillie 1989, Townsend et al 1990). This approach is technically easier than resection and carries less risk of perforation, while the duration of surgery is comparable. The menstrual results, at least in the short term, are also similar with amenorrhoea in 40–67% of cases. On the debit side, a roller-ball cannot be used to treat submucous fibroids which are so common in menorrhagic patients, so this technique must be considered less versatile than resection.

Complications of intrauterine surgery

As with all forms of surgical intervention regardless of the degree of invasiveness, complications are inevitable and often due to relative inexperience (Table 23.5). This is certainly the case with endometrial ablation where uterine perforation has been documented both in our initial series using the resectoscope (Magos et al 1989b) and that of Goldrath et al (1981), while radiofrequency thermal ablation initially resulted in two cases of vesico-vaginal fistulae (Phipps et al 1990a). Other complications include haemorrhage secondary to surgery that is too radical, which if not controlled by laser or electrodiathermy coagulation, can be effectively treated by the simple measure of inserting a 30 cc Foley catheter balloon into the uterine cavity, inflating it with sterile water, and leaving it in situ for 6–8 hours to produce tamponade. The literature includes a case of air embolism following TCRE (Wood & Roberts 1990), while postoperative infection is a difficult diagnosis and probably uncommon, although it is our usual practice to give one dose of antibiotics at the start of surgery for prophylaxis.

Most attention at least with respect to hysteroscopic endometrial ablation has been focused on the risks of fluid overload from the distension/irrigation fluid required for surgery. By necessity the non-compliant nature of the myometrium means that the uterine cavity can only be distended sufficiently for an adequate surgical view under relatively high pressures of 80–100 mmHg (Quinones 1984). This can be achieved by simple gravity, using a sphygmomanometer cuff, or more conveniently by means of a pressure-control pump such as the one designed by Quinones or the more expensive and complicated HAMOU Hysteromat (both manufactured by Karl Storz GmBh, Tuttlingen, West Germany). Simultaneously, the use of a continuous flow instrument allows for suction of the solution to ensure a clear operative view throughout surgery as well as the accurate monitoring of fluid balance.

In the case of laser ablation, 5% dextrose was initially used by Goldrath et al (1981) as the irrigation fluid, but subsequently with the realization of the risks of dilutional hyponatraemia, both he and others have generally changed to dextrose/saline or normal saline (Goldrath 1986, Lomano 1986). A minority have suggested using high viscosity dextran (Hyskon) to avoid the risk of fluid overload (Baggish & Baltoyannis 1988), but this can cause serious anaphylactic reactions so cannot be considered a totally safe alternative. The choice of irrigant is more limited with electrocautery as the fluid must be ion-free, and Hyskon (Neuwirth 1983, DeCherney & Polan 1983), 1·5% glycine solution (Magos et al 1989b) and more recently sorbitol have been the most widely used.

Absorption of large volumes of irrigating fluid is associated with the well known and potentially serious dangers of fluid overload, hypertension, hyponatraemia, neurological symptoms, haemolysis and even death, long known to the urologists as the TUR syndrome. There have in fact only been two reports looking formally at fluid dynamics during endometrial surgery. Morrison et al (1989) investigated 12 women undergoing laser

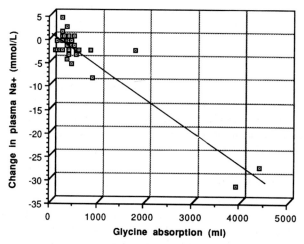

Fig. 23.6   Effect of absorption of 1·5% glycine solution during endometrial resection on plasma sodium. (Reproduced with permission from Magos et al 1990.)

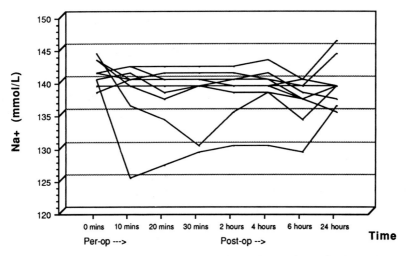

Fig. 23.7 Changes in plasma sodium during and after endometrial resection ($n = 10$).

ablation using 0·9% saline as the uterine irrigant. In their study the mean volume of uterine irrigant absorbed was 2·5 l (maximum: 10·5), fluid absorption being accompanied by a significant rise in central venous pressure and serum chloride, and significant decrease in plasma total protein, albumin and haematocrit.

Our figures for the absorption of 1·5% glycine solution during TCRE are summarized in Table 23.4, showing that the average (median) volume is only 350 ml, which is considerably less than reported in the above study. Further analysis revealed that tubal blockage was associated with a 20% reduction of the amount of irrigant absorbed during surgery (315 ml versus 400 ml), while biochemical studies established a direct relationship between the volume of fluid absorbed and, for instance, drop in plasma sodium (Fig. 23.6) (Magos et al 1990). Detailed intra- and post-operative monitoring of 10 women undergoing TCRE also showed that clinically significant changes in biochemical variables can occur within 10 minutes of surgery in the presence of excessive fluid absorption (Fig. 23.7) (Baumann et al 1990). In agreement with the data presented by Morrison et al (1989), changes in plasma sodium were paralleled by falls in the serum concentration of total protein, albumin, haemoglobin and packed cell volume. There was also evidence of delayed intravascular haemolysis but all parameters returned to normal spontaneously within 24 hours. Based on this information we now have strict guidelines concerning fluid balance as outlined in Table 23.6, which means in practice that fluid overload and all its sequelae is no longer a clinical problem as surgery would in theory always be terminated well before any danger to the patient (although this is rarely necessary). It goes without saying that the careful monitoring of fluid balance during hysteroscopic surgery is essential and requires a dedicated member of staff.

Table 23.6 Fluid balance guidelines for endometrial resection

Volume of irrigant absorbed	
1000 ml	Well tolerated by healthy patients
	Continue surgery
1000–2000 ml	Mild hyponatraemia likely
	Complete surgery as quickly as possible
> 2000 ml	Severe hyponatraemia/other disturbances likely
	Stop surgery

Finally, there have even been rare reports of fatalities associated with intrauterine surgery. Precise details are generally no more than a mixture of rumour and speculation, but it is clear that hysteroscopic surgery is not for the novice but should be an extension of basic skills learnt at diagnostic procedures. Hysteroscopy is technically quite different from laparoscopy, and expertise with the latter is no guarantee of success with the former. Training in hysteroscopic surgery, knowledge of the indications and contraindications, limitations and above all operative risks of the various techniques are essential prerequisites to ensure the safety and proper care of our patients.

Comparison of techniques

Accepting that TCRE is a more recent procedure with a shorter follow up, the results so far suggest that laser ablation and endometrial resection are of comparable efficacy in producing amenorrhoea and hypomenorrhoea. The same probably applies to radiofrequency induced thermal ablation with the proviso that this technique is restricted to treating those patients who have essentially normal uterine cavity in terms of size and shape. That aside, all the techniques have advantages and disadvantages (Table 23.7), but the ability to deal with both normal and abnormally enlarged cavities and fibroids the most efficiently, together with the faster operating time, and not

Table 23.7 Comparison of endometrial laser ablation, endometrial resection and radiofrequency-induced thermal ablation

	Laser	Resectoscope	RITEA
Precision	+ + +	+ +	+
Safety: Patient	+ + +	+	+ +
Surgeon	+	+ + +	+ +
Speed	+	+ + +	+ +
Cost	+	+ + +	+ +
Histology	+	+ + +	+
Fibroids	+ +	+ + +	+
Efficacy	???	???	???
	worst + <---> + + + best		

least in the cost conscious climate of the present health care system, the lesser capital outlay associated with TCRE must weigh heavily in its favour as the preferred surgical option. In the final analysis, however, the best technique is the one that the surgeon feels most confident with.

CONCLUSION

Endometrial destruction by whatever method is undoubtedly a very attractive alternative to both long-term drug therapy and hysterectomy for the management of menorrhagia for both patients and the health service, and there seems little doubt that these techniques are set to dramatically change everyday gynaecological practice (Magos 1990). All the current approaches are associated with a much shorter hospital stay, faster recovery, definite financial savings (Rutherford & Glass 1990), and menstruation is almost universally improved to a clinically meaningful degree. On the debit side, amenorrhoea cannot be guaranteed with any of the present techniques and long-term morbidity is as yet unknown, particularly with respect of the chance of unwanted pregnancy and potential malignant change within the uterine cavity. Of some concern are the findings of a recently published large retrospective comparison of transurethral resection of the prostate in men with open prostatectomy showing a small but significantly increased risk of dying from cardio-vascular causes for up to 8 years after the endoscopic procedure (Roos et al 1989). While the results of this study cannot be applied directly to hysteroscopic endometrial surgery, it is important to provide patients with all the facts. Ultimately, a formal comparison with traditional treatments must be the judge of the therapeutic role of endometrial destruction.

REFERENCES

Amin H K, Neuwirth R S 1983 Operative hysteroscopy utilizing dextran as distending medium. Clinical Obstet Gynecol 26: 277–284
Asherman J G 1948 Amenorrhoea traumatica atretica. J Obstet Gynaecol Brit Empire 55: 23–30
Asherman J G 1950 Traumatic intra-uterine adhesions. J Obstet Gynaecol Brit Empire 57: 892–896
Baggish M S, Baltoyannis P 1988 New techniques for laser ablation of the endometrium in high-risk patients. Am J Obstet Gynecol 159: 287–292
Baggish M S, Pauerstein C J, Woodruff J D 1967 Role of stroma in regeneration of endometrial epithelium. Am J Obstet Gynecol 99: 459–465
Baumann R, Magos A L, Kay J D S, Turnbull A C 1990 Absorption of glycine irrigating solution during transcervical resection of the endometrium. Br Med J 300: 304–305
Bergman P 1961 Traumatic intrauterine lesions. Acta Obstet Gynecol Scand 40 (Suppl. 4): 1–39
Burke L, Rubin H W, Kim I 1973 Uterine abscess formation secondary to endometrial cryosurgery. Obstet Gynecol 41: 224–226
Cahan W G, Brockunier A Jr 1967 Cryosurgery of the uterine cavity. Am J Obstet Gynecol 99: 138–153
Carmichael D E 1970 Asherman's syndrome. Obstet Gynecol 36: 922–928

Centerwall B S 1981 Premenopausal hysterectomy and cardiovascular disease. Am J Obstet Gynecol 139: 58–61

Cornier E 1986 Traitement hysterofibroscopique ambulatoire des metrorragies rebelles par laser Nd: YAG. J Gynecol Obstet Biol Reprod 15: 661–664

Coulter A, McPherson K, Vessey M 1988 Do British women undergo too many or too few hysterectomies? Soc Sci Med 27: 987–994

Daniell J, Tosh R, Meisels S 1986 Photodynamic ablation of the endometrium with the Nd: YAG laser hysteroscopically as a treatment for menorrhagia. Colposc Gynaecol Laser Surg 2: 43–46

Davis J A 1989 Hysteroscopic endometrial ablation with the neodymium-YAG laser. Br J Obstet Gynaecol 96: 928–932

DeCherney A H, Diamond M P, Lavy G, Polan M L 1987 Endometrial ablation for intractable uterine bleeding: hysteroscopic resection. Obstet Gynecol 70: 668–670

DeCherney A, Polan M L 1983 Hysteroscopic management of intrauterine lesions and intractable uterine bleeding. Obstet Gynecol 61: 392–397

DHSS 1985 Department of Health and Social Security and Office of Population Censuses and Surveys. Hospital in-patient enquiry 1985. London, HMSO: table, p1

Dicker R C, Greenspan J R, Strauss L T, Cowart M R, Scally M J, Peterson H B, DeStafano F, Rubin G L, Ory H W 1982a Complications of abdominal and vaginal hysterectomy among women of reproductive age in the United States. Am J Obstet Gynecol 144: 841–848

Dicker R C, Scally M J, Greenspan J R, Layde P M, Ory H W, Maze J M, Smith J C 1982b Hysterectomy among women of reproductive age. Trends in the United States. JAMA 248: 323–327

Dmowski W P, Greenblatt R 1969 Asherman's syndrome and risk of placenta accreta. Obstet Gynecol 34: 288–299

Droegemueller W, Greer B, Makowski E 1970 Preliminary observations of cryocoagulation of the endometrium. Am J Obstet Gynecol 107: 958–961

Droegemueller W, Greer B, Makowski E 1971 Cryosurgery in patients with dysfunctional uterine bleeding. Obstet Gynecol 38: 256–258

Eriksen J, Kaestel C 1960 The incidence of uterine atresia after post-partum curettage. Dan Med Bull 7: 50

Goldrath M H 1986 Hysteroscopic laser ablation of the endometrium. In: Sharp F, Jordan J A (eds) Gynaecological Laser Surgery: Proceedings of the Fifteenth Study Group of the Royal College of Obstetricians and Gynaecologists, London. New York, Perinatology Press, pp 253–269

Goldrath M H 1990 Use of danazol in hysteroscopic surgery for menorrhagia. J Reprod Med 35 (Suppl. 1): 91–96

Goldrath M H, Fuller T A, Segal S 1981 Laser photovaporization of endometrium for the treatment of menorrhagia. Am J Obstet Gynecol 140: 14–19

Grant J M, Hussein I Y 1984 An audit of abdominal hysterectomy over a decade in a district hospital. Br J Obstet Gynaecol 91: 73–77

Hallez J-P, Netter A, Cartier R 1987 Methodical intrauterine resection. Am J Obstet Gynecol 156: 1080–1084

Iles S, Gath D 1989 Psychological problems and uterine bleeding. Bailliere's Clinical Obstetrics and Gynaecology 3: 375–389

Jeppsson S, Mellquist P, Rannevik G 1984 Short-term effects of danazol on endometrial histology. Acta Obstet Gynecol Scand 123: 41–44

Klein S M, Garcia C-M 1973 Asherman's syndrome: a critique and current review. Fertil Steril 24: 722–735

Lefler H T Jr 1989 Premenstrual syndrome improvement after laser ablation of the endometrium for menorrhagia. J Reprod Med 34: 905–906

Lewis B V 1989 Hysteroscopy. In: Studd J (ed) Progress in Obstetrics and Gynaecology, Volume 7. Edinburgh, Churchill Livingstone, pp 305–317

Lockwood G M, Magos A L, Baumann R, Turnbull A C 1990 Endometrial resection when hysterectomy is undesirable, dangerous or impossible. Br J Obstet Gynaecol 97: 656–658

Loffer F D 1988 Laser ablation of the endometrium. Obstet Gynecol Clin North Am 15: 77–89

Lomano J M 1986 Photocoagulation of the endometrium with the Nd:YAG laser for the treatment of menorrhagia. J Reprod Med 31: 148–150

Lomano J M 1988 Dragging versus blanching technique for endometrial ablation with the Nd:YAG laser in the treatment of chronic menorrhagia. Am J Obstet Gynecol 159: 152–155

Louros N C, Danezis J M, Pontifix G 1968 Use of intrauterine devices in the treatment of intrauterine adhesions. Fertil Steril 19: 509–528

Magos A L 1990 Management of menorrhagia. Br Med J 300: 1537–1538

Magos A L, Baumann R, Cheung K, Turnbull A C 1989a Intra-uterine surgery under intravenous sedation: an out-patient alternative to hysterectomy. Lancet ii: 925–926

Magos A L, Baumann R, Turnbull A C 1989b Transcervical resection of the endometrium in women with menorrhagia. Br Med J 298: 1209–1212

Magos A L, Baumann R, Turnbull A C 1990 Safety of transcervical endometrial resection. Lancet i: 44

Morrison L M M, Davis J, Sumner D 1989 Absorption of irrigating fluid during laser photocoagulation of the endometrium in the treatment of menorrhagia. Br J Obstet Gynaecol 96: 346–352

Neuwirth R S 1978 A new technique for and additional experience with hysteroscopic resection of submucous fibroids. Am J Obstet Gynecol 131: 91–94

Neuwirth R S 1983 Hysteroscopic management of symptomatic submucous fibroids. Obstet Gynecol 62: 509–511

Phipps J W, Lewis B V, Prior M V, Roberts T 1990a Experimental and clinical studies with radiofrequency induced thermal endometrial ablation for functional menorrhagia. Obstet Gynecol 76: 876–881

Phipps J H, Lewis B V, Roberts T, Prior M V, Hand V W, Elder M, Field S B 1990b Treatment of functional menorrhgia by radiofrequency-induced thermal endometrial ablation. Lancet 335: 374–376

Quinones R G 1984 Hysteroscopy with a new fluid technique. In: Siegler A M, Lindemann H J (eds) 'Hysteroscopy: principles and practice'. Philadelphia, J B Lippincott, 41–42

Reid P C, Sharp F 1988 Hysteroscopic Nd:YAG endometrial ablation: an in vitro and in vivo laser-tissue interaction study. Presented at the IIIrd European Congress on Hysteroscopy and Endoscopic Surgery, Amsterdam

Roos N P, Wennberg J E, Malenka D J, Fisher E S, McPherson K, Andersen T F, Cohen M M, Ramsey E 1989 Mortality and reoperation after open and transurethral resection of the prostate for benign prostatic hyperplasia. N Engl J Med 320: 1120–1124

Rutherford A J, Glass M R 1990 Management of menorrhagia. Br Med J 301: 290–291

Schenker J G, Polishuk W Z 1973 Regeneration of rabbit endometrium following intrauterine instillation of chemical agents. Gynecol Obstet Invest 4: 1–13

Schenker J C, Sacks M I, Polishuk W Z 1971 Regeneration of rabbit endometrium following curettage. Am J Obstet Gynecol 111: 970–978

Schenker J C, Polishuk W Z, Sacks M I 1973a Regeneration of the endometrium in rabbits after curettage: I. Pretreatment with estrogens. J Reprod Med 11: 43–48

Schenker J C, Polishuk W Z, Sacks M I 1973b Regeneration of the endometrium in rabbits after curettage: II. Pretreatment with progesterone. J Reprod Med 11: 49–57

Siddle N, Sarrel P, Whitehead M I 1987 The effect of hysterectomy on the age of ovarian failure: identification of a subgroup of women with premature ovarian loss of ovarian function and literature review. Fertil Steril 47: 94–100

Studd J W W 1989 Hysterectomy and menorrhagia. Bailliere's Clin Obstet Gynaecol 3: 415–424

Taylor T, Smith A N, Fulton P M 1989 Effect of hysterectomy on bowel function. Br Med J 299: 300–301

Townsend D E, Richart R M, Paskowitz R A, Woolfork R E 1990 'Rollerball' coagulation of the endometrium. Obstet Gynecol 76: 310–313

Vancaillie T G 1989 Electrocoagulation of the endometrium with the ball-end resectoscope. Obstet Gynecol 74: 425–427

Wingo P A, Huezo C M, Rubin G L, Ory H W, Petersen H B 1985 The mortality risk associated with hysterectomy. Am J Obstet Gynecol 152: 803–808

Wood S M, Roberts F L 1990 Air embolism during transcervical resection of endometrium. Br Med J 300: 945

Zondek B, Rozin S 1964 Filling defects in the hysterogram simulating intrauterine synechiae which disappear after denervation. Am J Obstet Gynecol 88: 123–127

Index